SERVICE *on the* SKEENA

SERVICE *on the* SKEENA

Horace Wrinch, Frontier Physician

GEOFF MYNETT

RONSDALE PRESS

SERVICE ON THE SKEENA
Copyright © 2019 Geoff Mynett

RONSDALE PRESS
3350 West 21st Avenue, Vancouver, B.C. Canada V6S 1G7
www.ronsdalepress.com

Typesetting: Julie Cochrane, in Caslon 11.5 pt on 15
Cover Photo: Dr. Horace Wrinch, June 16, 1900. Courtesy Geoff Mynett.
Cover Design: Julie Cochrane
Front Matter Maps: Morgan Hite, Hesperus Arts
Paper: Ancient Forest Friendly Enviro 100 edition, 60 lb. Husky (FSC),
    100% post-consumer waste, totally chlorine-free and acid-free.

Ronsdale Press wishes to thank the following for their support of its publishing program: the Canada Council for the Arts, the Government of Canada, the British Columbia Arts Council, and the Province of British Columbia through the British Columbia Book Publishing Tax Credit program.

 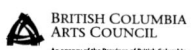 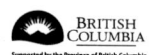

Library and Archives Canada Cataloguing in Publication

Title: Service on the Skeena: Horace Wrinch, frontier physician / Geoff Mynett.

Names: Mynett, Geoff, 1946– author.

Description: Includes bibliographical references.

Identifiers: Canadiana (print) 2019007129X | Canadiana (ebook) 20190071303 | ISBN 9781553805755 (softcover) | ISBN 9781553805762 (HTML) | ISBN 9781553805779 (PDF)

Subjects: LCSH: Wrinch, Horace. | LCSH: Physicians — British Columbia — Biography. | LCSH: Legislators — British Columbia — Biography. | LCSH: Judges — British Columbia — Biography. | LCSH: Clergy — British Columbia — Biography. | LCSH: Health insurance — British Columbia — History — 20th century. | LCGFT: Biographies.

Classification: LCC R464.W75 M96 2019 | DDC 610/.92 — dc23

At Ronsdale Press we are committed to protecting the environment. To this end we are working with Canopy and printers to phase out our use of paper produced from ancient forests. This book is one step towards that goal.

Printed in Canada by Island Blue, Victoria, B.C.

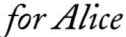

for Alice

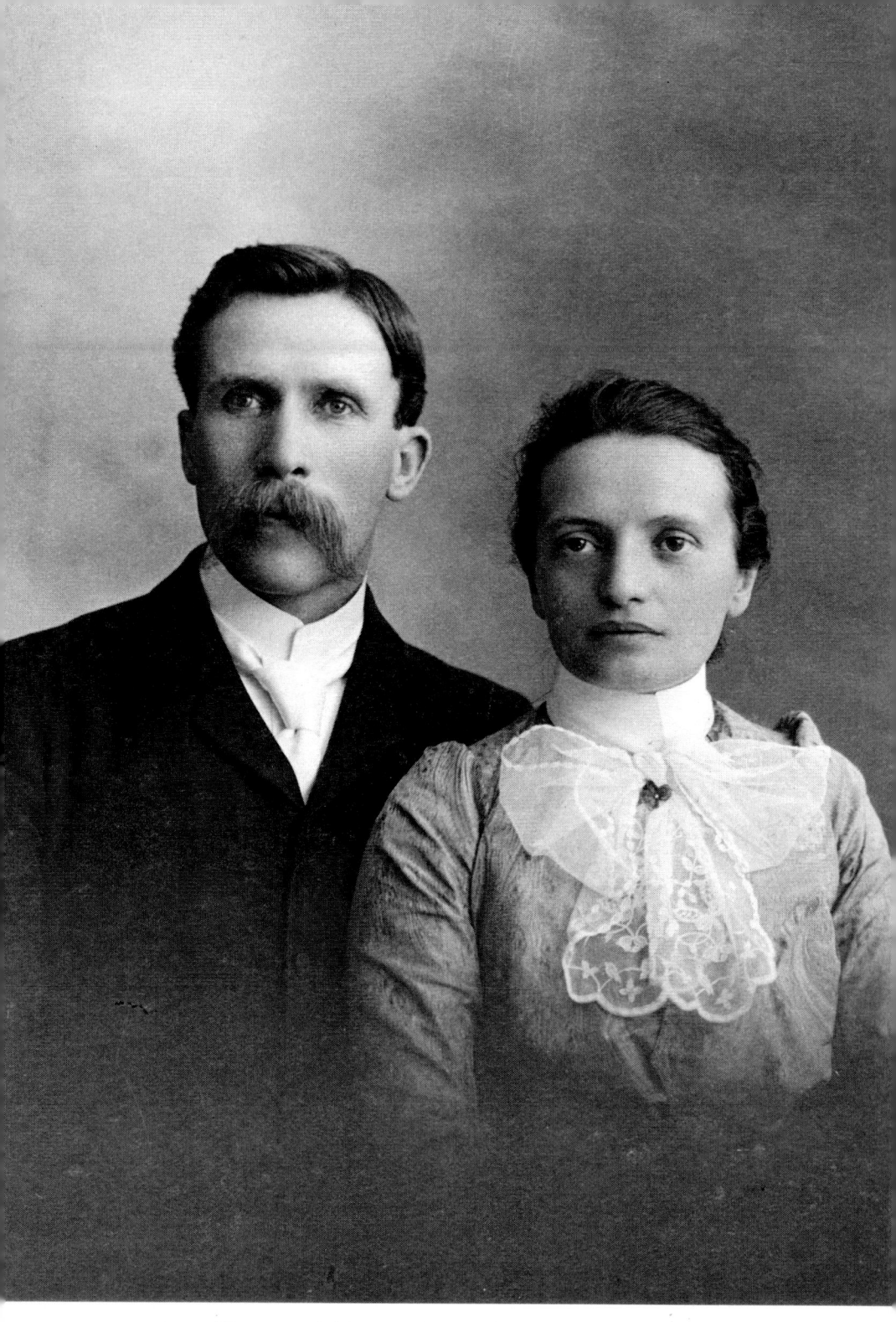

Horace and Alice on their wedding day, June 16, 1900.

CONTENTS

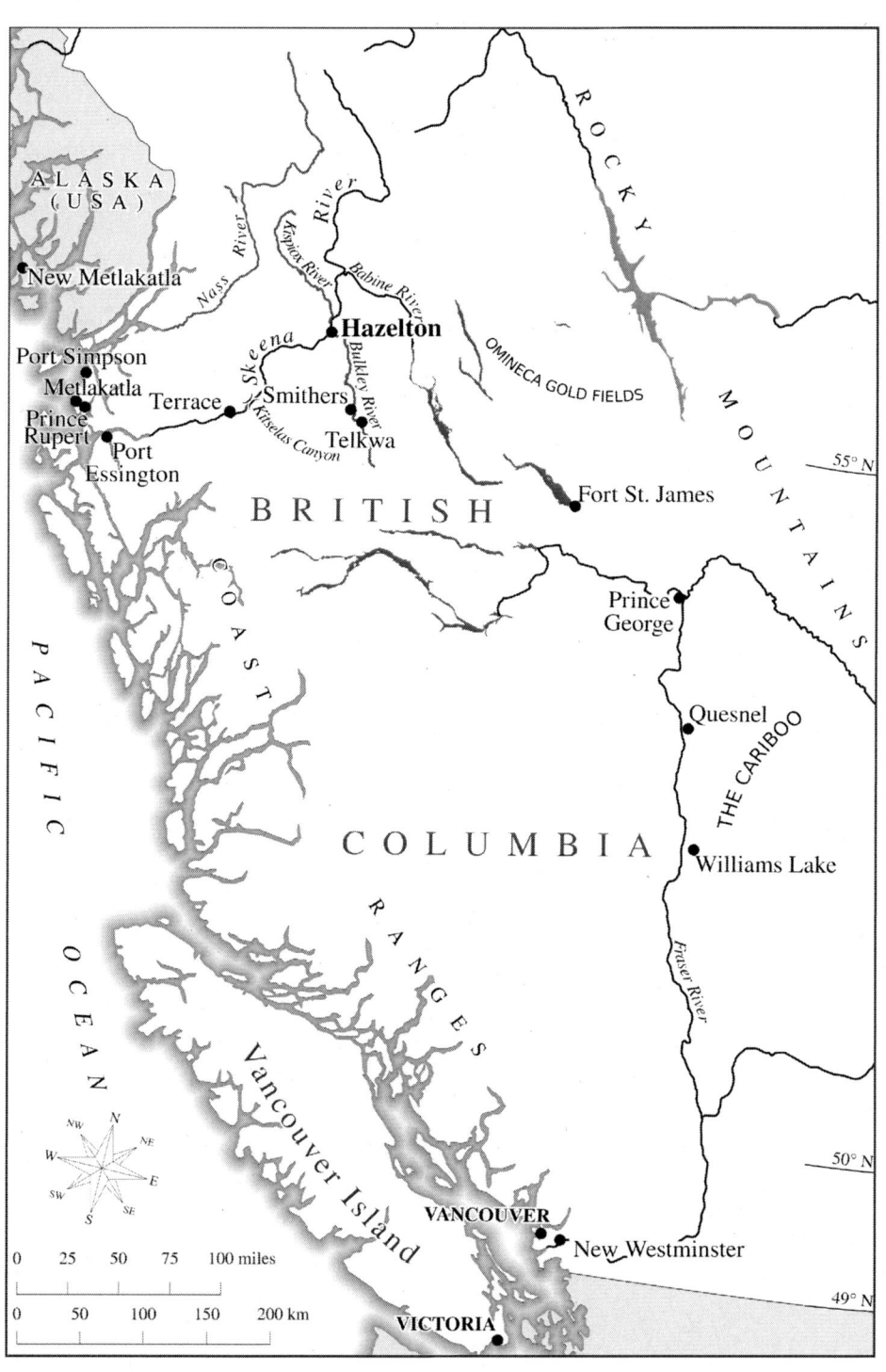

A L A S K A
(U S A)

New Metlakatla

Port Simpson
Metlakatla
Prince
Rupert
Port
Essington
Terrace

Nass River

Kispiox River

River

Babine River

Skeena

Kitselas Canyon

Bulkley River

Smithers
Telkwa

Hazelton

OMINECA GOLD FIELDS

Fort St. James

R O C K Y

M O U N T A I N S

55° N

B R I T I S H

C O A S T

Prince
George

Quesnel

THE CARIBOO

Williams Lake

C O L U M B I A

PACIFIC

R A N G E S

OCEAN

Vancouver Island

Fraser River

NW N NE
W   E
SW S SE

0   25   50   75   100 miles

0   50   100   150   200 km

VANCOUVER
New Westminster

50° N

VICTORIA

49° N

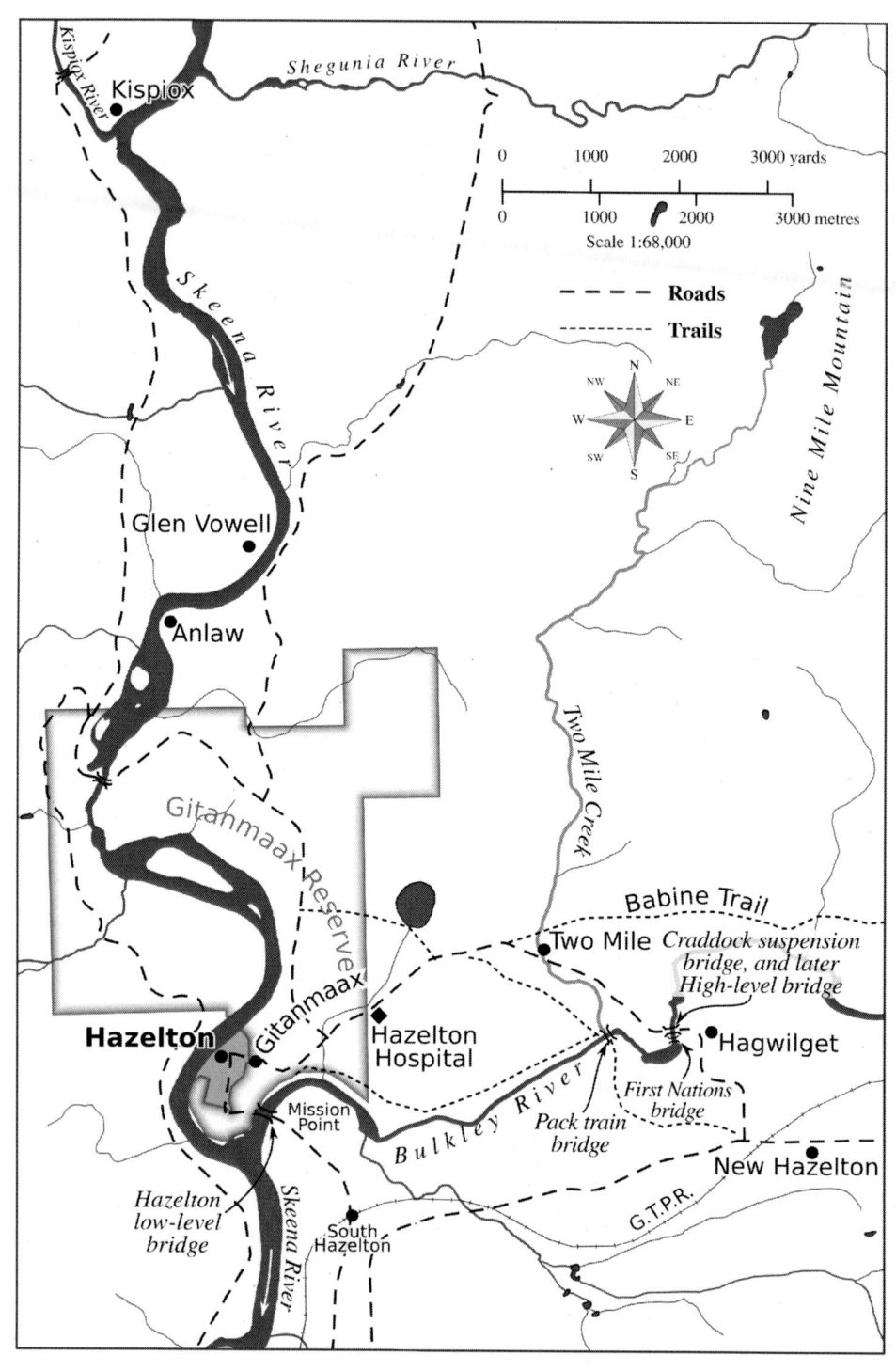

Kispiox River

Kispiox

Shegunia River

0   1000   2000   3000 yards

0   1000   2000   3000 metres
Scale 1:68,000

- - - **Roads**
········· **Trails**

N
NW   NE
W   E
SW   SE
S

Nine Mile Mountain

Skeena River

Glen Vowell

Anlaw

Gitanmaax Reserve

Two Mile Creek

Babine Trail

Two Mile   *Craddock suspension
bridge, and later
High-level bridge*

Gitanmaax

Hazelton Hospital

Hazelton

Mission Point

*Hazelton
low-level
bridge*

Skeena River

South
Hazelton

Bulkley River

*Pack train
bridge*

*First Nations
bridge*

Hagwilget

New Hazelton

G.T.P.R.

Introduction

WHEN HORACE WRINCH DIED in October 1939, the *Vancouver Sun* said he was "for forty years perhaps the best known and most beloved man in Northern British Columbia." Leading members of the community, prominent clerics and judges among them, attended his funeral at First Memorial United Church in Vancouver. Premier Duff Pattullo said he was deeply grieved to hear of his death. In Kispiox, where Horace had gone first, the Gitxsan held their own memorial service for him.

Although most people along the Skeena River have heard of Wrinch Memorial Hospital and many have had occasion to visit it, little is known about the man who built it and ran it for thirty-six years. Even less is known about the first thirty-four years of his life that he spent in England and Ontario before coming to British Columbia in 1900.

Horace was born on a farm in Essex in 1866, and travelled to Canada at the age of fourteen, seemingly on his own. After finishing his schooling at an agricultural college in Quebec, he farmed in Ontario for approximately ten years. Converted to Methodism, he became determined to serve as a medical missionary, and to that end qualified as a doctor and surgeon at Trinity Medical College, taking top honours. He married Alice Breckon, a nurse and schoolteacher, and someone as dedicated to service as he was. In 1900, they travelled to Kispiox in the Upper Skeena district in northern British Columbia. A couple of years later, they moved to Hazelton, where he built a hospital, founded a nursing school and started a hospital farm. It was the first hospital in the interior of British Columbia — from Atlin in the far north to the Cariboo in the south.

In 1907, to help fund the hospital and to create a sense of community around it, he established a basic form of health insurance. For a dollar a month, a member could obtain a ticket entitling him or her to medical and hospital services. This scheme lasted for several decades.

Horace was a magistrate for over twenty years, a community leader and a minister of the Methodist Church. Always interested in public health, he helped found the British Columbia Hospital Association in 1918 and served as its president for two terms. Drawn into politics in 1924, he served as an MLA, also for two terms. In the Legislature in Victoria, he became a well-known advocate for state health insurance. He introduced a motion for its adoption in February 1927.

"Mr. Speaker," Victoria's *Daily Colonist* recorded him as saying, "the necessity of health insurance legislation is a matter of vital importance for the people of this province. . . . In discussing the idea with sensible people, I have failed to hear one cogent argument advanced against the project." Continuing, he argued that the time had come for the House to commence the process of introducing province-wide health insurance for all citizens. His motion in the House propelled the train of events that led to the British Columbia Health Insurance Act. Given Royal Assent on April 1, 1936, this act was the culmination of many years of work by Horace and many others.

Horace did not stand for re-election in 1933. He retired from the hospital in 1936 after thirty-six years of service to his community.

This biography is based on his personal and professional letters and on contemporaneous reports in newspapers and journals. One problem in writing Horace's biography has been his reserve and self-effacement. In his letters and even in his short history of Hazelton Hospital, written in 1938, he hardly mentions himself at all.

Another problem has been what to call him. Should he be Dr. Wrinch? Or Wrinch? Or Horace? He was a formal, reserved person, seldom seen without a stiff collar and tie, and it might seem disrespectful to call him Horace. It would, however, seem artificial and isolating to call him anything else. In many ways progressive and tolerant of changing social mores, he might forgive the informality.

CHAPTER 1

The Farmer's Boy
1866–1880

HORACE WRINCH WAS BORN in the land of John Constable and died in the land of Emily Carr. The difference between the works of these iconic landscape painters illustrates his life. One was an apostle of nature and of the beauty inherent in the English countryside. The other was a painter of the forests and villages of the First Nations on the Skeena River in northern British Columbia. One was nineteenth-century romanticism, the other twentieth-century post-impressionism. Horace moved from Constable's settled, pastoral East Anglia, with its soft greens and open skies, its flat, arable lands and marshy inlets, to the raw, unsettled frontier reflected in Emily Carr's paintings of the Skeena River, with its mountains, dark mysteries and totem poles. From the farm, with its age-old rhythms moving in tune with the seasons, he moved to the angularity of life in a mission hospital. From the land of *Dedham Vale* and the *Hay Wain* and of open, light-filled skies, he moved to the dark forests of Gitanmaax and Kispiox, Kitwancool and Kitseguecla. Horace was born into the certainties and self-confidence of Victorian England but lived and died amidst the changing moral landscapes and doubt of the twentieth century. In East Anglia, he was in the settled middle; on the Skeena River, he was on the frontier.

John Constable, it has been said, was attempting not only to paint the scenery he saw around him but also to use landscape painting as a means of conveying ideas about morality and intellectual truth. Horace Wrinch, farmer, medical missionary, hospital builder, community leader and progressive politician, lived a life dedicated to his own conceptions of morality and truth. His motivation was religion; his execution, medicine.

———

On April 29, 1880, fourteen-year-old Horace stood at the rail of the SS *Sarmation* watching the Liverpool dockers cast off the mooring lines. He was travelling to Quebec, leaving behind him his parents and siblings on a farm in Essex. All the sights and sounds of the port would have been exciting and new to him. He would have felt on his lips the tang of the salt air and in his nose the smoke and grime of an industrial port. Around him towered the mass of ropes, masts and funnels of shipping in the busy harbour. On the dock, a crowd of people waved farewell to passengers, many of them also emigrants.

As the long, sleek ship with three masts and one funnel edged away from the dock, Horace was at the pivotal moment when one door was closing and another opening. He would have felt the presence of his home and family, but also that void that comes to travellers at the point of departure and before the next mental landscape opens. The enthusiasm of his siblings, the stifled emotions of his parents at the moment of parting, the walks around the farm to collect memories and say his farewells would still be fresh in his mind. Yet the uncertainty of the future and the enormity of what lay ahead would have loomed large for him, exciting and more than a little frightening.

Horace spent his boyhood on a farm in Essex, England. There he developed the practical streak that would serve him well all his life. With his family, he lived and breathed farming. He would also have learned to ride and care for horses, both of which were to be useful skills for him on the frontier. Few hands went idle on a farm. A young boy was expected to do many chores — from feeding chickens and collecting eggs to chopping wood. At harvest time, he and his brothers would have gathered in the fields with the local boys and used sticks and nets to catch the rabbits fleeing their sanctuaries in the crops as the binders approached. Wrinches had lived and farmed in Suffolk and Essex since the sixteenth century. Nothing in this heritage indicated that Horace would be anything but a farmer. The medicine, surgery, religion, hospital, community leadership and politics — all these came later.

Horace's father, Leonard, had married Elizabeth Cooper in Great Oakley in 1861. True to the family calling, he was a farmer. He and Elizabeth had a large Victorian family, all to be provided futures from limited resources. Horace, their fourth child, was born on January 6, 1866. Baptized into the Church of England at nearby St. Michael's, he had many siblings: Georgina, Leonard Edward, Marion Agnes, Walter, Frank Sidney, Warwick, John Alfred, Charles and Mary Evelyn.

This was the heyday of Victorian England. Prince Albert had died only a few years before, and Queen Victoria was settling into her deep and long mourning. The American Civil War had effectively ended at Appomattox the previous year. A few months after Horace was born, the two colonies on the Pacific coast of British North America came together as the one colony of British Columbia. The Dominion of Canada had not yet come into existence.

Leonard Wrinch, in the order of classes in England at that time, was a gentleman, but a member of the minor gentry rather than of the landed gentry. At the time of the 1881 census, he and Elizabeth were living with their children at Birch Hall, in Essex. Birch Hall was not as grand as it sounds, being a small but solid house of two storeys, with farm buildings clustering around a yard close by. Leonard leased a farm of 600 acres and employed fifteen men and five boys, as well as a cook and housemaid.

Birch Hall lies between the pleasant village of Kirby-le-Soken, stretching along the road two miles west of Walton-on-the-Naze, and Hamford Water, a small marshy inlet that leads into the North Sea south of the River Stour. Some of the Wrinch ancestors had lived in Dedham, a few miles away across the river, in what is now known as Constable Country. In such a rich farming area, agriculture should have been able to provide farmers with a good livelihood.

Leonard and Elizabeth engaged Miss Clarissa Golding, from London, as a governess for their children. When not learning their ABCs from her, the Wrinch children would have had time to explore the countryside. Hamford Water, a few fields to the north of Birch Hall, was an area of tidal creeks, mudflats, islands, salt marshes and splashy grasslands. To the children, these saltings — that is, lands flooded regularly by tides — would have been irresistible. This is flat land where the sky comes down to meet the low horizon, a land of water and grasses, of lights and mysterious sounds.

The time for formal schooling inevitably arrived and Miss Golding made way for a tutor. When he was about twelve, Horace was sent to Albert Memorial College. This school, now called Framlingham College, was a public (non-state) school in Framlingham in Suffolk. *Hazell's Annual Cyclopedia* for 1887 stated that Albert Memorial College devoted part of its curriculum to agriculture. Significantly, this school was one of only three in England to which farmers sent their sons to study agriculture, suggesting that Horace's father was at that time guiding him into farming. Here Horace was awarded a prize for French, and was presented with a book called, appropriately, *Self-Help.* This was probably Dr. Samuel Smiles's Victorian best-seller that contained moral tales about the benefits of thrift and hard work. Horace attended the school in 1879, leaving later that year or in early 1880 to journey to Quebec.

The Rev. W.W. Bird, the headmaster, who was leaving at the end of term to take over another school, addressed the boys. In his comments, he advised them "never to join in any undertaking upon which they could not invoke a blessing from Heaven." Possibly the "loud and hearty cheering from the whole school" after his remarks was more because it was the end of term or because the headmaster was leaving than for the urge to strive for blessings from Heaven. How many of the pupils were faithful to his direction later in life? Horace, for one, certainly was.

As the children grew, Leonard and Elizabeth would have wondered about their futures. Farming was what the Wrinches had always done and it was all they knew. No doubt the Wrinch girls, aware of family circumstances, knew that unless they could find husbands, being a governess like Miss Golding could well be their fate in life. In normal times, the boys would settle down and become farmers. Horace's brother Leonard would probably farm at Birch Hall. What should Horace do? Should he also become a farmer? If so, where? These were not, however, normal times for farmers in Essex.

Nostalgic memoirs, dreams of simpler times and greater glories, novels and romantic movies have cast a golden haze over rural England in the late Victorian period. It was, this picture tells us, a pastoral idyll — a time of bounteous harvests, smiling milkmaids, faithful cart horses and bulging hay wagons trundling home in the golden sunset. The reality of farming, though, was very different. English agriculture was in a severe depression with no end in sight.

"...the greatest single event of the 'seventies, fraught with immeasurable consequences for the future," G.M. Trevelyan wrote in his classic *English Social History*, "was the sudden collapse of English agriculture. From 1875 onwards the catastrophe set in. . . . The overthrow of the British landed aristocracy by the far-distant democracy of American farmers was one outcome of this change of economic circumstances."

And it wasn't only the aristocracy. Small farmers such as Leonard Wrinch were hit more severely than many others. Hard times for English farmers started in the 1870s and would continue well into the following century. Refrigeration, mechanization, new canals opening Chicago — the railhead for the American meat and grain business — to ocean shipping led to cheaper imports into England. This resulted in a collapse of prices for English farm produce. Essex was particularly hard hit because, with an ever-growing network of railways, it lost its competitive advantage of being so close to London. Bad weather in England in 1875, 1877 and 1879 spoiled harvests. In the decade after 1875, the acreage given to wheat in England fell by a million acres. By 1881, there were 100,000 fewer farm workers in England than there had been in 1871.

Farming in England was not, therefore, a promising career for the sons of Leonard Wrinch. Conceivably, Leonard and Elizabeth were starting to believe that farming was a dying way of life. Although it is not clear how deeply the farming depression affected them, they may have foreseen financial decline for themselves if they continued to farm in Essex. This could have played a significant part in the decision about to be made.

Since it contained all the farming news he needed, Leonard probably read the article in the *Essex Standard*, on September 6, 1879, which said:

> In the present depressed condition of agriculture and the gloomy prospects still before the farmers, the question of Emigration is sure to attract great attention amongst those, especially, those of small means. . . . It is natural and in many ways desirable that Englishmen leaving their own country should direct their eyes and feet to the Colonies, where their lot would be cast amongst their own flesh and blood, and they would live under British laws and institutions; and we are, therefore, not surprised to learn that the Government of the Dominion of Canada are making vigorous efforts to divert the stream of emigration to that great colony. . . . No more judicious course than this could be adopted.

Although Leonard was well-established in his community and set in his ways, it is possible that he may have been thinking that he and his family — or, if not him, his children — could emigrate to Canada and start afresh. He and Elizabeth, in any event, had commitments holding them back from emigrating. They both had aging parents who could not be abandoned. His mother, aged seventy-six, and her father, Edward Cooper, aged eighty-eight and still living in nearby Great Oakley, were both still needing filial care. If emigration was on his mind, Leonard may have suggested that they send one or more of the boys ahead to finish their education in Canada. The rest of them could follow later.

Not only did Canada advertise for immigrants but it also sent agents to Great Britain to foster enthusiasm for the new country and to facilitate immigration. In particular, Canada wanted farmers. British newspapers carried many articles about the activities of Canadian government agents. The campaign was successful. In October 1879, it was reported that 2,246 people left Liverpool for Canada, up from the 786 of September 1877. "The reports received of good and bountiful harvests in all parts of the Dominion have induced many persons to join their friends," it was stated in the press, "and the number of agricultural emigrants to Canada has greatly increased of late."

Leonard and Elizabeth made the decision: Horace would go to Canada. Listed in the *Sarmation*'s passenger list as a labourer and travelling in steerage, he left Liverpool on April 29, 1880, and arrived in Quebec on May 11. The fact that he was travelling in steerage speaks either to the state of the Wrinch funds or to Leonard's parsimony. There is no evidence to indicate that he was travelling with companions, although it is conceivable he was attached to some other family for the journey. At Liverpool, Horace would have had to find his way from the railway station, avoid the offers of help from those happy to separate innocent and unwary emigrants from their luggage, and, before being allowed to go on board, pass the medical inspection. The Allan Line was one of the main lines ferrying immigrants to Canada, and the *Sarmation*, carrying up to 900 passengers, was one of its most important ships. Two years previously, the new Governor General of Canada, the Marquis of Lorne, and his wife, had travelled on it on their way out to take up their new posts. Steerage would not, obviously, have been as luxurious as the vice-regal quarters.

When he arrived in Quebec, Horace could well have been helped by his maternal Aunt Emily and Uncle Thomas. In June 1876, Aunt Emily had married Thomas Springer Cole, from Great Oakley, the same village where she and her sister had grown up. Thomas had emigrated to Quebec a few years previously, then had come back home and married Emily. Returning to Quebec with his bride, he had resurrected the Young Men's Christian Association there in 1875 and for many years acted as its permanent secretary.

In about 1884, they moved to Toronto, where he became the Provincial Travelling Secretary of the YMCA and later an active leader in the Gideons movement. They could have been friendly faces to meet Horace on his arrival, providing a home for him and arranging for his schooling. Clearly the connection was strong. When Horace's brother Leonard arrived a few years later, Thomas loaned him some money to help buy land in Ontario. Later in life, Horace wrote of their aunt and uncle's kindness.

Here then is Horace: a farmer's boy, fourteen years old, setting out for Canada, leaving family and friends in a clean break. His parents and his siblings, the admonitions and teaching of the Rev. W.W. Bird, the village of Kirby-le-Soken, the pastures of arable Essex and its all-important seasons, the reeds and marshes of the saltings, and, above all, the practicality that farming taught and demanded — these were the influences that would have moulded the mind and soul of the young Horace.

As Horace wandered around the ship, standing at the railings and watching England fade into the distance, he must have wondered what life would hold for him in Canada. He would never see England — or his father — again.

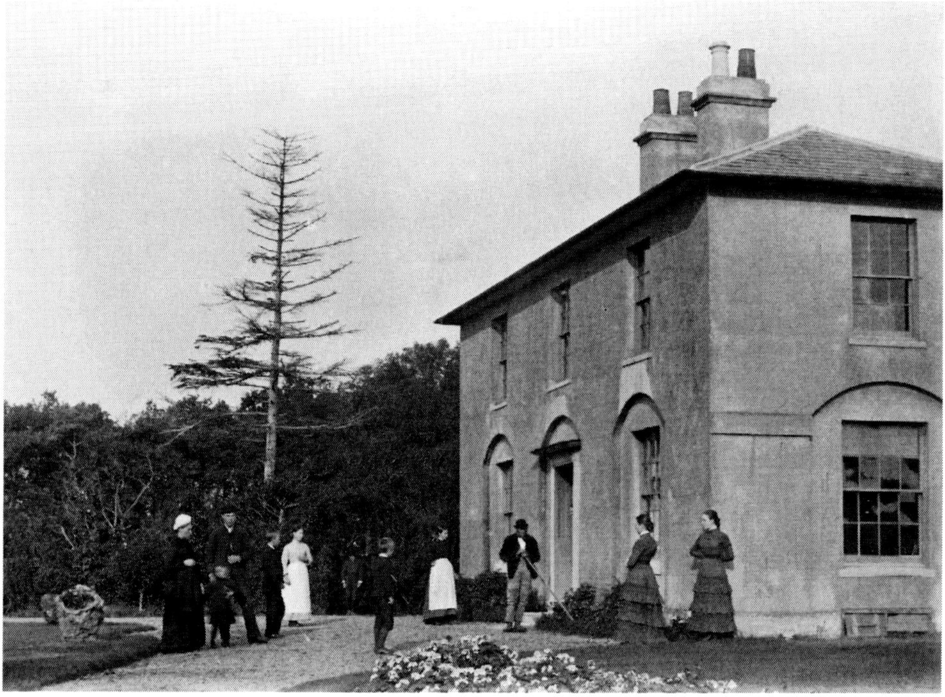

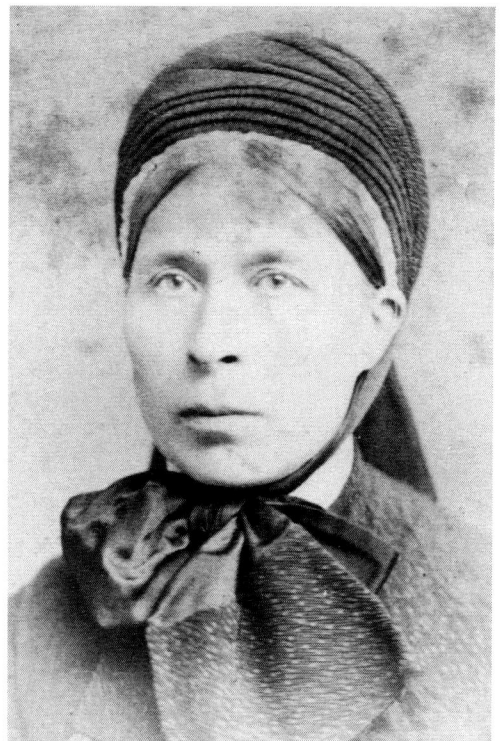

▲ The Wrinch family in front
of Birch Hall, Essex, England,
in about 1871–1873.

◄ Horace's mother
Elizabeth, in London
before 1885.

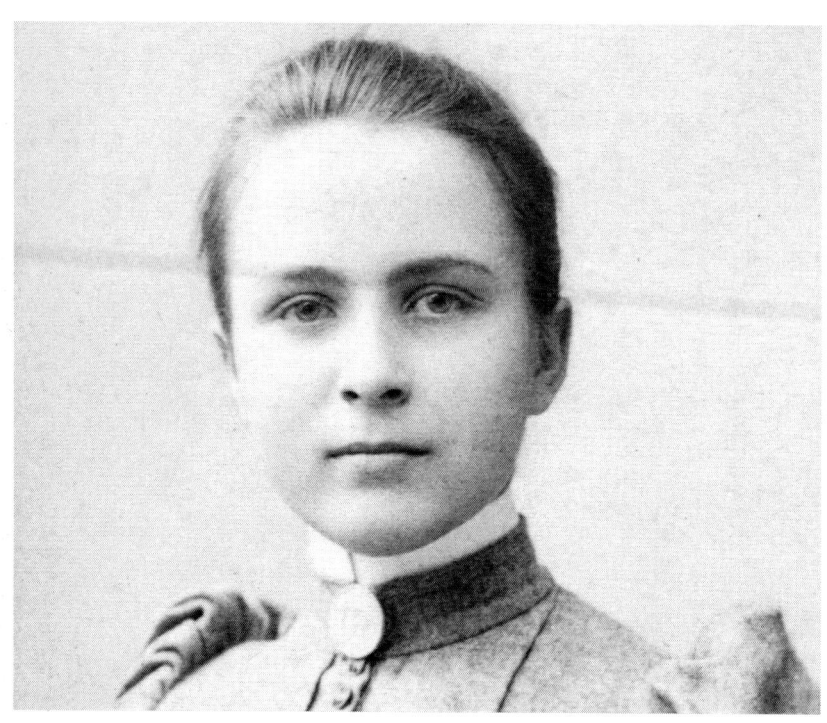

Mary Wrinch, Horace's artist sister, in 1892.

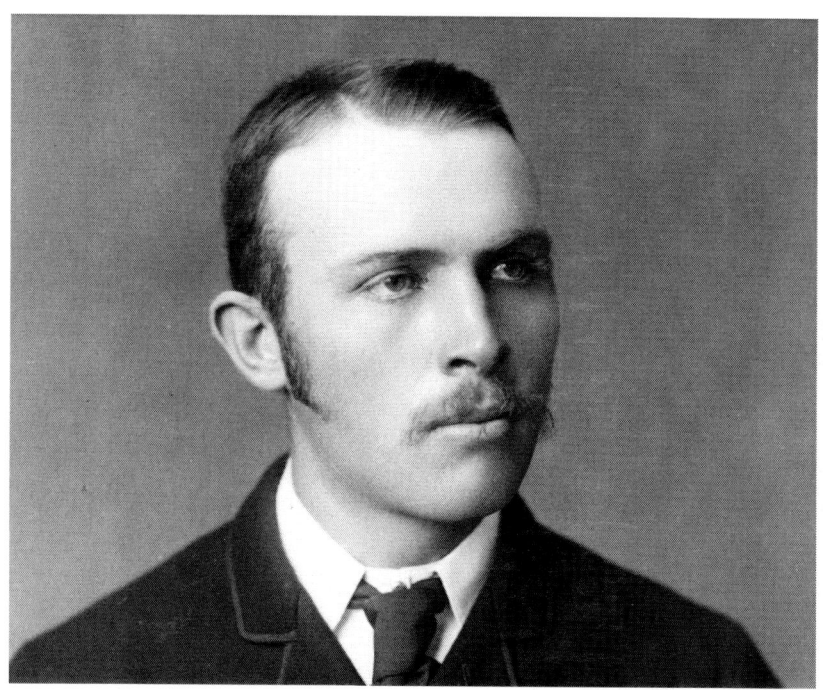

Leonard Wrinch, Horace's elder brother, in 1886.

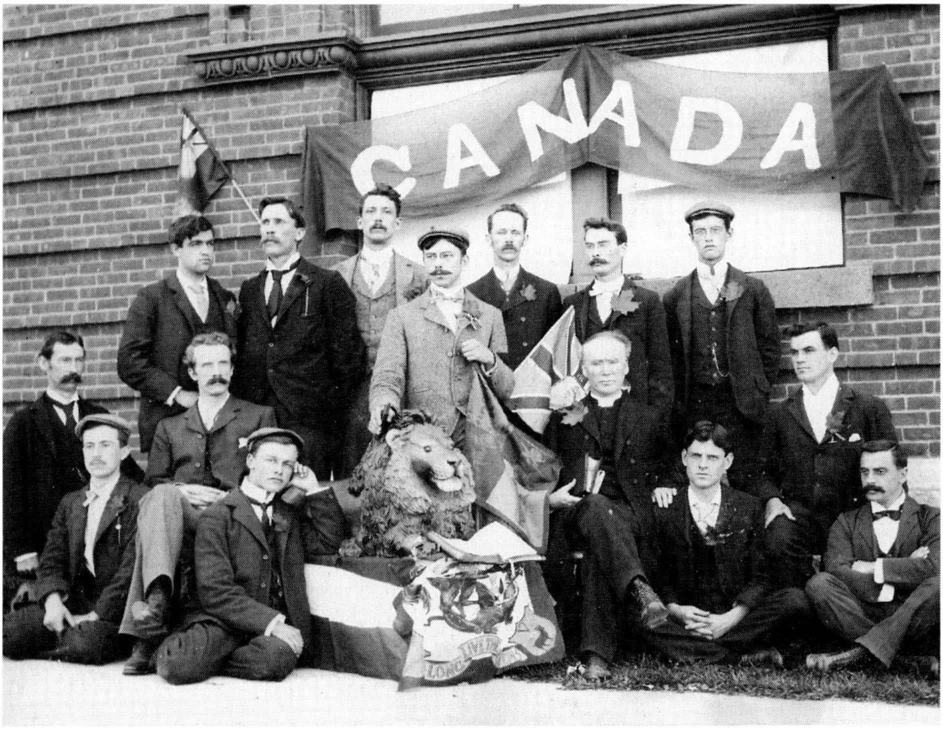

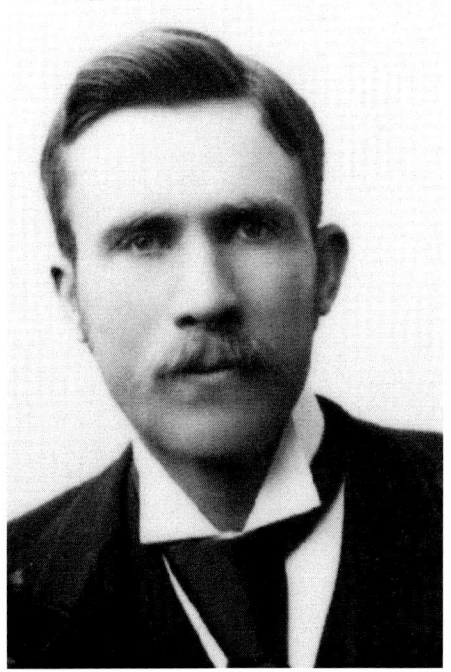

▲ Dominion Day, sometime before 1900. Horace, standing, is second from the left.

◄ Horace Wrinch in the early 1890s.

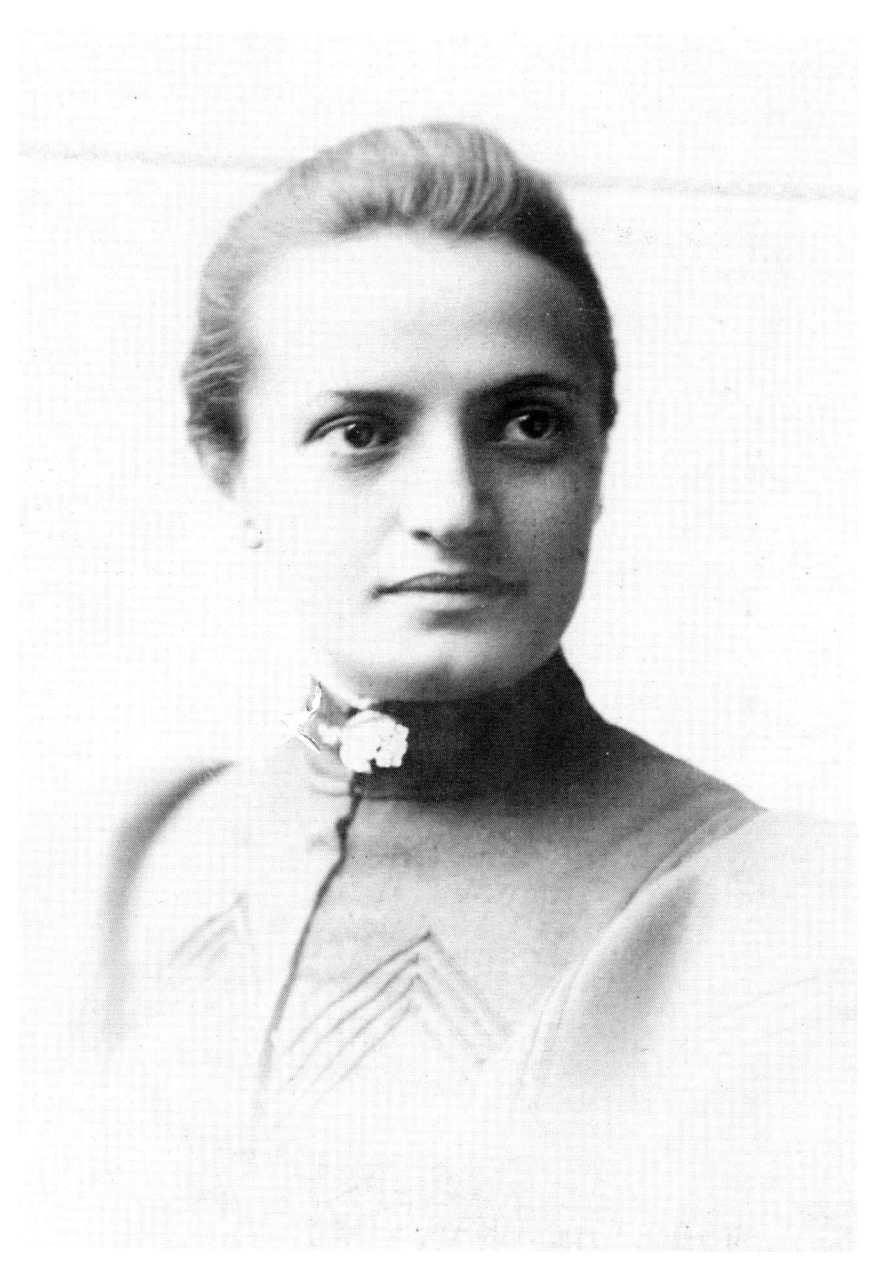

Alice Breckon, Horace's fiancée, a teacher, nurse and missionary.

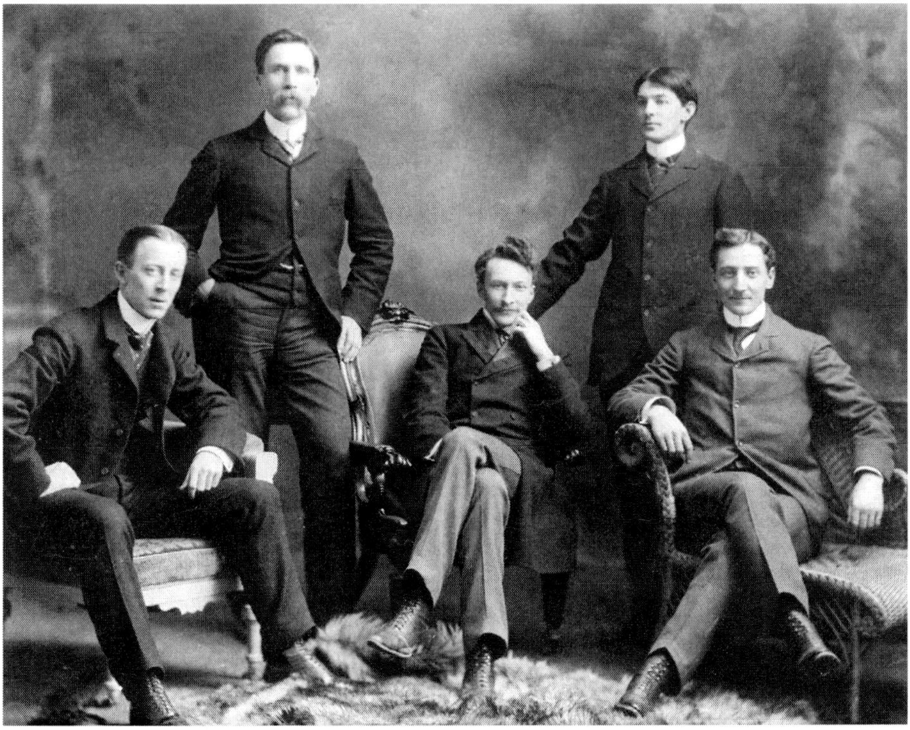

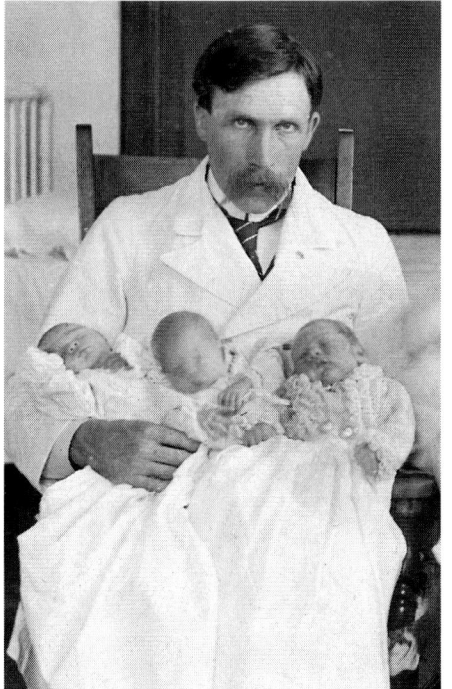

▲ St. Michael's Hospital staff
in 1899–1900. Standing, Horace
Wrinch and B. McKenna. Seated,
F.M. McNulty, B.J. Dwyer and
M. Crawford. (COURTESY: ST.
MICHAEL'S HOSPITAL ARCHIVES)

◀ Horace at St. Michael's
Hospital, Toronto,
1899–1900.

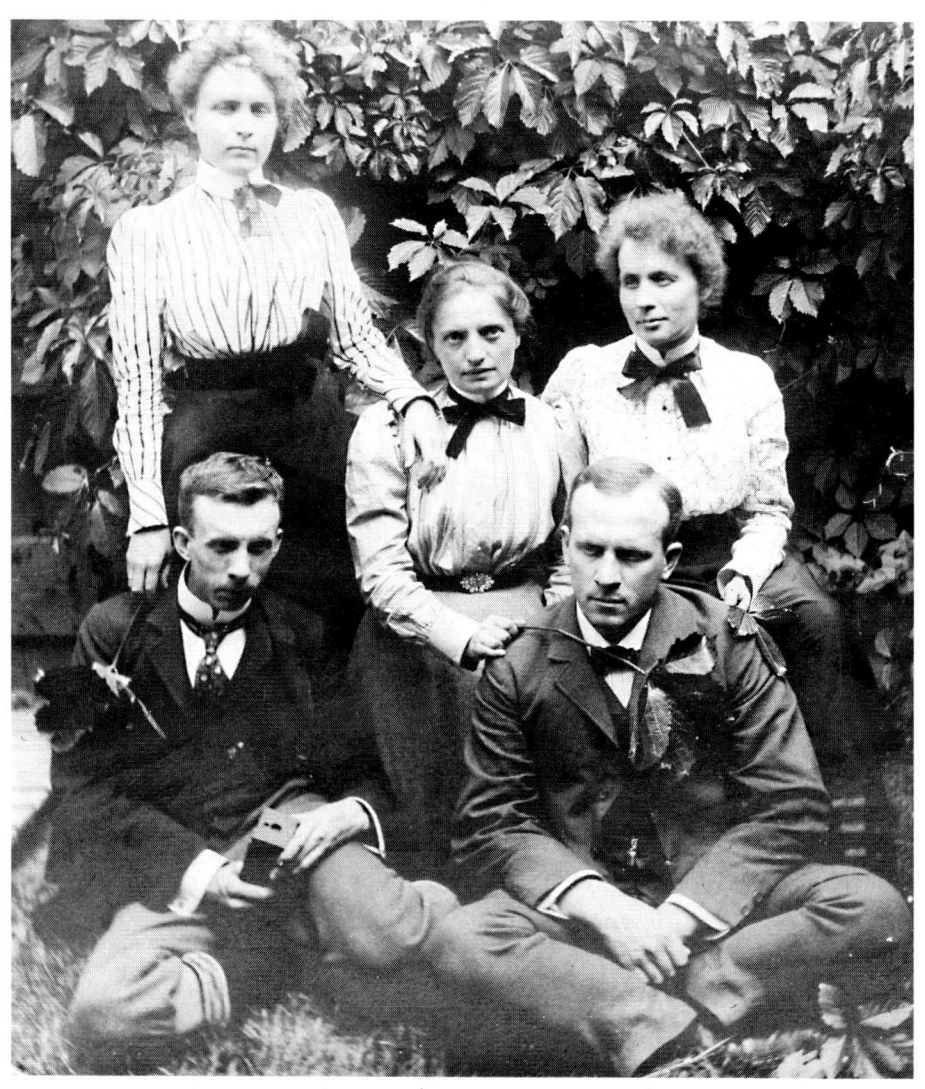

Alice, centre, with some of Horace's siblings in, perhaps, an engagement photograph. Mary Wrinch is standing on the left.

CHAPTER 2

Farmer, Missionary and Medic
1880–1900

FOLLOWING HIS ARRIVAL in Quebec, Horace enrolled at St. Francis Agricultural College in Richmond. This bilingual school was part of the larger St. Francis College and had opened only a few years previously. Situated just outside town, it was set on a high point of land overlooking the St. Francis River. A leafy, verdant place in summer, in winter it was exposed to winds moving along the river valley. For Horace, these winters in Quebec would have been much colder than winters he had been used to in Essex. After the main building of the college burned down in February 1882, a new college was built. Happily, though, the agricultural department had not been touched. During this period, the pupils had to make do for a year with lessons in the town hall and local churches. All but three of the fourteen boarders listed in the 1881 census were in their teen years, with Horace being the youngest. In this census, he was listed as belonging to the Episcopalian (Anglican) religion.

Students at the college got up at five in the morning. Horace, a farmer's boy and used to early mornings, would not have found this a great hardship. Work in the mornings varied. Sometimes he worked in the stables before breakfast. Other times it was straight to the classroom. At six he would come in to wash, have breakfast and then enjoy what the school was pleased to call "recreation time." Then there were prayers with the principal's family. After a day's work and supper, he had lectures to attend on some aspect of farming, followed by time for study.

He spent many days on the Beechmore farm, one of two farms the school managed. One was 203 acres and the other, the Model Farm, had eight fields of ten arpents (an old French land unit of about one acre) each. In addition, the school operated a vegetable garden. The students, helping the two farm labourers, worked on the farms and gardens. At this college, Horace would have come to understand all aspects of farming.

Horace's life here was rigorous. His courses had a theoretical side and a practical side. There was also remedial work in English grammar, mensuration, accounts, Canadian history and geography for those who were deemed to need it. On the theoretical side, Horace would have studied a variety of agricultural topics, municipal and rural law and veterinary arts; on the practical side, he would have been out working on the school's farms.

Nor was religion ignored. At one and the same time, the school professed to be non-sectarian and evangelical. It warned pupils that their morals and conduct would be watched so as to lead them into a virtuous and blameless life. In addition to two religious services each day, younger pupils such as Horace were required to recite portions of the scriptures, psalms and hymns every Monday morning. In case this was not enough religion, there was also the Young Men's Christian Association that Horace's uncle was so deeply involved in.

Horace spent the next three or four years at St. Francis. With his parents and siblings remaining in England, he would have become self-reliant. By necessity, he grew up quickly. In these years, Horace changed from a boy of fourteen into a young man of eighteen. When he graduated in 1884, he did so, as a contemporary account of his life records, with the Governor General's Gold Medal for academic performance.

——~~~——

Back home in Essex, Leonard and Elizabeth would have worried about Horace's welfare. They would also have been eager for news about Canada. Had they gone into nearby Ipswich one Monday in September 1881, they could have heard Rev. A.J. Bray from Montreal talk about "Canada as a Field for Settlement." The council chamber of the town hall that evening was full and many had to be turned away. The mayor, Alfred Wrinch, coincidentally Leonard's first cousin, introduced the speaker. Neatly noting that the sea passage to Quebec was about 1,000 miles less than the one to New York, Rev. Bray described the advantages of Canada as a welcoming place for immigrants.

His address was most likely part of the Canadian government's campaign to attract settlers. He expounded on the huge, empty, fertile spaces west of Ontario, where good land could be had for very little. Stretching the truth more perhaps than a clergyman should, he said that no climate was so good as Canada's and that, although there were some who had said it was cold there, "he had inquired of farmers in every part of the Dominion and had never heard one complaint of the severity of the winter."

Whether or not the Wrinch family was indeed planning to follow Horace, it was soon too late for Horace's father. In February 1881, perhaps aware he was seriously ill, Leonard made his will, and on April 9th of the following year he died. Nothing in this will·shows any evidence that he was thinking of emigrating. "As a mark of respect for the memory of the deceased," the local paper said, ". . . most of the farmers and residents of the parish and neighbourhood attended the funeral." Leonard's will was probated in May, leaving a gross estate of £2,317. If the family had previously decided to emigrate to Canada, his death might have caused a less resolute person than Elizabeth to falter.

As it was, Elizabeth carried on undaunted. Soon after her husband died, she gave up the farm. But she could not go yet. Leonard's mother, also Elizabeth, and her father, Edward Cooper, were still alive. When Edward died at the end of March 1883, he left four surviving children and a useful estate of over £24,000. Elizabeth knew that with her mother-in-law still alive and needing help, she herself could not yet leave, but there was nothing to stop the eldest of her children from following Horace to Canada. Leonard was the first to go, leaving Kirby-le-Soken the year after his father died. Set down in the passenger list as a "gentleman," he journeyed on the 3,500-ton SS *Montreal*, arriving in Quebec on May 22, 1883. Elizabeth had perhaps sent him on ahead to meet Horace and to buy some farm property in Ontario. Meanwhile, she could finish dealing with family affairs in Essex before joining them.

After her mother-in-law died in January 1885, there was no longer any reason for Elizabeth to stay. While she was wrapping up her affairs, Horace's brother, fourteen-year-old Warwick, left home and arrived in Quebec in May, travelling on the SS *Circassian*.

On April 30, 1885, on the instructions of Leonard's executors, Messrs. Spurling & Sons auctioned off "all the valuable Household Furniture and Effects." These included Brussels and other carpets, a mahogany telescope, a dining table, rosewood card tables, an eight-day clock in an inlaid case, feather beds and bedding, a hundred ounces of plate, a Derby tea service, a Copeland green-and-white dinner service and miscellaneous kitchen, stable and garden utensils. Elizabeth, it seems clear, was selling everything and leaving.

In the *British Farmer's Guide to Ontario*, issued by the government of Ontario in 1880 and designed to entice British farmers to immigrate, the advantages of farming in Ontario over farming in England were made clear. Apart from the fertile soil and bountiful agricultural products, these advantages included, it stated, the purchase of land for an amount similar to an annual rental of land in England: light taxes; no poor rate, "for there are few paupers"; no tithes or similar levies because there was no state church; and, for those who chose to rent, low rents and easy terms. Halton County, about thirty miles southwest of Toronto, was described in the *Guide* as being one of the older counties of Ontario. The *Guide* praised the fruits and, in particular, the strawberries that grew in abundance. The land was also well suited for grain and stock-raising. "Fewer counties," the *Guide* said, "offer greater attractions to old country settlers than Halton." It sounded safe and familiar. It sounded like home.

After he had finished his studies at St. Francis and after a short time working in a notary's office in Richmond, Horace joined his twenty-two-year-old brother Leonard in Ontario. In November 1884, Leonard bought a farm of a hundred acres from John Lucas, a pioneer in Halton County, for $6,000. He borrowed $1,600 from the Western Canada Loan and Savings Co. and, in 1885, a further $1,000 from his Uncle Thomas, giving mortgages to both. The farm was located just outside Bronte in the Trafalgar Township. Bronte, a fishing village on Lake Ontario, supported a flourishing shipbuilding industry that produced many of the fishing vessels and schooners sailing on the Great Lakes. Palermo was the next closest village, being only four miles away. After they arrived in August 1885 on the SS *Polynesian*, Elizabeth and her other children joined Horace, Warwick and Leonard on the farm and re-established the family home.

—*∿∿*—

The Wrinch family had settled in a populated, well-farmed area. Except for the First Nations, who had lived on the land for thousands of years and considered it theirs, most of Canada at this time would have seemed largely empty. It had a population of little more than 4.3 million, of which almost 2 million lived in Ontario, approximately 1.3 million in Quebec and 50,000 in British Columbia, with the others scattered around the country. Canada was still a predominantly rural society, having only thirty-seven towns and cities with a population of over 5,000. None of these, except Victoria, the capital of British Columbia with its population of 6,000, was west of

Winnipeg. Victoria itself was described as a "thriving city . . . [where] the scenery is marvellously fine; the climate salubrious, and sport abundant." More prosaically, it was also described by others as a quiet, muddy town at the southern end of Vancouver Island.

When Horace arrived in Canada, the country was younger than he was. After years of manoeuvring and discussion, of conferences and political strife, Ontario, Quebec, Nova Scotia and New Brunswick had come together in 1867 to form the Dominion of Canada. Although very much part of the British Empire — and passionately so as far as the British immigrants were concerned — it was starting to feel its own identity separate from Britain.

At the time British Columbia joined the Dominion in 1871, the Skeena River district, a sea of mountain ranges, wide valleys, forests, rivers and streams seven hundred miles north of Victoria, was still largely unknown. A few muddy mule tracks and narrow wagon roads, usually closed by snow and ice in winter, were the only routes on land. Only a few non-Indigenous people were to be seen, mainly some strategically located Hudson's Bay Company traders who dealt mainly in the fur trade, some determined missionaries and increasing numbers of ever-optimistic miners. Where the Skeena River merged with the Bulkley River is the point explorers and traders had called the Forks. On this point was a Gitxsan settlement called Gitanmaax.

A few years before, in 1866, the Hudson's Bay Company had sent Thomas Hankin and William Manson, two of its traders, to manage its post at the Forks. Situated on the flat land on the south side of the Bulkley River, the post was soon closed for being unprofitable. Hankin, though, had recognized the trading possibilities of the land across the river. In the spring of 1871, having left the Hudson's Bay Company, he set up a store on the riverbank there, close to Gitanmaax. On account of the hazel bushes growing so profusely on the bench above the settlement, he named the hamlet Hazelton.

This small community at first consisted of a few houses and a trading store or two, but it soon grew. The Collins Overland Telegraph was an enterprise to build a telegraph line to Europe, with the line going through British Columbia and then through Alaska to connect with one being built across Siberia. By mid-1866, the line had reached Fort Stager at Kispiox, a Gitxsan village approximately eight miles upriver from Hazelton, but was then abandoned after news of the completion of a telegraph cable across the Atlantic arrived. The community grew as some telegraph workers remained in the area to prospect for minerals. The discovery of gold in the Omineca Mountains brought more prospectors into the district in the gold rush of 1869–1872. Even after the rush petered out, many miners stayed to prospect in the hills in the summer, spending the winters in Hazelton.

These settlers and prospectors needed supplies. With the Skeena River being impassable for steamers at that time, the only ways to transport supplies to Hazelton were by canoe up the river in summer and by dog sled over the ice in winter. Some with mules and horses also found their way up the overland trails from the South, but that was a long and rough journey. In the early days, steamers could go up the Skeena River only a short distance from Port Essington at its mouth. Goods, including the mail, were taken as far as possible by steamer and were then unloaded and taken by canoe or mule train for the remainder of the journey to Hazelton, and then on to prospectors and settlers in the hinterland.

Although the first attempt to reach Hazelton from Port Essington by steamer had been made in June 1866, many more attempts followed. Even after the steamer *Caledonia* successfully reached Hazelton in May 1891, the river was navigable only from May to October. Ice in winter and variable water levels meant that until the railroad arrived in 1912 the Skeena River remained a formidable obstacle.

Farming, religion and, later, medicine dominated Horace's life between 1880 and 1900. Being a private person, though, he left no description of what he did during this time. Save for a few scraps of information in church and other archives, none of his papers from this early period has survived. Evidence of his progress can, though, be found in church minutes and college and missionary publications.

These years of growing up and farming in Ontario were critical to the formation of his character and the development of his abilities.

After he had joined his brother Leonard at the farm at Bronte, he bought a half interest in a hundred-acre lot from him, borrowing $3,000 to pay for it and then giving him back a first mortgage on the land. Horace, a farmer's boy and trained as a farmer in Quebec, then settled down to a farmer's life. He and his brother worked the soil together at Bronte for approximately ten years, with Leonard continuing there until 1919. In a number of places, Horace is called an excellent mechanic and he probably maintained the machinery on the farm. Here he also learned carpentry and cabinetmaking. Nothing indicated that he would be anything but a farmer all his life.

Then, reportedly in 1888, something happened that changed his life and set it in a completely different direction. The lightning bolt of religious conversion hit him. He became a fervent Methodist. Although he had been baptized into the Church of England, he now found a new sense of God. This was not a teenage crush on Christ; this was an adult adoption of a more deeply held faith and one that demanded action and good deeds as well as good thoughts. Horace became illuminated with the convert's zeal.

The family religion was now split. The 1891 census records Horace as farming at Bronte and living in the house of his brother Leonard. With them lived their mother, Elizabeth, now aged fifty, and siblings Agnes, Frank, Warwick, Alfred and Mary. While the others declared themselves as Anglican, Leonard, Horace and Frank declared themselves as Methodists. Horace's conversion was the most important event in his life. His actions thereafter were governed by his understanding of God and by the need to help others in body and in spirit.

Religion was all-pervasive in the last half of the nineteenth century. "No one will ever understand Victorian England who does not appreciate that among highly civilized countries," Sir Robert Ensor wrote in the Oxford History of England classic study *England: 1870–1914*, "it was one of the most religious that the world has known." This was largely true throughout the English-speaking world.

The Methodist Church in Canada had only recently come into existence, being the union of a number of like-thinking churches. It was, above all, a church that emphasized the duty to perform practical service for the community. Horace's religious zeal, a powerful motivation in many young people in the 1890s, was part of the religious nature of the age, an age where the Methodist philosophy of doing good for society was making the English-speaking world devout in a practical way. These were the years of evangelism and salvation by good works.

Leonard had a similar conversion experience. Together, he and Horace joined the Methodist church in nearby Palermo. Both being leaders, they soon bubbled to the surface of the small pool of a hundred or so Methodists in the district. The Recording Steward's records for Palermo show that as early as 1889 Leonard was active in the church and was a member of the parish board. By the following year, Horace was also on the board. In August 1892, the minutes recorded that Horris Wrench [sic] was elected a local preacher. In July 1894, they stated:

> Brother Horice C. Wrinch [sic], who has been a local preacher for more than six months and whom we deem called to separate himself entirely to the work of the ministry and qualified therefor, we therefore ask the Milton District Meeting to recommend him as a candidate for the itinerant ministry of the Methodist Church.

Later, when Horace was about to leave for the frontier wilderness of British Columbia, a fellow student from Albert College wrote:

> Dr. Wrinch was converted at twenty-two years of age, and united with [joined] the Methodist Church at Mount Pleasant appointment, Palermo Circuit, Milton District. He was recommended for the Methodist Ministry by the Palermo Quarterly Board in February 1894, but did not apply for admission on probation until 1899, when the recommendation was endorsed by the Central Methodist Church, Toronto, of which he was then a member and president of the Epworth League.

Ever practical, Horace involved himself in community causes. When, in 1891, nearby Appleby needed a community hall, he became a member of the committee set up to canvass the community, raise the funds, acquire the land (which was donated), plan the building and supervise its construction. The building was opened that same year. For the hall, the committee acquired 275 chairs at $31 per 100 chairs and installed carbide gas for lighting. Horace was thereupon elected one of the trustees. His work on the Appleby community hall was instructive because in a small way it taught him how to handle a community project and carry a building plan from fundraising to completion.

Between his conversion and his departure for Kispiox in 1900, Horace was active in church and mission circles. In addition to local preaching, he joined the Epworth League and the Sons of Temperance Movement. The Epworth League, named after the Lincolnshire village of Epworth, the birthplace of John and Charles Wesley, the founders of the Methodist movement, was an organization of young Methodists between the ages of eighteen and thirty-five.

Becoming active in the temperance movement, Horace attended meetings such as the ones at Palermo, Appleby and Prospect divisions in January 1893. The meeting was one where "great enthusiasm prevails," the local newspaper said, "and it is expected that one of the largest divisions in the province will be in Bronte. Many ladies were there to help in the good work, as in all good movements they are found." The Canadian Temperance Act of 1878 (the Scott Act) allowed municipalities to hold plebiscites on the prohibition of alcohol. A non-binding plebiscite in Ontario in 1894 had approved the prohibition. Temperance activism was almost a family concern. Leonard is often reported as organizing meetings and as being an active officer of the Sons of Temperance in the district. Their sister Mary was also involved, organizing, it was reported, a Sons of Temperance concert in 1892. However, she seems to have reverted because the 1901 census records her as being Church of England (Anglican).

Horace became ever more deeply drawn into church work. Perhaps inspired by the recommendation from the Palermo Board, in the early 1890s he decided to become a missionary. One unverified report credits the woman he later married, Alice Breckon, with persuading him to take up missionary work. In addition, he decided to become a medical missionary.

A local physician, Dr. Anson Buck, could well have been his inspiration and his role model. Dr. Buck had been the physician in Palermo since the 1850s. He was a much-beloved doctor and community leader and, significantly, a leading Methodist. He was an officer of the Sons of Temperance and also a teacher of medical students, with connections to Albert College in Belleville and Trinity Medical College in Toronto. Dr. Buck and Horace worked together on temperance committees. Neither a clergyman nor a doctor, Horace would have known that if he wanted to become a medical missionary, he would need qualifications. Dr. Buck could have inspired him, and opened doors.

Applying to become a student missionary, Horace filled out the application addressed to the Rev. Dr. Alexander Sutherland, secretary of the Methodist General Board of Missions. In answer to the question — what remuneration do you require? — he firmly, and perhaps wisely, wrote "none." Although he may have pondered a little about how best to answer the next question, which was about his convictions with regard to missionary service, he had no doubts. He wrote resolutely, "I believe missionary work to be the highest form of service in which one can engage. I have offered myself for that work for that reason." Then, ever practical, he wrote, "At present I do not know how much time I can give or when or whether I shall be able to give more than occasional meetings."

Until 1893, Horace continued to farm with his brother at Bronte. If he wanted — as he did — to become a medical missionary, he would first have to matriculate to qualify himself to enter medical school. Perhaps in need of money to pay for the next six years of study, he sold his share of the farm at Halton back to his brother for $4,200. He then moved to Belleville, Ontario, to take the matriculation course offered by Albert College.

This college, a good Methodist institution with strong connections to the missionary movement, granted diplomas in collegiate courses, music, finance, fine arts, commercial science and elocution, as well as teacher training, and preparation for the "Preliminary Examinations for the Methodist Church." Horace conceivably also took some religious studies there. The *Albert College Times* noted that the YMCA at the college had been "a powerful instrument in the development of the religious life of the students. Devotional meetings are held from nine to ten every Sabbath morning." The same issue noted the visit of Rev. Thomas Crosby, a missionary from British Columbia and a man very much connected to Horace's future decision to move there in 1900.

Horace was active in the Albert College community. He became the correspondence secretary for the college's Missionary Society, as well as participating in YMCA affairs both at the college and in Belleville. Of Horace, a contemporary wrote in 1900:

> From January 1894 to July 1895, he attended Albert College, where the writer first met him. He was recognized at once as a safe and strong leader, not only in Christian work but also in athletics and in the management of social and other college functions. His fellow students were always glad to honour him with office in all the college societies and he was a favourite committee member — in fact, wherever there was work to do which required good judgment he was in demand. He showed his exceptional mental ability by leading all his classes and taking the medal in general proficiency.

An undated and unsigned account of Horace's life "so far," in the United Church of Canada Archives in Toronto, relates that at Albert College he initiated the practice of meeting new students at the railway station, "thus giving them a hearty welcome and freeing them from the loneliness which comes to those away from home for the first time." It also reported that he had introduced the first "Albert College yell, which means so much in developing College spirits and in binding students together."

Between 1895 and 1900, Horace was active in a number of other church organizations. In addition to the Epworth League, the Sons of Temperance and the YMCA, he was also active in the Students' Missionary Campaign and the Young Persons' Forward Movement for Missions. These were overlapping organizations in colleges that promoted mission work and, as important, raised money to fund them. Horace became better acquainted with Rev. Dr. Sutherland, a man later to become instrumental in the establishment of the Hazelton Hospital. Sutherland, writing in the *Missionary Campaigner*, drew everyone's attention "to a missionary movement among the young people of our Church which is destined, if wisely prosecuted, to accomplish great good in promoting a missionary spirit in the Churches, and in developing true Christian liberality on the lines of systematic giving. It is becoming known as the "Students' Missionary Campaign. . . . The movement began about a year ago, and now some two hundred students, men and women . . . are ready for such service as they may be able to render."

Sutherland explained further:

The general outline of the plan is as follows: During the season of college vacation, the students will spend their time, chiefly in the districts in which they reside, and with the consent and co-operation of the pastors of our churches, in holding missionary meetings, giving information, circulating missionary literature, organizing the young people for missionary effort and systematic giving, and thus give increased momentum to the missionary work of the Church. When the vacation season is over, the work will not be abandoned, but those who return to college will still give such time as may be practicable to places within reach.

To promote this movement, a letter was sent to Methodist colleges in Canada, calling for volunteers to work as "missionaries" in their own neighbourhoods. In this campaign, planned for 1896, Horace was clearly a leader. He called for and instructed volunteers. He preached. He requested campaigners to assist in the missionary work of their local Epworth Leagues. Those in charge, a group that appears to have included Horace, issued instructions to them and exhorted them to greater endeavours. He wrote articles and leaflets with practical guidance for members. "Campaigners. Please Read this Carefully. Ten Timely Touches to Think out Thoughtfully," he wrote in one article. The ten steps included:

1. Use every available opportunity from now till college closes to get filled with missionary information and spirit. Read! Study!! Pray!!!

. . .

5. Urge the committee to get some missionary books, if only two or three, and circulate them amongst the members (not keep on a shelf to look at).

. . .

8. Don't criticise Home Missions nor speak of them as of minor importance in comparison with Foreign.

. . .

10. Cut this out and carry it in your pocket-book and refer to it before each address you give. Or, better still, carry a copy of this issue with you all the time. There are some other things in it you cannot afford to forget.

Horace was also instrumental in finding the money to enable prospective young missionaries to study at colleges. All in all, he was a zealous campaigner.

Now thirty years old, Horace's next step was to qualify as a doctor and surgeon. Consequently, after he matriculated from Albert College, he moved to Toronto. There he enrolled in Trinity Medical College, starting his courses in 1896 or possibly at the beginning of 1897. Becoming a missionary doctor at the time was neither cheap nor quick. A medical missionary had to be "at least as thoroughly prepared for practice as anyone who proposes practicing in a Christian country," a note in the *Missionary Campaigner* said.

Sad failures, it reported, had proved that a hurried medical training would not do for the mission field, where a man had to deal with disease in its most acute and chronic stages. Students were required to use even the vacations in the four-year course fruitfully. The vacation of the first year, the note said, should be spent in a drugstore, the second, assisting a medical practitioner and the third, at a hospital.

Although Leonard remained on the farm, Horace's mother and most of his siblings were now living at 619 Church Street in Toronto. For the duration of his medical training, Horace lived there with them.

Mary, his youngest sister, had started at Bishop Strachan School in 1889 (reportedly skipping classes to paint), but by 1893 she had finished and was studying at the Central School of Art (later the Ontario School of Art). As early as 1895, she was exhibiting at the Royal Canadian Academy of Arts Annual Exhibition. Horace was probably able to help Mary with an art commission because, in 1900, she illustrated a medical textbook of diseases of the nose and throat. "My mother and family backed me in everything from the start," she wrote.

In 1897, though, the year after Horace started medical school, their mother Elizabeth died. The family buried her in the nearby cemetery of St. James the Less, where over the years other members of the family would also be buried.

While studying medicine, Horace kept up his work for the Church. The *Missionary Campaigner* noted in November 1898 that of the seventeen or more men in Trinity Medical College who were intending to give their lives to missionary work, no less than eleven were connected with "our Methodist Church and would gladly enter the field in her ranks." Of Horace, it said:

> Mr. H.C. Wrinch, after getting the required matriculation standing from Albert College, entered directly upon his medical preparation for service. It is about seven years since he admitted the claims of God's neglected poor, and made it his purpose to minister to them. As to field, his preference is only that it may be one that might otherwise never be reached for the Master. His standing in the Methodist Church is that of a local preacher.

In his volunteer work for the Church, Horace went to communities around southern Ontario to talk to them about the Young People's Forward Movement for Missions. After each visit he recorded the details of the visit, how much literature he sold and their response to his message. On June 18, 1897, for example, he visited Davenport in Toronto West; on June 24, he visited the Britannia congregation, which had sixteen members and fourteen associates, and he sold to its members fifteen cents worth of missionary literature; on September 12, he went to speak at the Guelph District Convention, following which they endorsed his message of prayer and weekly donations; and on September 20, he visited Dublin Street and Paisley Street in Guelph, where he sold tracts and other literature for eighty-five cents.

While at Trinity, he was active in the college community. In 1898–1899, he was the president of the college YMCA. He was also vice-president of the Trinity Medical College Literature Society. Here he made a lifelong friend in Robert Peers, who went on to have a distinguished career in California as a tuberculosis specialist. Horace was a regular contributor of articles to the *Missionary Campaigner*. He was also now writing for medical journals. He wrote an article for the *Canada Lancet* of January 1900 entitled "A Case of Interstitial Emphysema." In the August edition, there is a note by him on "A Case of Incarcerated Ovary."

Horace graduated as a doctor and surgeon in 1899, taking honours in all four years and an overall Certificate of Honour. By 1900, he had accumulated an impressive list of qualifications. He was a Doctor of Medicine and Surgery (MDCM — *Medicinae Doctorem et Chirurgiae Magistrum*), FTMC (Fellow of Trinity Medical College) and also LCP&S, Ontario (Licentiate of the College of Physicians and Surgeons). Several good offers were made to him by eminent Toronto physicians, but he refused them all. A brilliant medical career in Toronto could have been his, had he chosen that path. He didn't. God, he believed, was calling him elsewhere.

After qualifying, Horace joined the staff of St. Michael's Hospital in Toronto as a house surgeon. Almost immediately he became secretary of the new Post-Graduate Medical Society that was formed to stimulate clinical and pathological research among house surgeons. At the November meeting, he delivered the evening's paper, which was "a very thorough study of a case of interstitial emphysema complicating pulmonary tuberculosis in the infant."

St. Michael's was exactly the type of institution to appeal to him. Although founded by the Catholic Sisters of St. Joseph, the hospital was resolutely non-denominational, necessarily so in the face of anti-Catholic prejudice in Toronto. Originally with a bed capacity of twenty-six, a staff of six doctors and four nurses (although it grew quickly in size), it had been established in 1892 in an old Baptist Church on Bond Street to care for the poor population in the south end of Toronto. In 1899, Horace was one of two (perhaps three) interns there, working with the long-time medical superintendent, Dr. Robert Dwyer. He would have taken careful note of the fact that the hospital also had its own nurses training school.

—————

Alice Breckon, three years younger than Horace, was a neighbour of the Wrinch family at Bronte. Alice's grandfather, John Breckon, had emigrated with his wife Isabella from Westerdale on the North York Moors of England in 1831. They had cleared the land, built a log home, farmed and raised a family. One son, Captain John Breckon of the Halton Rifles Militia, settled down as a strawberry farmer and became known as "the strawberry king." Another son, Ralph, married Martha Dynes, daughter of the Dynes who owned nearby property. Ralph and Martha Breckon named their eldest daughter, born on January 17, 1869, Alice Jane.

Alice grew up on the farm in this staunchly Methodist family. At the end of December 1886, when she was almost eighteen, she qualified as a teacher. The Third Class professional examinations she sat in the Model School in nearby Merton comprised a written examination in drawing, education (theory and methods), school law, physiology and hygiene, as well as an oral examination in practical teaching, drill and calisthenics. "Owing to the thorough training received," the *Acton Free Press* said, all students passed and Alice was awarded her teacher's certificate. In July 1890, the Toronto Public School Board announced a number of new teaching appointments. Among them was Miss Alice Breckon, who had been appointed to the relatively new school in Morse Street, which had approximately 220 pupils. She thereupon moved to Toronto and took up her teaching duties.

Neither Horace nor Alice left any record of when or how they met, or when they became engaged. They may well have built up an acquaintance during the time they lived close to each other in Bronte, or they may have spent time together along with other young Methodists in Palermo. It is equally possible that they met during their studies in Toronto, where they could have attended the same church and moved in the same proto-missionary circles.

Alice had not only force of character and leadership but also missionary fire. She was a speaker at the Christian Endeavour meeting in the Broadway Tabernacle in July 1894. She attended the annual convention of the Methodist Young People's Association in 1895, where she shared a platform with Rev. Albert Carman, long-time head of Albert College and one of the leading Methodists in Canada. She spoke at the convention on "Visiting and Relief." In March 1895, she gave a talk entitled "Missionary Work in the Epworth League" at Westby Church, a talk which a reviewer called crisp, interesting and very good. She also wrote and published a pamphlet on "Visiting and Relief" that was advertised in a number of issues of the *Methodist Magazine and Review*. In Alice, Horace had not only found his partner in life but had also met his match in evangelical zeal and missionary competence.

Clearly Alice took her religion seriously. She gave up teaching to study nursing, reportedly with a view to becoming a nurse-missionary. While waiting for an opening at Grace Homeopathic Hospital Training School for Nurses in Toronto, she took courses in deaconess studies, although there is no evidence that she actually qualified as a deaconess. In October 1898, she graduated from Grace Hospital with honours and a silver medal. Taking a certificate of honour with her was her roommate and friend, Helen Bone, who later was herself to play a part in the story of Hazelton Hospital.

In a photograph taken of the nurses at the time, Alice stands among the nurses, unsmiling, but with a look of quiet self-assurance on her face. A contemporary report states that, for the year before her marriage and while waiting for Horace to finish his own medical training, she acted as superintendent at the hospital. Even this brief period as an administrator would have served her well when, along with Horace, she was overseeing the hospital and nurses training school at Hazelton.

A flavour of the religious enthusiasm of the times is found years later in Alice's obituary in the *Christian Guardian*. The writer described the lodging house of young missionaries where she had lived when studying to be a nurse and preparing for missionary service:

About twenty five years ago [the 1890s] there appeared the beginnings of an intense missionary impulse among the students of Canada and especially among Methodist students. . . . In accordance with that youthful vision a number of students were domiciled in Toronto in a house where a missionary programme of limitless possibilities was the centre around which all other activities of that home revolved. Not one of those inmates possessed any money, not one could appeal to accessible resources of wealthy relatives or friends. Each was "on his own" and all were committed by the rigor of biting circumstance to high adventure in courage and faith. . . . Every morning saw the individual processes of prayer and Bible study, familiarly known as "the morning watch." After breakfast, morning prayers, where each in turn ministered in the office of priest presenting to the Father of mercies thanks and supplication, prepared for the labours of the day. The meal-time at noon and at evening almost invariably gave occasion for the discussion of some phase of missionary need or achievement, and indirect contact with the actual "fields" of the world was maintained by the presence of missionaries on furlough, who on the frontiers of civilization had been "breaking the road for the rest."

Significantly, perhaps, these missionaries on furlough included Richard Large, with his "infectious laughter and sparkling wit," Rev. John Jackson with his unquenchable zeal and Rev. Thomas Crosby — all well-known missionaries from the Pacific coast. From them, Alice and Horace, her fiancé, would have learned much about the wilds of northern British Columbia.

—◦◦◦—

Horace applied, and was accepted, for mission work. But where should he spread the Gospel? Where could he be most useful? Many Methodist missionaries, including many from the lodgings where Alice was living and from Horace's missionary circle at Trinity Medical, had gone to China. Horace's first wish was also to go to China, but he said he was ready to be sent anywhere. Alarming reports at that time, though, were coming out of China about a rebellion led by the Society for Harmonious Fists, known to history as the Boxers, whose aim was to rid the country of foreign influences and especially of missionaries, by force if necessary. The crisis and the accompanying violence in China were growing. Was mission work there too dangerous for a dedicated missionary, or would it be a greater challenge fit for a zealous Christian?

Missionaries from the northern coast of British Columbia at this time, however, were reporting to church authorities on the growing medical crisis on the Upper Skeena River. The Pacific coast was well served by missionaries and mission hospitals. As long ago as 1874, Rev. Thomas Crosby and his wife, Emma, had journeyed to the Hudson's Bay Company trading post at Fort Simpson (later renamed Port Simpson) to start a mission. In the crowded conditions of the fish canneries on the coast, disease spread quickly. He saw the urgent need for a doctor and appealed for help.

In answer to this call, Dr. Alfred Bolton, from Portland, Ontario, arrived on the coast in 1889 and quickly saw that he needed to build a hospital. Over the next ten years, he built four: one at Port Simpson, together with a house for himself and his family; two mainly summer hospitals — at Port Essington and Rivers Inlet; and a hospital at Bella Bella. To run the hospitals, he recruited Doctors Jackson, Large and Rush, all of whom would have been known to Horace from Trinity Medical College.

In his 1896 booklet *Medical Work Among the Indians*, Dr. Bolton described the medical suffering of the Tsimshian First Nations on the coast. He wrote of the missionaries' helplessness in the face of sickness and new diseases:

> Contact with whites brought the introduction of infectious diseases, smallpox making great havoc on different occasions; and other diseases, as tuberculosis more slowly, but not less surely, decimating the tribes. The "fire-water," too, has done its deadly work. Civilization at first brought little to counterbalance or cure its own ills, excepting that the strong hand of the law restrained to some degree the former bloody quarrels. . . . It is little wonder, then, that the workers on the Methodist Missions there should have asked that a medical missionary be added to their force. . . . In conclusion, I may state that parts of this district, as the west coast of Vancouver Island and the country around the head waters of the Skeena River, are as yet almost out of the reach of our medical mission.

The hospitals at that time were all located on the coast. There were no qualified doctors, let alone hospitals, in the interior. Missionaries, Indian Agents and anyone else who had a little medical knowledge did what they could. As long ago as 1888, three residents of Hazelton, one of whom was the Rev. John Field, had seen the need for a doctor in the district and written to the Indian Department requesting one, but nothing seems to have come from this.

In 1889, the Dominion government appointed Richard Loring as Indian Agent for the newly formed Babine Agency, a position he held for three decades. His charges were the Gitxsan and the

Wet'suwet'en in the Upper Skeena and Bulkley River regions. Inevitably, given his position between the First Nations and settlers and also between the federal and provincial governments, Loring was — and remains — controversial. Although not medically qualified, part of his job was to provide medical services to the First Nations in the district. "No medical man has yet been resident in this Agency," he wrote in a letter of 1896, "and though one has been seriously needed, I am much gratified to mention that common surgical work is attended to by me."

On occasion he was assisted by his teenage stepdaughter, Constance. When she was twelve, she reportedly administered chloroform to a man whose leg Loring was having to amputate. In his letters and requests for medical supplies, he dutifully sets out long lists of the names of those he vaccinated. Whatever the criticisms of his role as Indian Agent might be, his role in improving the health of the First Nations in the decade between his arrival and the arrival of Horace in 1900 was significant. Down the river from Hazelton at Meanskinisht, the Anglican Rev. Robert Tomlinson also provided medical aid to First Nations. He had studied medicine in Dublin but was not qualified as a doctor either in British Columbia or in Great Britain. Nor was he a surgeon.

Many of the Gitxsan working in the salmon fisheries on the coast took infections they had picked up there back to their villages. The winter period was especially difficult for them. The need for medical help in the Upper Skeena district had become urgent. In his short *History of Hazelton Hospital*, Horace wrote:

Transportation from the coast being entirely by water, there was a period of six or seven months every winter, when the rivers were frozen, or breaking-up; when no one travelled either in or out. The suffering and mortality of the people during those closed-in periods can readily be imagined. When Dr. Bolton and Mr. Crosby were in Toronto attending the General Conference in 1896, they told of these distressing conditions, and begged the Mission Board to send a doctor to Hazelton. The need was made clear enough: and it was not for lack of sympathy that no doctor was sent at the time. But the Board had already sent out as many missionaries as their income could take care of. They made it very plain to the applicants for more help that only as the missionary income was increased could any appointments be made to our mission fields.

After the few Hudson's Bay Company traders, the missionaries were among the earliest non-Indigenous residents of the district. In 1895, Rev. W.H. Pierce went to Kispiox as the Methodist missionary, taking over from Rev. Spencer, who had already been there for four years. He reported on the disease and sickness among the Gitxsan and appealed for a doctor. In fact, Pierce claimed credit for diverting Horace from his earlier intention of going to China. When in Toronto in early 1900, Pierce had spoken in a church about the need for medical services for the Gitxsan. "Dr. Wrinch was then preparing to go out as medical missionary to China," he wrote, "but after hearing these stories he told me at the close that he had decided to go to the Upper Skeena and open up medical work there." This life-changing meeting between Pierce and Horace likely happened at the annual meeting of the Methodist Women's Missionary Society on March 13, 1900.

Thomas Crosby, though, also claimed the credit for changing Horace's purposed mission from China to the Upper Skeena. "When attending General Conference in Toronto in 1898," he wrote, "I met Dr. Horace C. Wrinch, who then intended going to China where the numbers are so great. I argued with him that he could find on the Skeena River all that one man could do. He is a man especially qualified for this work, being strong and having a practical knowledge of carpentry and farm work."

The truth of why Horace went to the Upper Skeena and not to China may be even less clear-cut. Whatever Horace's own inclinations may have been, the Methodist Missions Board in Toronto had its own ideas. It had been considering sending a medical missionary to the Upper Skeena for some time, having already, on October 14, 1899, sent the matter to its executive committee for further consideration. With Pierce's help, the Gitxsan had reportedly submitted a petition asking that a doctor be sent to them and for a hospital to be built. That November, Dr. Sutherland, the Secretary of the Methodist Board of Missions, wrote to a colleague:

> For some time we have been thinking of Dr. Wrinch as a suitable man for some part of the Indian field and unless some unforeseen contingency arises, we hope to be able to send him out immediately after the next Annual Conference. If this project is carried out, we will be willing to have his name associated with the Picton and Belleville Districts. . . . The thought at present is to send him to a point on the Upper Skeena where the presence of a medical missionary is very much needed. . . . I would suggest in the meantime the Leagues proceed rigorously with the work of collecting funds that may be available when the proper time arrives. It will cost $250 or $300 to send Dr. Wrinch and his wife to the place I have indicated; then the first undertaking after his arrival will be to erect a house. What will the cost be is difficult to tell. The salary will be at least $800.

Sutherland was not one to rush into decisions without checking his facts first. On November 9th, he wrote to Loring, saying that the Rev. Pierce had requested a medical missionary and had quoted Loring, as being confident that the provincial government would provide financial assistance. Was this true? And was there really such a need for medical help as the Rev. Pierce had said? "As the undertaking will involve considerable expenditure, the Missionary Board cannot well take definite action till they know what amount of assistance can be relied upon."

Apparently, he received a favourable reply because, soon after, events came together. Dr. Bolton on the coast saw the urgent need for a doctor in the Upper Skeena district. Thomas Crosby saw the need for a missionary there, and Horace wanted to go where he could be of most use. The Missions Board was now prepared to send a medical missionary to the Upper Skeena but still lacked sufficient funds to pay for one. Horace thought he could raise the money, and so he agreed to go. The Upper Skeena it would be.

To find financial support, Horace went back to his friends at Albert College. The Young Students of Picton County, of Albert College and of the Epworth League found the money. "He was accepted by the Toronto Conference last year and is at present time a probationer of two year's standing," the *Missionary Outlook* reported in 1900. "He has been appointed this year by the British Columbia Conference to Kishpiax, on the Upper Skeena, where it is expected he will establish a medical mission station."

As always, Horace's religious zeal was tempered by his common sense and practicality. Medical missionary he may be, the site of his Mission he may have agreed to — but what exactly was he to do and what help would he get from the Missions Board? In a letter of April 12, 1912, he recalled the marching orders that Sutherland had given him:

> We are sending you out as a medical missionary. Upon reaching the field, you medical men generally think you require hospitals. The Missions Board will not become responsible either for erection or maintenance of a hospital at Hazelton. If you need a hospital there, you must find ways and means locally for its erection and maintenance.

Bluntly put, Horace was being sent to the wilds of the Upper Skeena to build a hospital, but the initiative of buying land, finding the money and building the hospital rested on him. The Missions Board would encourage him, praise him and pray for him — but would not promise financial support. Only later did it relent and provide a grant.

Horace and Alice were a poster couple for missionary service. In addition to being a qualified lay preacher, Horace was a farmer, doctor and surgeon. Alice was a teacher and nurse, with some deaconess training. Both were proven leaders and highly competent. Both were fired with the zeal to do God's work by serving people in body and mind and bringing them to Christ. They even looked the part.

The photograph taken on their wedding day shows them serious and unsmiling, looking perhaps to the distant horizons of Canada and the unknowns of Christ's service. Both show firm resolve on their faces. On June 1, 1900, Dr. Sutherland wrote to a colleague at Albert College that "Dr. Wrinch, who is going to British Columbia and whom you support in part, is one of the strongest men we have sent out. He is a credit to you, and every cent raised for his support is well invested."

The spring of 1900 would have been a busy one for Horace and Alice. They were uprooting their lives, ending employment relationships, saying farewell to friends and relatives, packing what they thought they could take, disposing of what they could not, and, amidst all this, planning for their wedding in June. At this time, they might have been asking themselves questions and looking for answers. For how long would they be gone? Would they ever return home? Should they have gone to China? It is unlikely, though, that they had doubts about their decision to become missionaries. A committed couple, they were married on June 16, 1900, in a "pretty house wedding" at her brother Ralph's farm in Merton.

At a farewell meeting held for them a few days later at the Holloway Street Church in Belleville, Rev. McIntyre addressed the congregation that had come to pray for their mission and wish them well. He said he had personally recommended that Horace be allowed to choose his own posting in the missionary service and that Horace had replied that he had no desire to go except to a hard place where others were not willing to go.

Perhaps a few doctors in the congregation silently lamented that Horace was throwing away a brilliant career to work in a place in the wilderness no one had ever heard of. Why hadn't he just accepted a position at one of the big hospitals in Toronto where he could do some real good? Several good offers had indeed been made to him, but he had turned them all down.

"We will want to read our papers as regularly as we take our meals," McIntyre said. "Yet Dr. Wrinch could be shut out from the outside world and have no mail from November until May, except what was brought in by dog train." (Perhaps there were those in the congregation who thought he was exaggerating for rhetorical effect. He wasn't.)

"I am making no sacrifice," Horace replied, befittingly modest, "for there is no sacrifice in giving up the lesser for the higher, and although I could make a living in Toronto among hundreds of other doctors, I wish to go to where I can be of greater service and what in life can count for more."

They were going to British Columbia with the good wishes of the medical fraternity. An item in the *Canada Lancet* reported:

Dr. H.C. Wrinch (Trin' '99) of last year's House Staff, St. Michael's Hospital, was married recently to Miss A.J. Breckon, of Merton. Dr. and Mrs. Wrinch leave this week for British Columbia, where the doctor will labour as a medical missionary to the Indians in the Skeena River District. A man of sterling worth and ability, we wish him the same success in his new field that has attended him in the discharge of his duties in Toronto.

Their marriage vows exchanged, their mission determined, they began their life's journey. On July 17, they boarded a Canadian Pacific train to cross the country. Their destination was the mission post in the Gitxsan village of Kispiox, where Rev. Pierce was the resident Methodist missionary. This journey Horace could not have made when he arrived in Canada because the railway had not yet been built. It would, moreover, take longer than the journey from Kirby-le-Soken to Quebec.

Once again, Horace was leaving his home and his family. Leonard was farming in Halton. Warwick was starting in business. Frank, at the University of Toronto — he would soon leave for Princeton —

had published his *A Contribution to the Psychology of Time*. Mary, who was to become the most famous of his siblings, was establishing herself as an artist. For this departure, though, Horace had not only his life's companion with him but also his God.

CHAPTER 3

Up the Skeena River to Kispiox
1900–1902

HORACE AND ALICE STOOD on the deck of the MV *Queen City* as it wound its way up the British Columbia coast. The ship, a stubby black-and-white-hulled steamer with two masts and a tall, thin funnel, was under the command of the attentive Captain Edward McCoskrie. Where it stopped on its 700-mile journey on the way up the coast from Vancouver, Horace had met many of his new colleagues, including the Rev. J.C. Spencer in Bella Coola and Dr. Richard Large, his old friend from Trinity Medical, in Rivers Inlet. Soon, he and Alice would be arriving at Port Essington, at the mouth of the Skeena River.

Horace thought back to their arrival in Vancouver on July 22. On their five-day train journey, they had crossed the near-endless prairies, seen the majestic Rocky Mountains appear on the horizon and then envelop them with snow-capped peaks and mighty slabs of granite, and had come at last to Canada's west coast. Here they had checked in at the still new Commercial Hotel on Hastings and Cambie streets. Vancouver was a youthful, irreverent town. Fresh and exuberant in the Pacific sunshine, it bustled with new people and new ideas. Its population had grown from 1,000 in 1881 to over 20,000 by the turn of the century and would go on to 100,000 by 1911. How old and well-established Toronto must have seemed!

Horace had gone first to report to the chairman of the Indian District. Then he had taken a ferry to Victoria to visit the province's superintendent of Indian Affairs, from whom he had managed to obtain a supply of medicinal drugs for indigent First Nations. He and Alice then spent some time in Vancouver buying personal and medical supplies sufficient to last the entire winter. Horace had photographed Alice in Stanley Park, as she stood demurely in a black skirt, white blouse and straw hat beside the impossibly large trees. Having joined up with a number of missionary colleagues, they then boarded the *Queen City* on August 9 for the journey north.

The first stage of their journey would take them to Port Essington, and the second stage would take them upriver to Kispiox. Soon this would become a familiar journey for them, but now, entranced, they were seeing everything for the first time.

The Pacific Coast would have been a revelation to them of God's grandeur and beauty. The August seascape, fused by light, was all blue waters and deep greens of the steep shores. Above the forested slopes was a fringe of mountains, many still snow-capped. The light of the summer sun brought the sea and the water together in shimmering harmony, dark where the shore met the water and hazy in the distance. White heads of bald eagles dotted the trees. They would have had tantalizing glimpses of the fins of orcas and porpoises slicing the swells. Huge Haida canoes passed them on trading voyages. Steam tugs chugged by, pulling rafts of huge trees — larger than anything they had seen before — to sawmills in Vancouver.

The passengers on board the *Queen City* reflected the missionary nature of the North. Many had likely been attending the annual summer Methodist camp at Chilliwack, which had been particularly "wet and disagreeable" that year, with poor attendance. In addition to the lushly bearded Thomas Crosby, the passengers included Rev. Robert Whittington (the recently appointed superintendent of Indian and Chinese Missions in British Columbia), Rev. George Raley and Mrs. Raley from Kitimat, Miss Jackson who was going to the hospital in Bella Bella, and Mrs. Ardagh, wife of Dr. Ardagh from Metlakatla. Mrs. William Dudoward and Miss A.A. Dudoward, relatives of the Tsimshian chief, Alfred Dudoward, were also on board, probably heading for Port Simpson.

Almost thirty years before, Alfred Dudoward and his wife Kate had requested the Methodists in Victoria to send a missionary to Port Simpson. Not long after that, in June 1874, Thomas and Emma Crosby had arrived there to start their missionary service. Horace knew that this formidable group of missionaries and their wives would have been assessing him. In return, both he and Alice had been taking the opportunity of learning as much as they could about their new home.

Tearing himself away from the view, Horace went below to the saloon cabin. There Thomas Crosby was gathering the passengers together to make a surprise presentation to McCoskrie. Horace found a place for Alice to sit amongst the ladies, from whom Crosby was collecting final signatures to his letter.

Captain McCoskrie, invited from the bridge down to the saloon cabin, came in a little uncertainly, not sure as to whether he was about to listen to a career-limiting complaint. Crosby asked him to sit down and then told him on behalf of those present how much they had all enjoyed the six-day journey from Vancouver. As a token of their keen appreciation of the marked kindness and courtesy they had received at his hands and indeed from all the ship's company, he said, they wanted to present him with a letter of commendation. "Nor have we heard anywhere," someone said, "a single coarse word or rude remark from any of the crew." (Doubtless the captain had warned them of the presence of missionaries on board and instructed them not to swear.) To a round of applause, Crosby then presented him with the letter signed by the saloon passengers.

McCoskrie expressed his complete surprise at the address. "I have only followed my usual custom," he said. "I feel this is the duty of every master of a steamer or of anyone having the welfare of others entrusted to him."

Horace and the captain likely talked about Kispiox. Horace would have shared with him his plan to build a hospital there. The captain would perhaps have told him that Kispiox was absolutely the wrong place for a hospital. Hazelton was a far better location for everyone, First Nations and settlers alike. A hospital there would be closer to where the river steamers tied up, and it would be more convenient for the First Nations from downriver and from across the Bulkley River. Moreover, Hazelton was going to expand along the riverbank between the First Nations land and the Hagwilget Canyon. The captain would have told Horace he himself had rights to land in Hazelton (or was planning to acquire them) and intended to develop a townsite between Hazelton and the First Nations bridge across the Bulkley River at the Canyon. This acquaintance had consequences when Horace was acquiring land for the hospital.

—∿∿—

Horace and Alice arrived in Port Essington on August 14, 1900. From there they would start the next and most dangerous leg of the journey, up the Skeena River to Kispiox. Before that, though, Horace stayed on the *Queen City* with Whittington and Rev. S.S. Osterhout to go to Port Simpson on the Nass River, a few miles farther up the coast. The Church had a problem there, and Whittington wanted to assess the situation. Although there is no evidence either way, it is likely that Alice went with them. They left the *Queen City* and spent a day or two at Port Simpson, visiting also the canneries at Mill Bay. They probably met there the Rev. William Hogan, a friendly Irish missionary, affectionately known as Father Hogan, although he was Anglican. There too they would likely have met his daughter, May, still with an Irish lilt in her voice, who was preparing to celebrate her nineteenth birthday. Later, she would play a part in Horace's story.

The reason Whittington wanted to visit the Nass River was to see how urgently a medical missionary was needed. In fact, there had been some talk of diverting Horace from Kispiox to fill this need. But Sutherland and Whittington held firm. "To have changed your appointment at this date would, in my judgement, have been a calamity to the Upper Skeena river work," Sutherland wrote, though, he added, it would have been a boon to the people on the Nass.

Now they had to get back to Port Essington. Because there was no other ship going there, they decided to go north to Ketchikan, Alaska, to catch a ride back south on the MV *Tees*, which was scheduled to call in there to collect a load of salmon. On August 18, Whittington, Osterhout and Horace (and, if in fact she was with them, Alice) went across the border into Alaska, arriving the following day, a Sunday. That morning turned out to be a lively one in Ketchikan.

Walking along the wooden planks of the wharf, they found themselves stepping through fresh blood. Farther on, they saw a dead man lying stretched out on a door, his blood still dripping onto the ground in a congealing pool. Since there was no preacher in town, the saloon keeper, seeing two, asked Whittington to bury the dead man the next day. "He's got no friends," he said, "but we don't exactly like to bury him without anything."

Whittington was told that the body was that of a desperado, Dan Robinson, a cannery boss, who, after breaking United States Marshall E.C. Hasey's ribs and arm, had been coming after him with a rifle. In the gunfight just before the clerics had arrived, Hasey had shot Robinson dead. As a medical man, Horace could well have been asked to give medical help to the injured Hasey. A fine welcome to the United States, he might have thought!

The MV *Tees* was in fact too heavily loaded with salmon from another cannery to come to Ketchikan and never did arrive. The clerical party was then forced to wait for two days for the next southbound ship. While waiting, they took the opportunity to go to New

Metlakatla to visit the veteran — and even then controversial — missionary, the increasingly authoritarian William Duncan.

Rev. Whittington and Horace finally arrived back in Port Essington on Sunday, August 26, and stayed with Rev. Jennings. By now, Horace and Alice had, no doubt, heard many stories about the Skeena, how unpredictable it was and at times how dangerous. How true were all these stories about the wildness of this river? (They were true.) Would the town of Hazelton, with its population of traders, miners and packers, be as wild, as sinful, and as booze-soggy as reports said? (It was.)

Now that they were so close to their journey's end, their heads must have been buzzing with questions. How would the Gitxsan of Kispiox and Gitanmaax receive them? How would they actually get on with Pierce? Would they manage to survive in such isolation? Were they as prepared as they could be? And how well could they, when it came right down to it, spread the Gospel and do the Lord's work in healing bodies? With what excitement and apprehensions, they must have loaded their supplies onto the river steamer! They would though, despite such possible misgivings, have been eager to reach their final destination and get to work.

—∿∿—

Horace and Alice would have known that British Columbia was huge, with a land area approximately seven times larger than England. As they would have already seen on their journey up the coast, it was largely a land of forests and mountains with few towns or villages. The Skeena, rising in the mountains to the east of Hazelton and flowing approximately 350 miles to the sea, comes from a basin of approximately 21,000 square miles. Innumerable rivers and streams feed into it. One, the Kispiox River joins the Skeena approximately eight miles above Hazelton. Another, the Bulkley River leaves a wide, fertile valley and pounds through the long, deep Hagwilget Canyon before joining the Skeena at Hazelton.

Until the arrival of the railroad in 1912, the Skeena River was the highway to Hazelton. In winter, when the river was frozen or too dangerous, the only way in to Hazelton was by horse from the South or East or by a difficult overland route from the more navigable Nass River to the North. Hazelton was, as Horace called it, a "little shut-in" community.

Unlike the gentle Stour in Essex or the Saint Francis River in Richmond, Quebec, the Skeena was wild, unpredictable and dangerous. With a reputation for being one of the toughest rivers in North America for navigation, it drops more than 800 feet in the 180 miles from Hazelton to Port Essington. In the early summer, it is prone to high water and sudden floods. In the Kitselas Canyon, not far from present-day Terrace, it can rise (and fall) seven or more feet in a day. Huge shifting whirlpools could drop a steamer suddenly onto rocks. The pebbly shoals were always moving.

A steamer captain could not rely on his observations even from the previous voyage to guide him. The journey upstream from Port Essington to Hazelton could take between three-and-a-half days and two weeks (or more). It could take no more than one day to go downstream. First Nations canoes took at least fifteen days to go up and one day to go down.

On the journey up the Skeena to Hazelton, a steamer passed through a dozen rapids and canyons. The rapids had descriptive names such as Hardscrabble Rapids, the Devil's Elbow, the Sheeps Rapids, where the white water resembled "a flock of sheep on the rampage" and the Hornet's Nest, where the entire river was "studded with submerged boulders and the water [was] very swift." The worst spot was the Kitselas Canyon, a bottleneck where large rocks and islets in the middle of the river presented a formidable navigational challenge. To help steamers navigate these rapids, ringbolts were attached to canyon walls or onto the islets, and steamers pulled themselves through using long hawsers.

In a letter of July 1901, Horace wrote that the river steamers were very comfortable and able to carry forty to fifty passengers, though they often carried more. Made with flat bottoms — able to float on dew, some said — and with a large paddlewheel at the stern, they could actually navigate in two to four feet of water, depending on whether they were loaded. The river was powerful. Engines sometimes were not powerful enough, though, and occasionally a steamer would whirl away downstream until it could recover its traction. The Skeena was also a killer. The newspapers frequently recorded canoes being wrecked and bodies found in the river.

The river steamers operated from May until October, when freezing stopped navigation. Even in the summer months, steamers could not navigate the river when the water was too high or too low. There were only two mail deliveries each winter and even these carried no parcels or heavy packages. Soon after Horace and Alice moved from Kispiox to Hazelton, the number of deliveries in winter doubled to four and service improved.

Usually the first full mail of the new season — the one with all the parcels, journals, packages of drugs and other medical supplies — arrived on the first steamer in May. By September, therefore, Horace had to make sure that all the supplies he needed for the following seven or eight months had been ordered and actually were on their way to him. Even when he could travel, his journeys to Victoria or Vancouver, a distance of almost 800 miles, took the better part of a week, with the return journey taking even much longer.

On August 27, 1900, Horace and Alice, accompanied by Whittington and Jennings, walked up the gangplank onto the MV *Monte Cristo*. Whittington, who went with them upriver to Kispiox, wrote an excited report on the journey for the *Western Methodist Recorder*:

> On Monday Bro. Jennings, Dr. and Mrs. Wrinch and myself started up the Skeena for Kish-py-ax. For six days and a half we stemmed the rapid current, twenty-nine times the steel wire hawser three thousand feet long was used to pull us through the worst places, and three times it snapped and left us whirling downstream to smoother water. Nerve tension as great sometimes as hawser tension. A sail up the Skeena must always be one of thrilling interest. Visited all our work on the

Upper Skeena, and on Wednesday September 5, in the early morning, started down river again. What a mad rush, landscape whirling all around us, now shooting a rapid, sometimes bumping the bottom, but always flying swiftly along. The upward toil of six and one half days was retraced in the downward rush of one. The Skeena is the sail of a lifetime.

A year or so later, Whittington recalled this first journey to Kispiox: "My first journey from Port Essington on the old *Monte Cristo* was one succession of struggles with the rapids. . . . So great was the fascination that all day long the passengers stood at the front of the boat watching the straining hawser as it wound us slowly up these whirling rapids." Horace and Alice would have been among those passengers standing on deck, admiring the scenery, for every river bend, every rapids, every vista would have been new and exciting. And they would have been looking forward to seeing Hazelton, and their new home at Kispiox.

—⁓—

Horace and Alice would have stared eagerly as Captain Bonser steered the *Monte Cristo* around the last corner and Hazelton came into view. Here was a wide river valley, with low, tree-lined cliffs on either side. From the right, tumbling over the stones and pebbly banks flowed the Bulkley River. From the left, a little more sedate but flowing strongly, was the Skeena. As he turned the steamer upstream and into that last bend, the captain, as usual, sounded the ship's horn.

Rounding the point, they would have seen the tumble of settlers' houses, shacks and warehouses lining the Hazelton riverbank. On the bench immediately behind was Gitanmaax, the Gitxsan village, with houses stretching out above the newly completed St. Peter's Anglican Church. The Gitxsan cemetery — the City of the Dead, as it was called, with its elaborate grave-houses — lay on a second bench above.

The arrival of the steamer was a big day in town. The passengers would have spotted boys running excitedly along the riverbank to meet them. Dogs were everywhere — all of them barking. Some said there were as many as 500 in town. These were working dogs, used to pull sleds in winter, but in summer they ran loose. They were always hungry and killed any chicken they could find, hence the perennial shortage of eggs. More than once, it was said, the dogs had torn the shingles off the roof of the Hudson's Bay Company warehouse and stolen bacon and ham.

First Nations canoes were pulled up on the rocky bank. A crowd of Gitxsan boys, settlers, the managers of the trading houses and others were waiting to greet the passengers and making preparations to unload the goods. The steamer tied up alongside the Hudson's Bay Company warehouse — there was no wharf here — and the gangplank lowered.

The Rev. Pierce from Kispiox likely was there to greet Horace and Alice. He would have shown them round the few streets in town. For a town with only about forty non-Indigenous inhabitants (but with many transients — miners and packers, mainly), Hazelton had a large number of stores. There were three main trading houses, each with its own warehouse. This made sense to Horace because he knew that all supplies for the Northern Interior were brought here, warehoused and then taken on by mule train.

The area for which Horace was to be the sole doctor and surgeon was even larger than the Skeena River basin. It stretched north to Atlin on the Yukon border and south to the Cariboo region. The need for medical care was great. The nearest doctors to the east were in Edmonton. To the west, the closest doctors and hospitals were on the coast. Far away to the south at Williams Creek was the three-room Cariboo Hospital, established in 1863 to serve the needs of the miners at Barkerville. The resident population of Hazelton was small, but it was growing and, with the increase in mining and with the much-talked-of railway, would soon quickly increase.

Hazelton was at its busiest in the winter months. In the summer, the villages emptied as the Gitxsan went down to the coast to work in the canneries, went out hunting for long stretches of time or worked in the mines. Transient miners often stayed in town during the winter and prospected in the mountains in the summer. The pattern was for a prospector to find a stream with gold in it and try to keep the secret but fail, which led to a rush of other miners arriving to stake claims.

Many seams and placer deposits were not rich enough for major exploitation and quickly became exhausted. The prospectors then moved on to the next find. Other prospectors started seeping in from the South. One of the routes to the Klondike, albeit one of the least successful, was up the Skeena River and then overland. Many gave up and stayed to prospect for gold in the mountains in and around Hazelton.

The Klondike Gold Rush showed the need to connect the Yukon to the rest of Canada by telegraph. The Dominion government, therefore, decided to build a line from Quesnel in the South to Atlin in the North. Construction started from both ends in 1899 and the line was completed in 1901. It reached Hazelton from the South in 1900, and a subsidiary line was quickly run to the coast. Relay cabins were built every twenty to thirty miles, with two men staffing each cabin. Pack trains took in supplies to the telegraph operators each summer. This telegraph connected Hazelton to the outside world.

Horace would have known that God's work had not been ignored in the Upper Skeena. Missionaries of the main churches had in fact been active in the area for several decades. Despite some rivalries and some disputes, the three denominations co-existed, at times appearing not to want to encroach upon each other's territory but at other times bickering. Generally speaking, Hazelton was Anglican, and Kitwanga, Kitseguecla and Kispiox were Methodist. The Catholics, of whom Father Morice was the most famous, had settled in Fort St. James and were so successful that across the Hagwilget Canyon the Wet'suwet'en were largely Catholic. The Salvation Army, with attractive bands, banners and uniforms, came into the district and upset the balance. It was often seen as poaching the converts of the others. A dispute in Kispiox between the Methodists and the Salvationists led to the partition of reserve land, with the Methodists staying at Kispiox and the Salvation Army settling on land at the new village of Glen Vowell. It is hard to know what the First Nations thought of these disputes between the Christians.

―⁓―

Horace and Alice arrived at Kispiox, about eight miles up the Skeena River, in mid-September 1900. The long journey they had started in Toronto in July was over. In reality, though, their journey had begun when, individually or together, they had decided to become missionaries seven or eight years before. Now, as they stood on the riverbank, looking at the forests, Gitxsan houses and totem poles, listening to the wind in the trees and the rushing of water over stones, their dreams and aspirations met reality. All the prayer meetings, all the missionary castles in their imaginations, all their hopes of bringing the Gospel to the less fortunate finally met the hard facts of missionary life.

They must have looked at their new home with some satisfaction, some enthusiasm, but surely also with some trepidation. It wasn't China, but it was almost as inaccessible. One journey had finished. But another was about to start. Horace was thirty-four; Alice was thirty-one. They had been married for less than three months. The rest of their lives started here, on the stony banks of the Skeena River.

At the end of their first three weeks at Kispiox, Horace wrote to Rev. E.R. Doxsee, a professor at Albert College, and recounted their experiences so far. For the first few days, he said, he and Alice had stayed on Mission Point across the Bulkley River with Mr. Cole, the Methodist teacher. He and Whittington had spent some time looking for possible locations for a hospital, without, though, coming to any definite conclusions. Optimistically, they believed they would be able to start building the following year. Whittington, his pastoral visit over, then went down the river and back to Vancouver.

Kispiox was situated at the point where the Kispiox River tumbles over shallow rapids to join the Skeena. A Gitxsan village of totem poles set along the riverbank among the forests and mountains, it was known to the Gitxsan as An'sp'ayaxw, which means "people of the hiding place." Here were Rev. Pierce's Methodist Mission, church and school. Apart from the often bedridden Margaret Pierce, Horace and Alice would be the only non-Indigenous residents.

In September 1901, Pierce described Kispiox:

This Indian village, the farthest north of our missions on the Skeena River, is situated in one of the most beautiful valleys in our Great Mountain Province. Not many years ago the whole village was heathen. Wild dances, pot-latching, dog-eating and tribal wars were continually carried on. Today there are forty good comfortable dwellings, a saw mill, two Epworth Leagues, co-operative stores, and a hall 40 x 25, built and paid for by the native Indian Epworth Leaguers.

A few days after their arrival in Kispiox, Horace received an urgent message from Charles French, the Hudson's Bay Company agent at its post at Babine. He and his wife Jennett, who was "congratulating herself upon the good fortune in having a doctor so near," had shared the excitement and dangers of the journey upriver with Horace on the *Monte Cristo*. Several members of the Babine First Nation were sick, and they had asked French to see if the new doctor could help them. Could Horace come at once? Horace wrote of this trip to his friend Rev. Doxsee at Albert College:

My travelling company consisted of a guide, a saddle-horse for each of us, and a third horse to carry our tent, provisions, cooking apparatus, axe, medicines, etc. Babine is about sixty-eight miles from here . . . so we were in doubt whether we could make it in two days each way. We got rather a late start on Tuesday morning as we had to get one horse shod before starting and then make them swim across the Skeena River before loading up our pack horse and getting the other horses saddled. However, we made pretty good time all the day and on Wednesday at about 6 p.m. as we were looking out for a good place to camp, we came round a point from which we could see a large valley with a lake winding along through it, and going a little further we could just distinguish some horses at its upper end . . . and we were somewhat undecided whether to go on or to camp. My companion suggested that he thought it was about three or four miles. He had never been over the trail before but as he knew the country pretty well I did not dare suggest that I thought it was more. So we decided that we would try to finish our journey that night.

As Horace feared, the journey turned out to be much longer than the guide had estimated, proving to be about eight miles. Night had fallen and the path had become a dangerous mass of stones, mudholes and tree roots. They eventually reached the Hudson's Bay Company palisade at half past nine, exhausted and famished. The next day, Horace tended to the patients, leaving some medicines and instructions with them.

On the Friday morning, after having rested the horses for a day, they started back, stopping only to shoot half a dozen grouse on the way. It rained hard on the Saturday, though, and the horses were slipping all about the trail. When Horace and his guide arrived back at Kispiox that evening, they had to swim their horses across the river again. Not, he wrote, a ride he would want to make every week.

Horace and Alice moved into the two front rooms of a new frame house. This they rented for $1 a week from Edward Sexsmith, a Gitxsan and Methodist lay preacher at the Kispiox mission. After settling in, Horace set up a dispensary and built a lean-to at the side of the house for treating patients. He soon grappled with the need to learn more about the people amongst whom they had settled.

The Gitxsan (then sometimes called the inland Tsimshian) lived in a territory that comprised most of the Skeena River basin upstream from Kitselas Canyon. The centre of the Gitxsan district was Gitanmaax, on the bench above Hazelton. The district included numerous other Gitxsan villages, including Kispiox, Kitwancool,

Kitwanga and Kitseguecla. The Tsimshian people lived on the coast and up the Skeena as far as Kitselas Canyon, with communities around Port Simpson, Port Essington and up to Alaska. On the Nass River to the north, lived the Nisga'a Nation.

The Wet'suwet'en, a branch of the Carrier Nation and very different from the Gitxsan and Tsimshian, lived in a territory that stretched from the Hagwilget Canyon up the Bulkley River valley. The canyon was the dividing line between the two nations. There were two Wet'suwet'en villages at the canyon, one at each end. Hagwilget was, as a result of an agreement between the two nations, actually on Gitxsan territory on a low bench close to the famous First Nations bridge. The other Wet'suwet'en village was thirty miles upstream at the narrow point of the canyon at Witset, then known to some as Moricetown and to others as Lach-al-sap. This is where the Wet'suwet'en stood on slippery rocks with nets or long poles to gaff salmon jumping upstream to spawn.

The First Nations along the Skeena, Bulkley and Nass rivers guarded their trading rights jealously. Some of the hostility to the encroachment of traders and miners into their lands was based on the justified concern that their rights would be disturbed and taken from them. They traded furs and eulachon oil. The eulachon (or candlefish) were small fish of the smelt family.

Rich in oil that was a food, an energy supply and a sauce used at every meal, eulachon migrated up the Nass each spring by the million. They were a highly valuable commodity and used as a major trading item. The tracks over the mountains to and from the Nass were known as "grease trails." One such trail came up from the Nass and down to the Skeena at Kitwancool and another, the Cranberry Trail, came over and down into the Kispiox Valley. In pre-contact days, these grease trails were the main overland routes for travelling around the interior.

There were approximately 3,000 members of the Gitxsan Nation in the Hazelton district. They had their own clans and houses, their own culture, traditions and language, and their own ideas of spirituality. They also had a rich medical tradition of their own. Their lives were ones of hunting and fishing, of trading and spiritual ceremonies. What must they have thought when the first missionaries came to change their ways, the first settlers came to take their lands and the first prospectors came to take their resources?

There was, inevitably, a clash between their culture and that of the settlers who came to live among them in ever-increasing numbers. Their experiences when the two cultures met were all too often unhappy. In particular, First Nations spiritual values and the new Christian values clashed. The missionaries wanted to bring the First Nations to Christ, to save their souls for eternal life. For the missionary, eternal life was not an abstract concept but a very real place with the risk of damnation and literal hellfire. Saving Gitxsan souls meant persuading them to give up what the missionaries (and most others) believed were heathen beliefs and practices.

Horace, in common with most Christians, would have shared these beliefs. He was a Christian of his times — righteous in his knowledge of religious truth, well-intentioned and paternalistic. He would have believed that by encouraging the First Nations to give up their spiritual ways, embrace Christian grace and joy, and join the brotherhood of Christ, he was helping them to eternal life. This was his Christian duty. He was, moreover, a doctor and surgeon. He wanted to heal their bodies as well as their souls. Better sanitation reduced disease and brought them closer to God's grace. So better sanitation there should be. Healing their bodies helped heal their souls. So medicine should be provided for them. By relieving their pain and setting the example of a good Christian life, he was, he would have believed, doing God's work.

This he would spend his life doing. Few, if any, are recorded as criticizing him for doing anything less than his best for all his patients: First Nations, Chinese, Baptists, Catholics and atheists alike. Of him, a First Nations patient is reported as saying, "He treated us like people. When he gave us medicine, he wrote on the bottle how to take it. And then he wrote, God is Love."

After Horace and Alice arrived in the district, the number of Gitxsan remained fairly constant, but the number of non-Indigenous people increased. He saw the settlers, miners and packers as needing God and spiritual salvation as much as — in some ways perhaps more than — the First Nations. He would have believed they should be setting good examples of sobriety, Sabbath attendance, godly language and the Christian life, which, all too often, they did not. Horace never lost his faith or his Christian ideals, but, as time went on, he appears to have become less of a missionary and more of a doctor and community leader.

—◦〜〜◦—

Horace and Alice would have wasted no time in exploring their new home. Walking around Kispiox meeting people in their first few days, they would have seen a village of about 225 Gitxsan, half of whom were Christian under the pastoral care of Pierce, himself half-Tsimshian. Horace reported that there were thirty-five children of school age and "much more could be accomplished if the children were home all the year, but they go with their parents to the fisheries in the summer, and often to the hunting grounds in the winter." The Gitxsan in Kispiox operated a co-operative store and a sawmill, which the previous year had made a profit of $300. Dr. Wrinch, Pierce reported, would soon be establishing a hospital and would carry on his work through that.

"To give my present geographical position," Horace wrote to a correspondent a week or so after he arrived, "I may say that I am 600 miles up the coast from Vancouver, and 200 miles inland up the Skeena River, and so almost as inaccessible at times as if in Central China." Hazelton, he said, was "more central for medical work and may yet be our permanent location." He wryly noted that the *Monte Cristo*, after fourteen journeys to Hazelton that summer, was now stuck on a rock in the river and *hors de combat*. He confirmed to his correspondents back east that only two mails came in winter and during that time the carriers would not accept newspapers, magazines or even thick letters.

Horace was the district enumerator for the 1901 census. This gave him an excellent way of becoming acquainted with the district's inhabitants, their families, their religion and their state of health. In Kispiox, he would have met and become acquainted with such community leaders as Robert Wilson and the twenty-four-year-old John Tait. There was also the intelligent and competent storekeeper Simon Johnson, a well-respected hunter, who had a farm downriver towards Hazelton where he kept the animals for his small pack train. His Gitxsan name was Gunanoot. Then there was Aleck Morrison, destined to be the first patient in the hospital — Patient No. 1.

The Missions Board in Toronto, ever short of cash, was not generous. In a letter of September 1900 to Whittington, Sutherland wrote that Horace would have to take enough supplies with him to last a year. The board would not pay for his medicines — the provincial government and the federal Indian Department would have to do that. Horace even failed to persuade Sutherland to reimburse him for the $40 he had spent on medicines in Vancouver and Victoria. "Thus far we have not," Sutherland wrote, "supplied any of our Indian missionaries with medicines and you will have to try and recoup this outlay by charging moderate fees to both Indians and whites."

Horace also had to provide his own furniture as well as his own supplies and all the hardware for his house. Missionary that he was, Horace was going to have to work hard for his and Alice's own survival and maintenance. Little would have been easy for them in these early years. He had wanted the most challenging place for his mission, somewhere no one else wanted to go. Finally, here he was.

Alice, the public health nurse, at once set to work visiting Gitxsan homes and helping new mothers with sanitation and medical needs. She also taught them how to use a sewing machine. For some reason, sewing machines held a fascination for the Gitxsan. Years later, Harold, Horace's youngest son, recalled walking to school in Hazelton through the Gitxsan cemetery on the bench above the town.

Peering into the grave houses, he often saw sewing machines and other household objects of value placed around the graves as tokens of identity and status.

Pierce wrote in January that Alice was active in the community and being very helpful. A Ladies Aid group had been formed that already had $43 in its treasury. On December 28 it organized a picnic outside in the snow. "Our Christmas passed off very well — everybody seemed to be happy and glad. On that day we held two services. In the morning seven were baptized, and in the evening eight joined the Epworth League." In this letter of January 5, 1901, Pierce wrote that "During the week, too, we organized a Junior League with Mrs. Wrinch as superintendent. There are forty-six names on the roll to start with. Dr. Wrinch and his wife are doing good work among the Upper Skeena people."

Pierce seemed to approve of Alice. Of her he wrote in his memoirs, "The girls she taught various kinds of needlework and knitting. A folding organ that she had brought with her from the east added interest to the musical part, not only in these small gatherings, but also in the church services on the Sabbath."

Horace, though, had a problem. Before officially being able to practise medicine in British Columbia, he was required to qualify by passing exams set by the Medical Council. These were to be held, probably in Vancouver, in late March or April. The problem was this: the Skeena River was not yet navigable. The Nass, however, was. The only way to get to Vancouver in time to take the exam was to walk over one of the grease trails, probably the Cranberry, and then on down to the Nass.

One morning in late March, therefore, he laced up his boots, arranged his pack and snowshoes comfortably on his shoulders and set out to walk the 125 miles over the mountains. On the Nass he found a canoe to take him sixty miles downriver to Kincolith, and then he went on by steamer to Vancouver. This was a journey of almost 1,000 miles. "Dr. W. came down over the trail, via the Naas River and reports everything at Kispiax and Hazelton [is] in flourishing condition," the *Western Methodist Recorder* stated. Later it was re-ported that Horace had "successfully passed the examination of the Medical Council of British Columbia."

On March 26, he took the Canadian Pacific SS *Charmer* to Vic-toria. While there he visited the provincial Legislature and listened to the debates among the representatives. He mentioned that there was a good deal of discussion in the House about building a railway to Hazelton. He also attended a meeting of the District of Indian Missionaries at the Metropolitan Church. Whittington and Carman, leading Methodists in the province and country respectively, were also in attendance. There, Horace was advanced in his position as a probationer for the ministry, one of the steps towards ordination.

In their early years in the district, Horace and Alice spent much time in canoes in and around Kispiox and Hazelton. Canoes were the means of transport when roads were bad and bridges almost entirely non-existent. These were not fragile birch bark canoes, light and speedy, but heavy dugouts often made of cedar by the Haida First Nations on Haida Gwaii or carved by Gitxsan from the local cot-tonwood trees. The largest ones were between thirty and fifty feet long, and could carry five or six tons of freight and six passengers.

The captain sat or stood at the front, while the passengers sat between him and the freight, which was placed in the centre of the canoe for balance. The crew often chanted as they paddled or poled. "They are each made out of one log," Horace wrote in 1901, "but are well shaped, and are not easily upset. Five men form a crew for these. Where the water is smooth they use paddles and sometimes sails. Where it is rapid they keep in close to the shore, and either use poles to push themselves along, or jump out on the shore and tow the canoe by means of a rope."

In Kispiox, Horace assisted Pierce with his religious duties. The Report of the Indian Department for the year that ended on June 30, 1902, noted that Horace was helping Pierce with the new church "during the spare moments from his arduous duties professionally." While Alice was helping Gitxsan women with public health or teaching Sunday School, Horace ministered to his patients, often riding on horseback, accompanied by his dog carrying medical supplies on its back.

Dogs were commonly used for carriage of goods. "In winter, when the rivers are frozen," Horace wrote, "a very pleasant and rapid method of travelling is by dog-sled or toboggan. I have a Newfoundland dog, which I trained to pull this past winter, and allowed him to pull me to Hazelton and back, occasionally, when the ice was good. It is surprising how much a dog will draw in proportion to its size. Generally, three or four dogs are hitched up together, always one in front of the other." One needed two good dogs, he said, to draw one man at satisfactory speed. "Weather conditions were not always favorable," Pierce wrote, "but the doctor never failed to keep his appointment."

At least once a week Horace went into Hazelton, usually walking the approximately eight miles each way. From there, it was more convenient for him to provide medical services to Gitxsan and the settlers living there and to the Wet'suwet'en from over the Bulkley River from the villages of Hagwilget and Witset (Moricetown). Soon he found somewhere in Hazelton, reportedly a stable, where he could store drugs and other medical supplies, eliminating the need to carry them on his weekly visits.

In the summer of 1901, Horace and Alice went down the Skeena to Port Essington to assist Dr. Bolton with a medical crisis. In November, Bolton wrote:

We were fortunate in having with us part of the summer Dr. and Mrs. Wrinch, of the Upper Skeena Mission. The doctor's assistance in the surgical cases cited and in others was almost essential, and the aggregate amount of work to be done was more than one should attempt alone. I did almost as much by myself in the preceding summer, but I would not wish to repeat the experience. I was also able to take a few holidays, which I never could do when alone without neglecting my work.

While Horace was at Port Essington, he and Dr. Bolton operated on two female First Nations patients with tumours, the second, he said, being "rather larger than a goose egg." He and Dr. Bolton wrote up their detailed case notes for an article in the November 1901 edition of the *Canada Lancet*. This operation was, reportedly, "the second operation of the kind ever performed in Canada." The patient was said to have made a good recovery. In September of the following year, Horace wrote:

> The smallpox outbreak at Port Essington last summer, at the height of the fishing season, gave a great deal of extra work and the vaccinating in connection with it made our aggregate of attendance somewhat high. The following is the record: for three months in association with Dr. Bolton, 4,115 [people]; balance of the year in our own work, 2,291; our highest single day's attendance at Port Essington exceeded two hundred.

In his autobiography *From Potlatch to Pulpit*, Pierce was generous with his praise of Horace. Nevertheless, across the years one senses the possibility of some friction between them. He was not pleased at Horace's being away from Kispiox that summer. Writing in June 1901, when on a visit to Vancouver, he complained at length to Dr. Sutherland:

> After the fishing is done, I cannot understand why two missionaries stay at Essington under full salary; there is hardly enough work for one. I was very sorry that there was no one at the Upper Skeena to help the people: both Whites and Indians are without one. . . . If I only had known Dr. Wrinch was going to stay at Essington with Dr. Bolton this summer, I would never have thought of coming down. What makes it look very bad, Dr. Wrinch and his wife went up on the steamer for Kishpiax three weeks ago according to our plan. They only got to Hazelton, and came back on the same boat. If his wife is going to be sick, why not leave her at Dr. Bolton's hospital like all other missionaries? He will be away six months from his work here before he goes back.

What Pierce did not yet know, perhaps, was that Alice was pregnant. Since she was over thirty and this was her first child, this could well have been an anxious pregnancy. She and Horace may have thought that it would be safer for her to be in the more settled conditions of Port Essington, where there was the additional medical help of Dr. Bolton and experienced nurses.

Difficult pregnancy or not, their son Leonard was born at Port Essington on September 3, 1901. "I was very much pleased to hear of Mrs. Wrinch's recovery," Dr. Sutherland wrote, "and congratulate you and her very heartily on the new 'head of house' which has come to cheer you." The pregnancy, illness and responsibilities of a mother in a frontier community as well as the growing need for nursing help in his work indicated to Horace that he needed assistance. In September 1901, he wrote:

> Admittedly, medical work loses much of its efficiency unless backed up by intelligent and skilful care in carrying out necessary treatment. In this work Mrs. Wrinch contributed very materially towards what success we obtained; and will gladly continue in it to the full extent of her ability. Even if we should not, this year, get any building into which we might take patients, we still feel that we ought to have someone before next winter to help along the lines indicated. The work for the present might be classified as either nursing or deaconess work, but the one who might be sent to us for this would of course be expected to fall into line in regular hospital nursing as soon as we can get accommodation for taking in patients.

The word went out. The Women's Missionary Society agreed to help. Miss Anne Sherwood, a good Methodist nurse, was found in the East and arrived some time before the Skeena became unnavigable in the following autumn.

—◦◦◦—

Horace started to make his mark early. On September 29, 1900, a few weeks after he had arrived, Richard Loring, the Indian Agent, reported to A.W. Vowell, the superintendent of Indian Affairs for British Columbia in Victoria, about "the acquisition of a doctor to the district in the person of H.M. Wrinch, M.D. [sic] of Toronto, an attendee of the Methodist Missionary Society. His abode pro. tem.," Loring wrote, "will be at Kispiox, calling Wednesday of each week in order to furnish medical treatment to those of us here [Hazelton] and the neighbourhood." He went on to say that "already the benefits of this doctor's mission have become most gratifying."

A year later, he was writing that Horace's "services are invaluable to the Indians. The lives of many were saved by surgical operations with the desired effects in every instance of successful termination." By then, Horace was under contract with the Department of Indian Affairs to supply medical services to the Gitxsan and Wet'suwet'en on the basis of $75 a month. The payment arrangements were complicated by the fact that the department paid him for surgeries (and, later, hospital treatments) on a different basis.

Horace did not let the absence of a hospital prevent him from conducting surgeries. In these early days before he had built his house and hospital, he sometimes operated on his patients as they lay on the kitchen table in Sexsmith's house and sometimes he went to the patient's home and operated there. Before November 1902, when Anne Sherwood, his first trained nurse, arrived, he was assisted in his operations by Constance Hankin. Alice herself, although a fully qualified nurse, was busy and had less time to spare for nursing: she had a new baby to look after as well as her social work in the community to attend to.

Reputed to be the first non-Indigenous girl born in Hazelton, Constance was the daughter of the Thomas Hankin, who had given Hazelton its name, and Margaret MacAulay, who was herself half-Tlingit. After Hankin's death, Margaret had married Richard Loring and was his principal interpreter for many years. Inheriting this facility for languages from her mother, Constance, who could speak several languages, was useful as an interpreter. On one occasion when her services were needed, she met Emanuel R. (Ruxton) Cox, whom she later married.

Many years later, Constance spoke of her experiences assisting Horace in his operations. Her first major surgery was for cancer of the breast, and it took place in the home of Richard Loring. The patient was her own mother. It was October 21, 1901. Constance was just twenty-one, but already familiar with simple surgical procedures from her times helping her stepfather. This operation, being for breast cancer, was more serious. Horace had placed a door on the table to provide a flat surface and had rigged up carbolic sheets (sheets soaked in carbolic which was a commonly used disinfectant) to provide as anti-septic an environment as possible. Dr. Wilson had come up from the coast to assist in the operation. They had a dry run the day before so that Constance would know what to do.

Before the operation, as was his habit, Horace knelt and prayed for God's blessing on their work. "A human life is placed in our hands," Constance recalled him saying. "We must have God's help if we are to do our best work. Let us pray together." Perhaps she knew that Horace felt the presence of his God, who he believed had created this body. The operation was successful. "In conclusion," Loring wrote a few days later, "I here must now report that Mrs. Loring, on 21st inst., underwent the operation in removing the cancer from her right breast by Drs. Wrinch and Wilson, and is, thank God, doing well at present writing."

"Dr. Wrinch himself really did most of the nursing," Constance said. "He could go without sleep for twenty-four hours." There was no laughing or irreverence here. Horace spoke quietly while operating, she said, and did not like to repeat himself. Not wanting to let him down, she never allowed herself to forget any of his instructions. To ask for a repetition of an order would be the same as "bringing herself down before him."

She recounted that when necessary, as in her mother's case, Horace used to do surgeries in people's homes. Later in life, she recounted that nearly every operation required some carpentry. "He had just a door with two trestles and when the question came for a patient to have his head lowered he propped the feet up with a bit of cord wood. He used the stable for his dispensary. And he packed the door and the trestles around with him." She recalled that "the doctor was a wonderful carpenter, probably learned on the farm on which he had been raised in Ontario. . . ."

———ᨍᨍ———

That Horace would build a hospital on the Upper Skeena was very much part of the plan. Building this hospital, therefore, was his next task — but where, how and with what? The three players were Horace, living in Kispiox; his immediate superior, Rev. Robert Whittington, head of Indian Missions for British Columbia, based in Vancouver; and Dr. Alexander Sutherland, who was dealing with the Methodist Missions Board in Toronto. Sutherland shepherded the proposal for establishing the hospital through the Board. "Dr. Wrinch was sent as a medical missionary to the Upper Skeena," Sutherland wrote to Whittington, "and it was understood that in addition to a house to live in, it would be necessary at no distant date to have a hospital."

In connection with the establishment of the hospital, he wrote that, "On the Upper Skeena you and Dr. Wrinch will require the wisdom of the serpent and the harmlessness of the dove; and, as Mark Twain observes, 'about an ounce of dove to a pound of serpent' will be the right proportion."

Even before Horace had arrived on the Skeena, the Hazelton community was aware that he was coming and that he would be building a hospital close by. Some in the community were already thinking about where the hospital could be. Loring wrote in a letter in July 1900 to Dr. Bolton, "Incidentally, I learned that it had been decreed to locate the doctor to be sent, and their hospital to be established on the Skeena, at Kispiox." He then went on to criticize Kispiox as a location for a hospital. Compared with Hazelton, he said, Kispiox was totally isolated.

He continued that he knew of "lovely and ideal building sites away from town." One of these was "on the Two Mile Creek, two miles to the south east of here and on common lands." The land described appears to be where the hospital would later be built.

There was likely also strong pressure from the settler community, which would be paying for it, to locate the hospital closer to Hazelton than at the more remote Kispiox. However convenient it might be for missionaries to preach religion to the Gitxsan there, Kispiox was unsuitable as a place to build a hospital. In any event, Horace, pragmatic and wise as the serpent as he had to be, would make up his own mind, in his own way.

Horace worked quickly, but he did not act alone. The residents of Hazelton, willing and eager to help, were supportive. In the first few weeks after his arrival in the district, he appears to have met with both First Nations and settlers to discuss plans. In his report of September 29, 1900 — a few weeks after Horace had arrived — Loring wrote:

> It has been fully deliberated upon to establish an hospital somewhere in the environment of Hazelton during next spring, but the exact locality of said institution has not yet been decided. . . . The hospital is no longer an interesting speculation but a pressing necessity and the forwarding of this all-important subject cannot too speedily be brought into action.

In early December 1901, a group of fifteen residents, including Richard Loring and Horace, met to discuss plans for the hospital. Richard Sargent, a resident since 1891, described by his previous employer, the Hudson's Bay Company, as "bright, capable but young and too independent," was one of the leaders in the community. He had his own store, and over the next forty years his name would become almost synonymous with Hazelton. There were also the Rev. John Field, the Anglican minister, whose church, St. Peter's, had only recently been completed, and Charley Barrett, superintendent of the government transports, who also ran the Diamond D ranch down the Bulkley Valley and who became one of the largest pack-train operators in the district. Edward Charleson was the purchasing agent for the telegraph company.

Also probably there were Robert Cunningham who ran the Cunningham store and William Larkworthy, the ambitious clerk from the Hudson's Bay Company. Larkworthy became one of the leading storekeepers and prominent citizens of Hazelton. He played a part in the acquisition of land for the new hospital. Perhaps James Kirby, the provincial constable, who had arrived in town the previous May, would also have attended. He was a veteran with many years' service in India with the South Wales Borderers. More recently he had been the constable in Port Essington. All these people would play their part in Horace's future.

This group of Hazelton residents was not, however, a happy family of co-operative settlers. As Sutherland had predicted, Horace needed all the tact and diplomacy he could summon to bring them together to support his project. The problem was that a deep feud separated two of these leading citizens and their adherents. On the one hand was Richard Loring and on the other was Richard Sargent. The former was the Indian Agent and federal government representative, with wide powers over First Nations matters. The latter was a magistrate appointed by the provincial government and manager of one of the largest trading stores in Hazelton, one that sold the liquor so widely consumed in town. Sargent was often supported by William Larkworthy and the Rev. John Field, all three being Anglicans.

The feud, which started well before Horace had arrived, had flared up in January 1900. It lasted several years and was deep and very personal. In April 1901, Loring wrote that he and Sargent were "not on speaking terms." Loring accused Sargent of selling whisky to the First Nations on the Gitanmaax Reserve, and of sending his men to set free a whisky seller Loring had arrested. Sargent accused Loring of abusing his authority and of interfering with Anglican Church Missionary Society activities with the Gitxsan.

Loring was so annoyed by this that he wrote a five-page letter of complaint about the Rev. Field and Sargent to the Church Missionary Society in London, England. Loring thought it wrong that Sargent should be one of the main sellers of liquor in town and at the same time be the magistrate in charge of enforcing the liquor laws. It made Loring's job of trying to keep liquor away from the Gitxsan difficult. Each faction sent petitions to the Attorney General, requesting the government to dismiss the other. This dispute even arrived on the desk of the deputy minister for Indian Affairs in Ottawa, who sent admonitory letters to the government in Victoria about the constitutional clash between federal and provincial powers. It was all very divisive.

Horace had to bring these diverse groups together at the same time as not being too hasty in accepting their advice on where to locate the hospital. They had, he knew, a vested interest in having the hospital as near to Hazelton as they could. Whatever Horace's own views, he would have known that he had to be diplomatic and yet make up his own mind. Everyone present at this meeting would almost certainly have agreed that a hospital in Kispiox was not viable.

Loring, who wrote an account of the meeting, recorded that a committee was struck to make the plans and that Dr. Wrinch would be giving advice and guidance. Since Horace was the only one who knew anything about hospitals, clearly he was going to be the guiding spirit behind the whole enterprise. It would be built, Loring wrote confidently, "in a splendid locality on the Two Mile Creek, to the south-east, at the distance indicated . . . and readily accessible to the Kit-Ksan [Gitxsan] of the Skeena below and above here and to the Hagwilget to the south-west a little." The estimate of cost, he reported, was $5,000 and a further $2,400 for equipment and annual maintenance.

Loring may have been precipitate in his identification of the site. For one thing, Larkworthy had already filed pre-emption rights to that lot, and would have to be persuaded to surrender his rights to the government. Horace, despite much advice from many quarters, was still looking at alternative sites early in 1902. In a letter of mid-August 1900 — written before Horace had even arrived in the district — Sutherland had cautioned him that he had better make a careful survey of the ground up and down the river and afterwards decide where to locate the hospital.

He drew Horace's attention to the fact that Henry Martin, the teacher Pierce had left at Kispiox while he was away in the South, had written to him that Hazelton had no water supply other than the river, and even that was not reliable for some parts of the year. Since the hospital absolutely had to have a reliable water supply, perhaps Hazelton was not, therefore, the most suitable location? It would certainly influence the decision. Sutherland wrote again to Horace in March 1901:

> Respecting a permanent location for your work and the best place for the hospital, I have been waiting for definite information from Bro. Whittington. In other words, if you and he are agreed as to the best point there can be no doubt that the Executive Committee will confirm the locale as soon as they are informed of it and you may proceed on that basis as soon as you like. I think Bro. Pierce told us that the Indians [of Kispiox] would donate the lumber for the hospital, but perhaps they will not be so ready to do that if you decide to locate at Hazelton. Nevertheless, the best location should be selected whether we get the lumber or not.

Since Whittington was in Vancouver, it was in fact entirely up to Horace to review all the possible sites and decide which one was the best. "The first important question confronting us," Horace wrote accordingly, "was to decide where to locate our permanent station, and where to live in the meantime."

As early as December 1900, though, it was clear that Horace was agreeing with Loring that the medical mission clearly could not be at Kispiox. The only advantage of building there would be free lumber. Kispiox was at one end of a wheel spoke, with all the other Gitxsan and Wet'suwet'en villages being at the end of other spokes; the hospital had to be situated near the centre of the wheel, and that meant the Hazelton area. A patient from, say, Moricetown or Kitselas, being rushed to hospital should not have to find a canoe in Hazelton to make another journey to Kispiox. Being practical, Horace would also have understood that it would cost substantially more to bring building materials as well as medical and other supplies from the coast, and then unload and reload them for the journey by wagon and canoe from Hazelton to Kispiox.

In a letter to the *Missionary Outlook* in September 1902, Horace reported:

> The growing white population, and the desire from that quarter for a hospital, has made the question somewhat more involved than would be the [case in] providing hospital accommodation simply for our Indian work. Our Church's interests have to be guarded, as also the interests of the Indian work. On that account deliberation of movement has been necessary. We have negotiations under way with both Provincial and Dominion Governments with good prospect of being able to arrive at an arrangement this year whereby an adjustment may be made suitable to all interests.

Since it was becoming clearer every day that the hospital would be built somewhere near Hazelton, Horace soon realized that he and Alice should move there from Kispiox. Already, the store of drugs and medical supplies he had kept in Hazelton had burned down once. Moreover, Horace and Alice now had a son. In Hazelton, it would be easier for Alice to obtain help when needed.

When Horace moved from Kispiox to Hazelton, he was moving away from an inward-looking mission community to a small town grappling with the encroachment of the modern world. Other missionaries kept to their small communities, many of which did not change. William Duncan had moved from non-Indigenous communities to found Metlakatla and later, after conflict with the authorities, to New Metlakatla, both as Christian communities, pure and uncontaminated by the iniquities of settlers, traders, miners and packers. Robert Tomlinson had moved to set up Christian villages for the same reason.

Duncan and Tomlinson had both moved away from the modern world; Horace moved into it. This was a crucial difference. Horace moved to a place where he could deliver medical care and express his conception of God's message to Gitxsan, Wet'suwet'en and settlers alike. This gave him full scope for his character to express itself in the community, first as a hospital-builder and administrator and ultimately as a contributor to the greater good of the province.

CHAPTER 4

Building Home and Hospital
1902–1905

WHEN HORACE AND ALICE moved to Hazelton from Kispiox in the summer of 1902, they were, relatively speaking, moving into the city. Several families of settlers lived there, with a number of transient miners and packers coming and going, giving a settled resident population of between thirty and forty. The small but busy little town had the ubiquitous Hudson's Bay Company store and trading post, two other general stores and trading posts, the Dominion government Indian Agent, Dominion government telegraph operators, a provincial government constable, Church of England missionary (John Field), two restaurant keepers, one hotel keeper, a carpenter, teamsters and others. The transient population was made up of prospectors, pack-train employees and telegraph line employees. Many miners wintered there, and amongst these were a number of Chinese. Though there was a large Gitxsan village on the benches above the town, Horace's practice also included a large number of non-Indigenous patients. He now went to Kispiox once a week, keeping a stock of medicines there. He and Alice rented a Gitxsan house on the bench above the town from Arthur Nelson. Horace was then thirty-six years old and Alice thirty-three.

Where the Bulkley River joins the Skeena is a low-lying point of land, with a succession of benches rising behind until they merge into the mountains. Rocher de Boule Mountain, with its tumbling rocks and sporadically worked mines, forms a dramatic view to the south. Downstream the jagged peaks of the Seven Sisters stand firm in the distance. On the second bench above the town is the Gitxsan cemetery, a quiet place of beauty and peace. In the early 1900s, the graves were covered by small wooden houses, with brightly painted roofs, windows and gables, furnished with numerous objects of value and status.

Horace and Alice walked down from their home on the bench into the scattering of houses on the banks of the river, and along to the point where the rivers merge. The river there slides smoothly over stone and gravel bars. Picking their way over the stones, Horace and Alice walked out onto the point. They stopped and looked around. A light breeze rustled through the cottonwood trees. Cotton from the trees was bursting from the over-ripe fruit and floating gently through the air like warm, friendly snow and gathering in airy clumps on the ground.

Off to their left was the slough, a narrow but dangerous waterway that separated a small island from the bank. This island was a spiritual place for the Gitxsan, full of legends. Purple and mauve splashes of fireweed among the tall grasses lined the riverbanks. The only noises were the raucous squawks of ravens, dogs barking in Hazelton a mile along the bank, and the rustling of leaves in the aspen trees, the breeze making them shimmer in the morning light.

Hazelton, laid out in 1871, was surrounded by the river on one side and the Gitanmaax Reserve, established in the 1890s, on the other three sides. As a consequence, Hazelton itself had no space to grow. This delineation of its boundary settled its future. Within this confined space, it opened to the outside world in a number of steps, including the aborted Collins Overland Telegraph of 1866, the Omineca Gold Rush of 1869, the arrival of the steamer *Caledonia* in 1891, the arrival of the Yukon Telegraph in 1900 and the coming of the railway in 1912. The presence of the hospital would bring a focus to the district and play no small part in its successful growth.

Soon Horace and Alice became better acquainted with the residents of the town and the surrounding district. They were a colourful group. Many, such as Sargent, Loring and Field, they already knew well. Other settlers were arriving in town, and the number of transients was increasing. Miners continued to stream into the mountains in the summer. Surveyors and planners for the railway came through. Government engineers came as the government started to construct wagon roads and bridges.

Frank Chettleburgh came to open a coal mine. Sperry Cline, a young veteran from the Matabele and Boer Wars, arrived in Hazelton while the hospital was being built. Before settling down as a provincial policeman in 1914, Cline tried his hand at many things, including mining. For a while, he ran the winter mail sleds to the coast for Richard Sargent, who, in addition to his other jobs, was the Hazelton postmaster.

Wiggs O'Neil typified many of the entrepreneurial types. He had spent the early 1900s in Hazelton, first as a purser and steward on the river steamers. After bringing the first motor launch to town, O'Neil started the automobile coach service between Hazelton and Telkwa. Much later he was appointed a General Motors dealer and spent many decades in the Bulkley Valley.

Horace, as the only doctor and surgeon in the Northern Interior, had a busy practice to maintain. In September 1902, he noted he had already that year attended to 2,956 patients. Already under contract with the Department of Indian Affairs, in 1902 he was appointed by the provincial government as the resident physician for Hazelton at a stipend of $500 a year. The province further added to his responsibilities in December 1902 by appointing him a justice of the peace, a position he held until 1922. Although a newcomer in town, Horace was already well known and was on his way to becoming a community leader.

—◦◦◦—

In the winter of 1901–1902, Horace drew up several plans: ones for his home, for the hospital, for the farm and for everything that would have to go with them. The first and most important question was, where he should build the hospital. Although he knew he would not build it at Kispiox, he had not yet decided exactly where in the Hazelton area he would. His experience at St. Michael's and Alice's experience at Grace Hospital had given them both insight into the realities of running a small hospital. They no doubt realized that the challenges of building in a place where there was no access to the outside world for six months of the year were daunting. All but the most basic building materials and all supplies of medical equipment and drugs would have to be brought up from the coast before winter.

However supportive Whittington and Sutherland were from afar, Horace, necessarily, had to do the actual work. After the necessary land had been acquired, it would fall to him to determine the order of tasks — to decide on the floor plans, to employ the necessary labour, to acquire the building materials, to install the heating and plumbing and to find sources of power. He had to be confident that he could run the hospital and that he would be able to raise the money to keep it in operation. He also had an absolute need for a reliable water supply, and for this it was imperative that he keep digging until he found sufficient water.

He also had to secure a regular food supply. Patients and staff had to be fed through the winter, and he could not trust an unreliable supply chain. With the river closed for so many months of the year, this meant he would have to establish a farm. With twenty-five years of a farmer's life behind him, he had the experience necessary to set up a farm, not only for dairy products, fruits and vegetables but also for grains for bread and fodder for animals.

Many questions required answers. How large should the hospital be? How many beds should it have? Then he had to think about staffing. How many nurses would he need? How could he pay for them? Who would handle the maintenance and who would work on the farm? He also had to find the time for numerous trips to Vancouver to purchase supplies. With the site, water, money, buildings and farm to plan — not to mention continuing to attend to his medical practice — he had more than enough to keep him busy.

—∿∿—

Horace decided on the location for the hospital in early 1902. Although the settlers of Hazelton — who would, in part, be paying for it — were advocating persuasively for a site close to Two Mile, the decision was by no means a foregone conclusion. On the one hand, such a site would be convenient for Hazelton residents and for the Gitxsan in Gitanmaax. Larkworthy, however, already had pre-emption rights there, although this problem could probably be overcome. At this time, the only ways across the Bulkley were by canoe (or over the ice in winter) or by an elegant but fragile First Nations bridge across the Hagwilget Canyon. Crossing this bridge was a nerve-racking experience at the best of times let alone for someone hurrying to the hospital in a medical emergency.

This suggested that the hospital should be on the Hazelton side of the Bulkley. On the other hand, the railroad, when it came, would undoubtedly run south of the Skeena and Bulkley rivers. A new town would grow up there and hemmed-in Hazelton might well wither. A site south of the river would have been more logical had there been a reliable bridge. There it would be more convenient for the Wet'suwet'en across the Hagwilget Canyon and settlers up the Bulkley Valley. Moreover, the Church already owned suitable land for a hospital and farm on Mission Point on the south side of the Bulkley

River. There were also wild cards. Could Horace find a reliable water supply on the Two Mile site? When would a secure bridge be built over the Bulkley River, and where? Horace weighed these considerations and made his decision. He decided that the hospital would be built on the flat ground between Hazelton and Two Mile.

Horace's next tasks were to acquire the land and raise funds, while keeping his Mission Board superiors informed. As early as April, he had sent plans for the hospital to Sutherland. By July 1902, Sutherland was writing that he was "going over as carefully as I can Dr. Wrinch's plans of the proposed hospital."

At the same time, Horace purchased some land of his own between the proposed hospital site and Two Mile. Since he had been away at Port Essington for much of the previous summer, this was fast work by any standard. The only things holding him back were the state of negotiations with the provincial and Dominion governments about funding and the bureaucracy of the Methodist Church in Toronto.

Horace went to Victoria in April 1902 to buy supplies and equipment. He also had meetings there with Whittington and provincial government officials. A journalist from the *Daily Colonist* in Victoria interviewed him and wrote:

Amongst the guests at the Angel Hotel is Dr. H.C. Wrinch, one of the medical missionaries of the Methodist Church in the Skeena River district. It is now two years since the doctor and Mrs. Wrinch came out from near Burlington in the province of Ontario to take up their present work, part of which time has been spent at Essington and the remainder at Hazelton, from which point the doctor has just come down. This trip down the Skeena though arduous, was not a very dangerous one, as already a good deal of the ice is out of that turbulent stream, and what was left afforded more toil through portaging than it did risk to the travelers on their 180 mile trip out to civilization, or rather the outside world, for though Hazelton is one of the outposts of settlement, even its Indian population is becoming fairly well advanced in some of the arts of European life. . . . The doctor describes the townsite of Hazelton as exceedingly picturesque. It is situated on a flat a few feet above the river, being backed by a succession of benches that rise at last to quite a considerable height. One great disadvantage, however, stares it in the face. Its area is but twenty acres or so, and the little plot is quite hemmed in by the river on two sides, and an Indian reservation on the remaining ones.

Horace took steps to acquire the land. Larkworthy was persuaded to surrender his pre-emption claim on the chosen lot in exchange for another lot. Part of the selected land was acquired from the provincial government and part was a donation from the Gitxsan Band of Gitanmaax. He also credited Captain McCoskrie, who now owned pre-emption rights to the land along the river from Hazelton to the Hagwilget bridge, for donating a portion of his land for the hospital. Horace also had to negotiate with Father Morice, the Catholic missionary across the Bulkley, for the conditions on which Father Morice would allow the largely Catholic Wet'suwet'en to donate money for the building of the hospital.

During this period, Horace had also been soliciting money to pay for its construction and operation. He attacked the problem with his usual vigour. With Whittington's help with the Province, and Sutherland's with the Dominion, he applied to both governments for financial support.

In September 1903, Horace noted that the Methodist Missions Board in Toronto had, despite its earlier refusal, authorized a grant of $1,000, conditional on other amounts being raised. He wanted also to raise $1,000 from local residents, and reported he already had furnishings of at least $150 and a subscription of $952, of which $468 had already been paid. The Indian Department had indicated that it was giving careful consideration to a request for $1,000. "We confidently hope," Horace wrote, "within a few weeks to hear favourably from this source, and also from the Provincial Government, from which we are asking $2,000."

The bureaucratic wheels of the Dominion government, though,

turned slowly. His first application in April 1902 had been turned down. His second and more detailed application in November was given qualified approval (the Department may consider the matter . . . and may put it into Supplementary Estimates . . . still subject to Parliamentary approval). In the debate on the Estimates in the House of Commons on October 12, 1903, Prime Minister Wilfrid Laurier said, "We have medical men in different parts of the province. . . . In the Babine Agency there is a medical attendant at Hazleton, Kishfyak and Hagineyet [sic]." Laurier then went on to mention and recommend to the House the approval of the Methodist Missions Board request for a $1,000 grant for the hospital at Hazelton. Thereupon the government issued the cheque for $1,000 but would not release it until satisfied that the provincial government had made its donation, which did not happen until July 1904.

In November 1902, after some months of negotiation and transactions, the Methodist Church acquired title to the land. This, the site near Two Mile, was on the bench above the mists of the river valley, about one and a half miles outside Hazelton on the trail to the Hagwilget Canyon. Horace would have been eager to get onto the land and start working. His faith in the project was such that he had acquired the land and was well on the way to completing the hospital before he even received the government money.

The key decisions it should be noted, were made in a single year. All that remained was to execute the plans, something which, with his busy medical practice, he had to do in his spare time. He had spent 1902 doing the preparatory work. The following year, 1903, he could start to build, first his home and then the hospital.

———

Horace had already taken steps to find staff. Anne Sherwood, his first trained nurse, had arrived in the early autumn of 1902. In her missionary zeal, she was enthusiastic and happy to be at Hazelton. "To me it seems hardly possible that the expectations of the more intelligent years of my life have been realized," she wrote enthusiastically, "and I am at last at my chosen work. To have reached a definite place and a definite work is indeed a pleasure to me." She taught a Bible class to Hazelton children on Sunday afternoon, and Horace conducted a Bible class for their parents in the evening. Dr. Wrinch, she wrote, expected to have the hospital ready towards the end of 1903. In the meantime, "whenever it is possible we have the patients come to the office, but very often we have to operate or give treatment in an Indian house, which entails a good deal more preparation than in an hospital."

Seventeen-year-old Helen Dean, a probationer nurse, came to join them in 1903 and stayed three years. Many years later, she wrote, "You took your life in your hands going up that river. . . . Of course there was no hospital then. We had many operations on Dr. Wrinch's kitchen table. No water laid on. No electricity. Oh my, what a doctor. You couldn't have a better doctor or surgeon. We were on duty twenty-four hours a day. We had to be. There was no money for extra staff."

—–⁓–—

Having taken possession of the site for the hospital in November, Horace was unable to commence construction owing to the onset of winter. There was, however, much he could do to prepare. He had time to clear the site, dig for a well (when the ground was not frozen), assess where to place the buildings, plan the farm, obtain seeds and animals, and revise and double-check the building plans.

That winter was a hard one. At one point, Horace wrote, the thermometer had dropped to thirty below zero (Fahrenheit or −34 degrees Celsius). He wrote that the snow on the ground lasted until the first week of April, and that there was still ice in the river. Old-timers, though, were saying the climate was changing dramatically. Everybody at that time was speculating — bets were placed on this in the bars — when the first river steamer of the year would arrive.

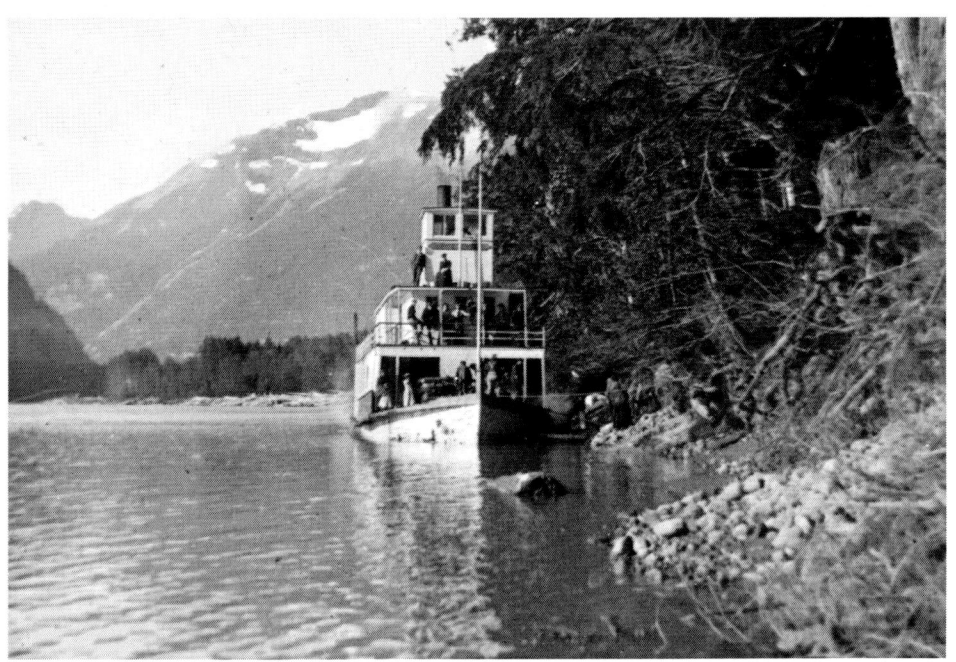

Sternwheeler *Monte Cristo* on Horace's journey up to Hazelton in September 1900.

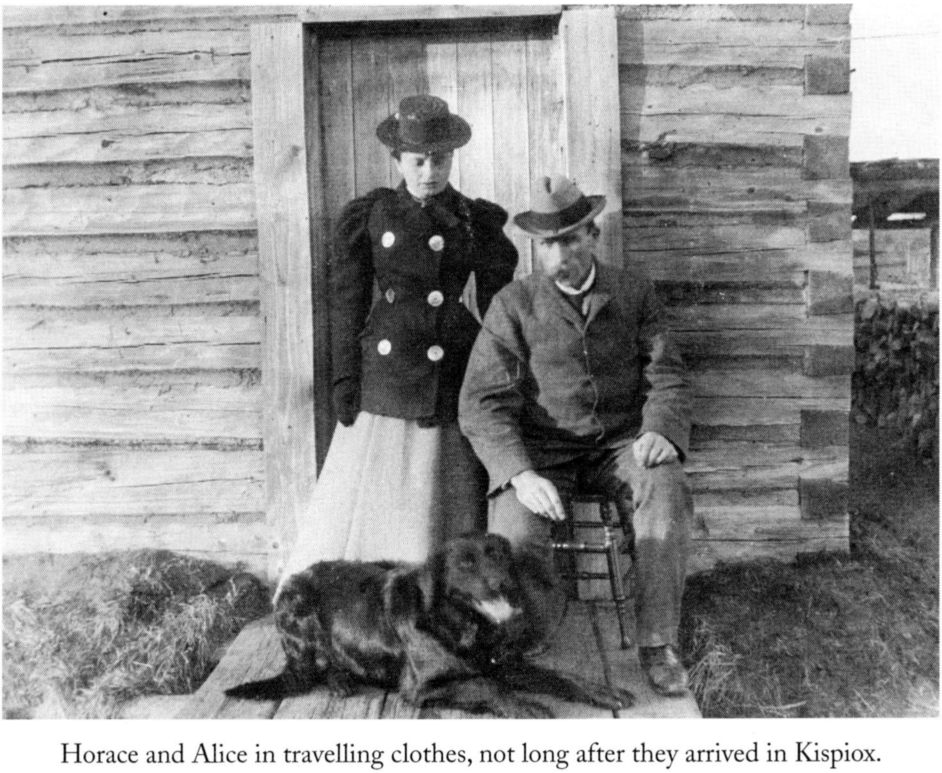

Horace and Alice in travelling clothes, not long after they arrived in Kispiox.

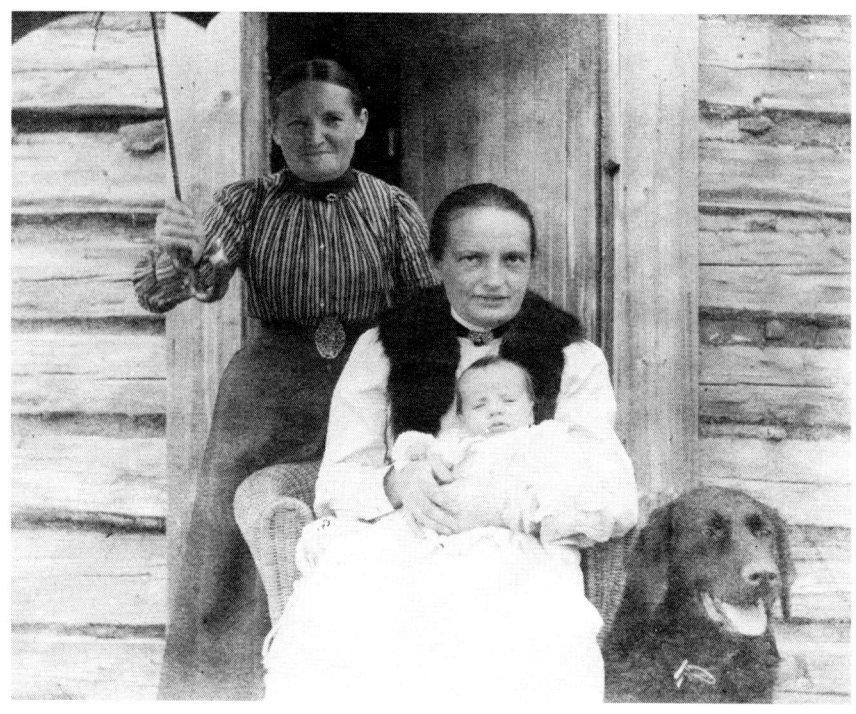

Alice with Leonard, who was born in Port Essington in 1901.

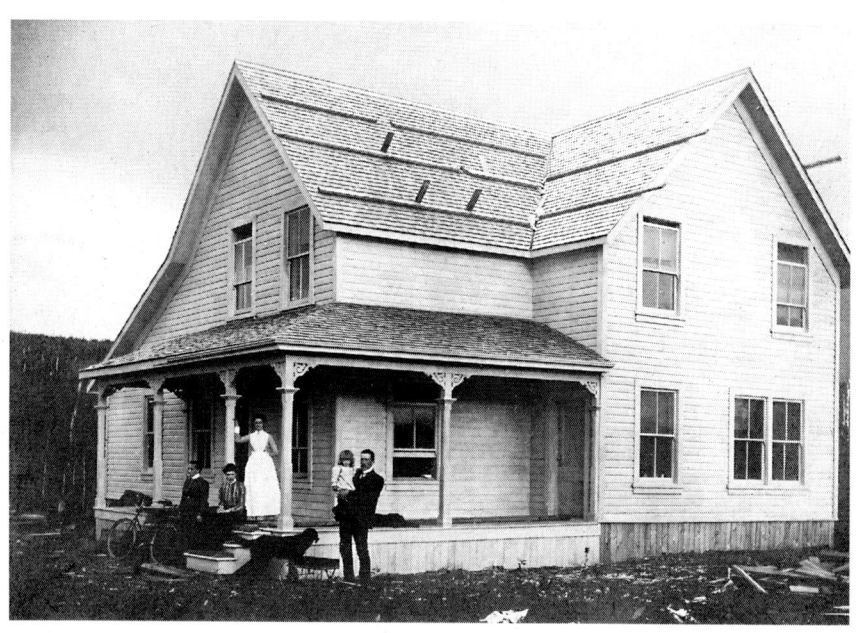

Horace and Alice, second from left, outside their
new home in the summer of 1903.

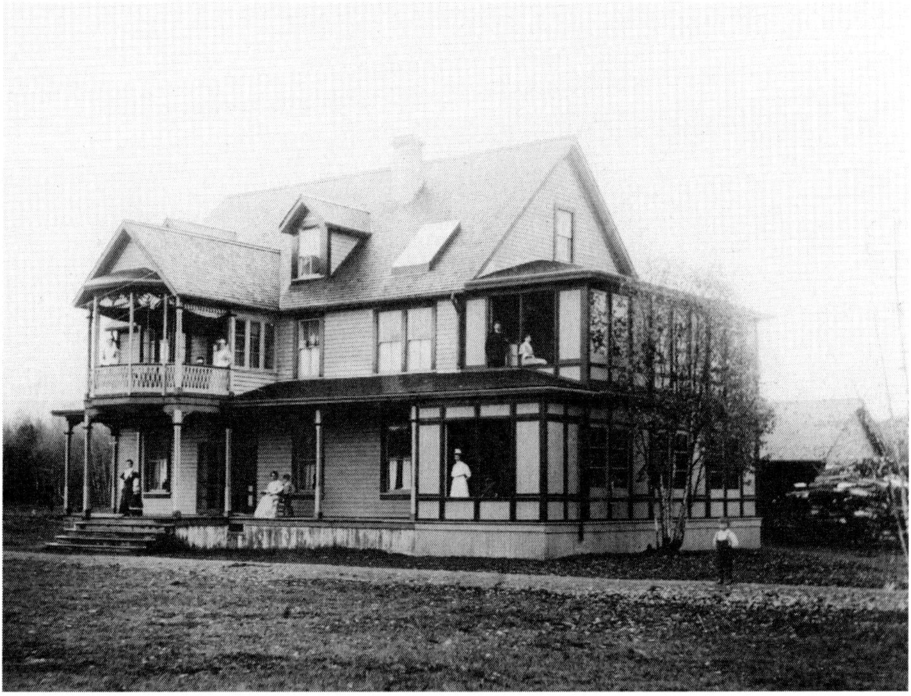

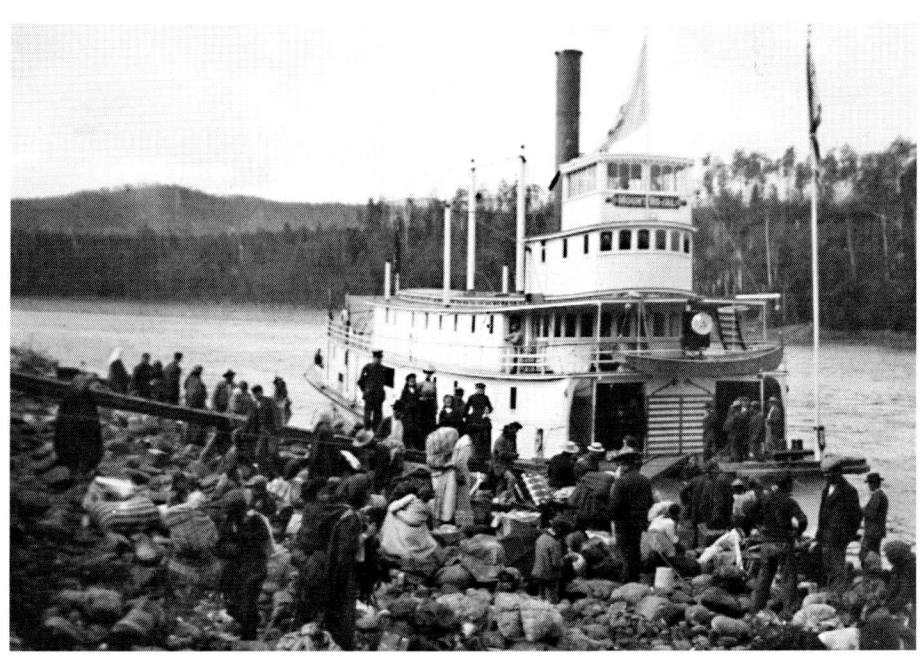

Hazelton Hospital, with 1907 extension on the right.

Sternwheeler *Mount Royal* at Hazelton.

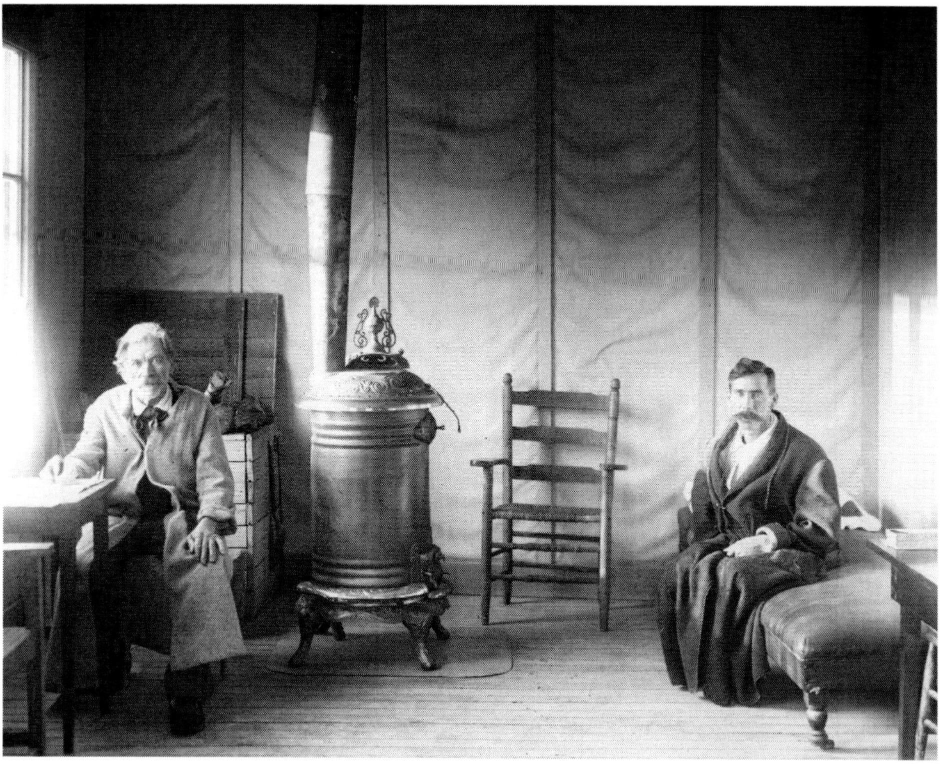

Patients inside the hospital.

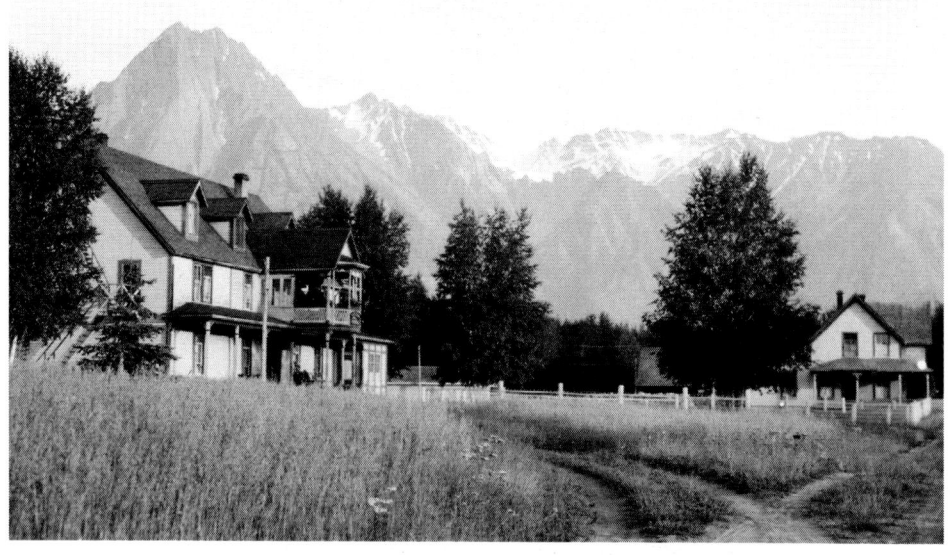

Hazelton Hospital on the left, the Wrinch home on the right and
Rocher de Boule Mountain behind them.

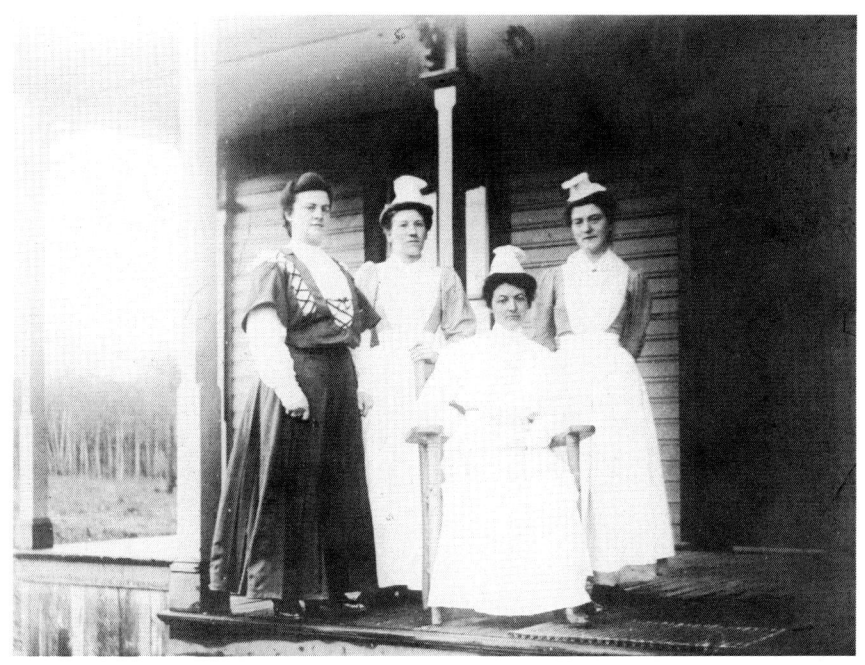

Matron and nurses in the early days of Hazelton Hospital.

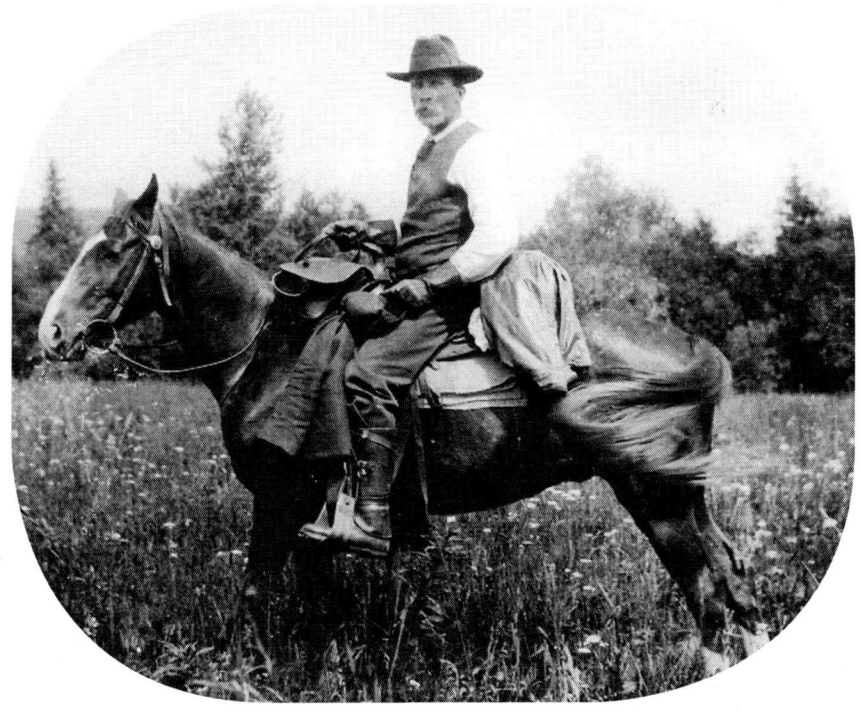

"A frontier physician on his rounds." Horace Wrinch in about 1905.

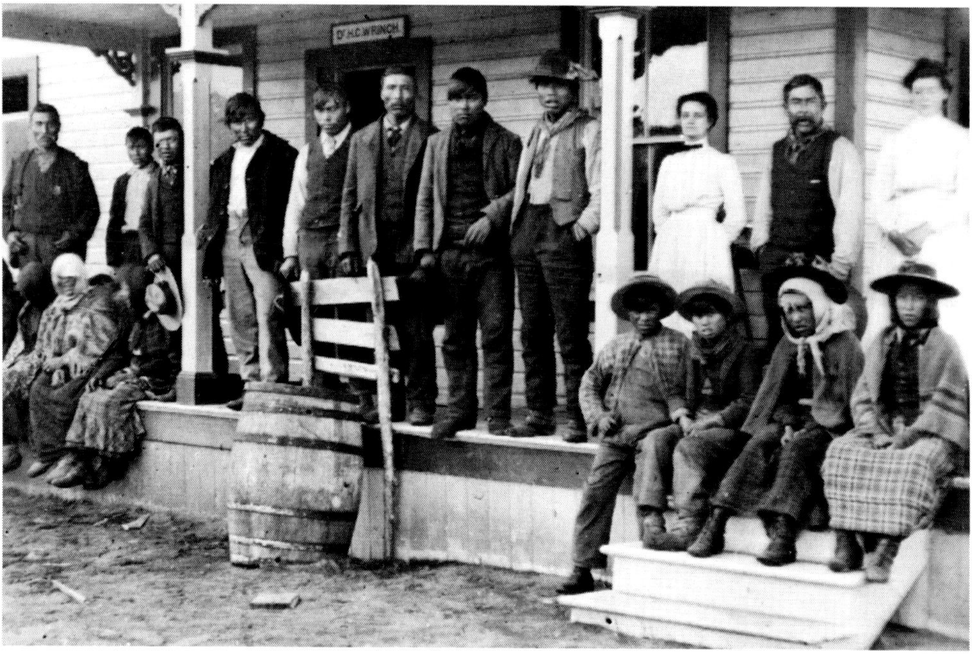

Patients waiting for Dr. Wrinch.

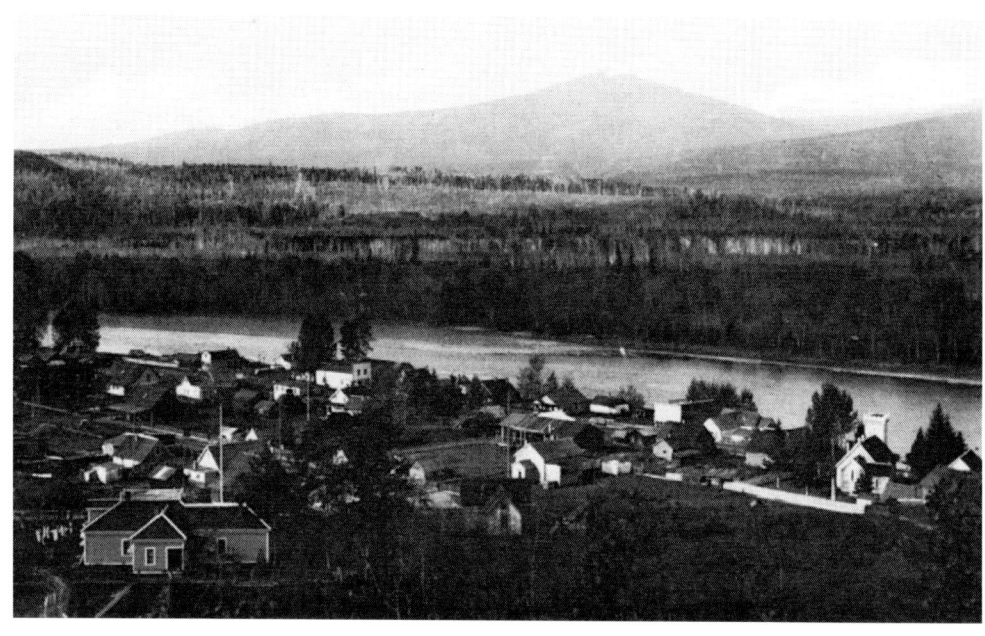

Hazelton, with St. Peter's Church on the right.
The Skeena River flows from right to left.

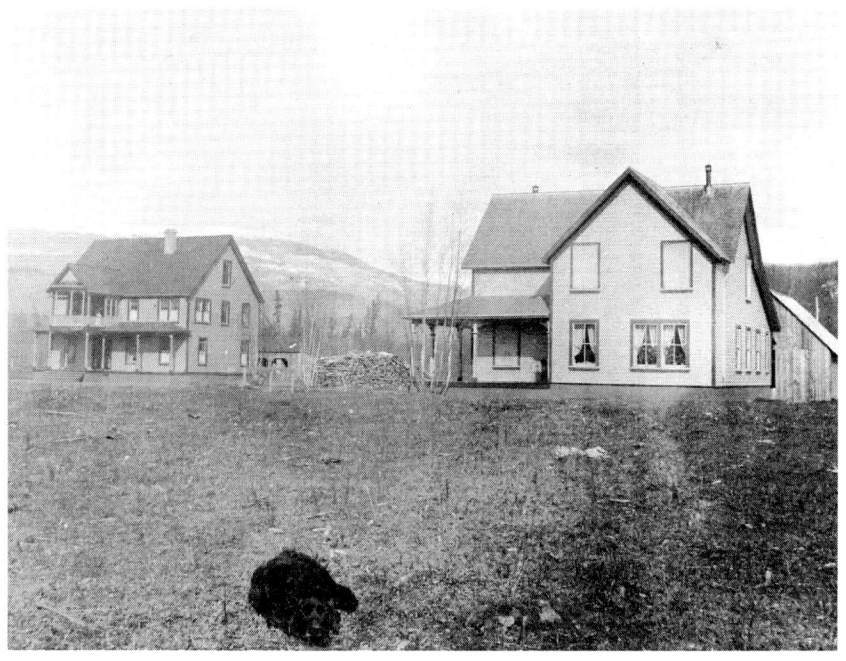

Wrinch home in the right foreground, with the hospital on the left.

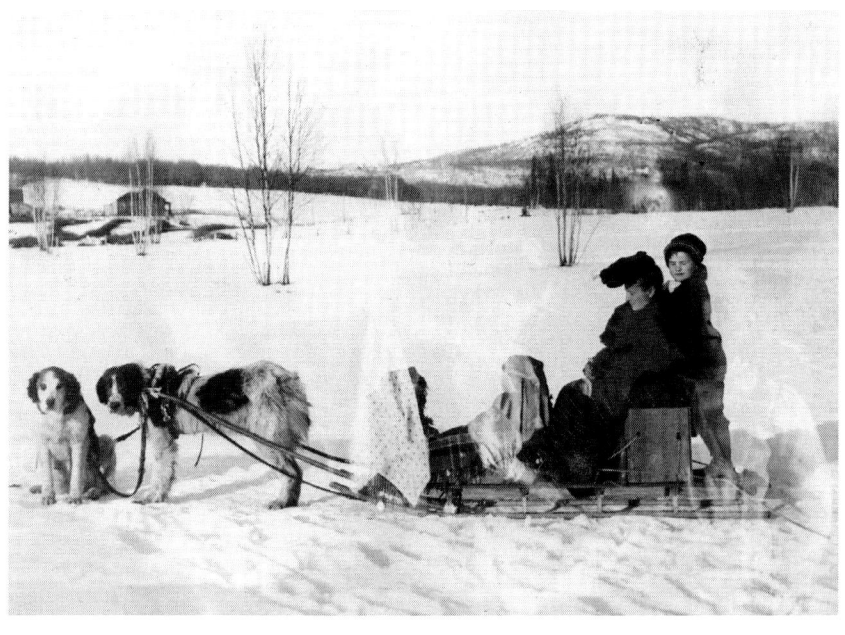

Alice Wrinch and children using winter transport.

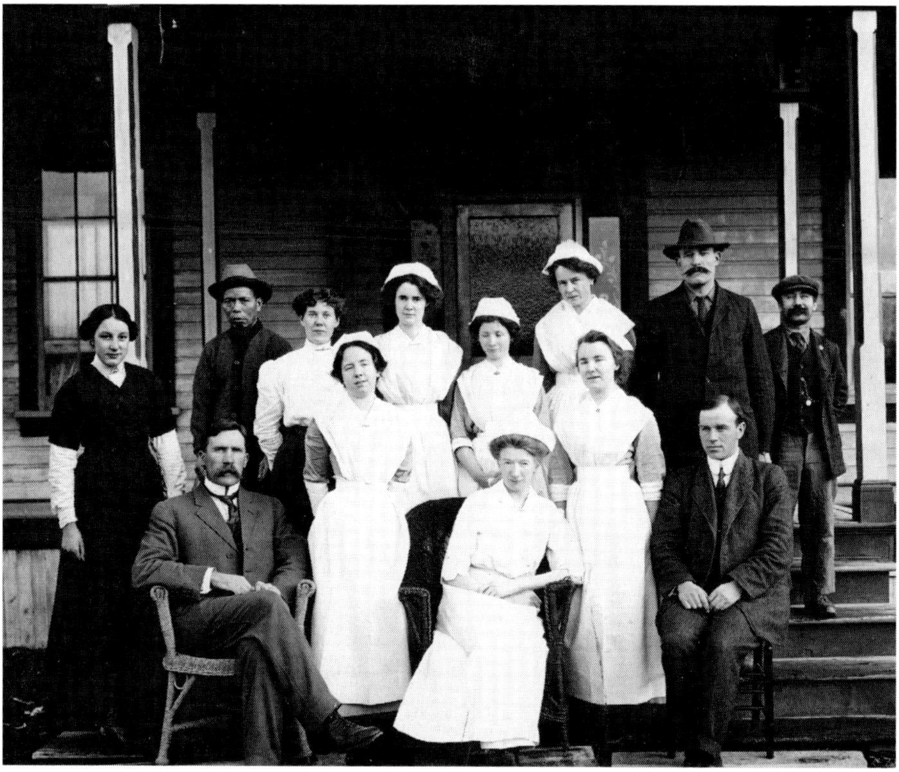

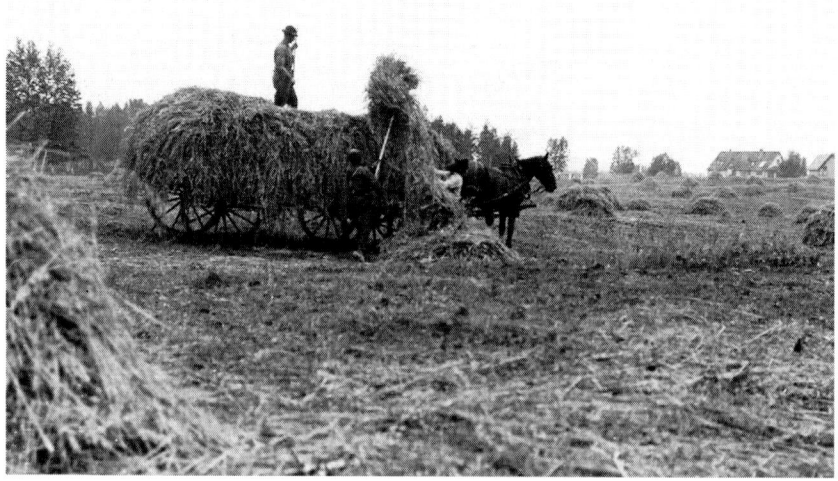

Hospital staff, 1912–1913. Horace is seated on the left, May Hogan, the matron, is centre and seated, and Dr. C.G. MacLean is on the right.

The hospital farm, with the hospital in the background.

Horace bemoaned the fact that eggs were $1 a dozen (if you could get them) and on occasion $1.20 a dozen, and never less than fifty cents in summer. Hay had become scarce on account of the snow staying so long. There were, he wrote, some very thin horses around.

In the spring of 1903, Horace was finally able to start construction of his own home. He had to employ carpenters, builders and well-diggers, and he had to buy supplies, both locally and, when necessary, from Vancouver. The land was cleared, the cellars dug and the site laid out. The Tomlinson sawmill at Meanskinisht supplied the lumber for both home and hospital, and this had to be brought upriver and then hauled up to the site. Meanwhile, Horace and Alice were still living in a rented house, from which he was maintaining his medical practice and conducting surgeries.

After construction work started, every day Horace went to the site one and a half miles away from their rented home to keep an eye on how things were going. After the workers had cleared about six acres of the brush and timber, he was able to say that it did not feel so much as if they were living in the bush.

Anne Sherwood, reporting on the progress of the building to her correspondents, excused her delay in replying sooner by saying that they'd had only four mails since the previous November. "You will be glad to learn that the building of Dr. Wrinch's residence is being pushed as fast as possible. . . . At present the house we live in [she was probably living with Horace and Alice in Arthur Nelson's house] is rather small and inconvenient. . . . We dine in our sitting room and sit in our dining room." Significantly for the hospital, she noted that the second attempt at digging a well had been rewarded by striking a copious spring.

For Horace, though, it was not merely a matter of giving instructions to builders and watching them. He was a skilled carpenter himself, coming from his days on the farm in Ontario. Cabinetmaking, a friend once said, was one of his relaxations. If only to save money and the cost of transport from Vancouver, he himself made much of the furniture for both their new home and the hospital. He also worked on the fabric of the building. "He then built the house . . . doing much of the work himself," a colleague recalled a few years later.

One day a man rode onto the grounds. With raging pain in his gums from a tooth infection, he slid off his horse, hitched it to a rail, splashed some water on his face from the rain barrel and looked around for the doctor. The place was still clearly a building site, with fresh lumber and mud everywhere. Someone above him was hammering in shingles, making a noise that sent a jar through his infected tooth with every hammer blow. The man asked one of the Gitxsan workers where the doctor was. The worker merely pointed upwards.

There, perched on the roof, hammering in the shingles, was Horace himself. This story illustrates his character: he had the skills needed to build a house, and he used them. "I can imagine," Horace's son Harold, who recounted the story, said, "that it would be with some misgivings that [the man] allowed my father to attend to the tooth."

The house went up. He had the outside painted by the carpenters, but the inside he and Alice thought they would try to do themselves in "spare moments." In early August 1903, Horace and Alice moved with great relief and pleasure into their new family home. After that they were busy making bedsteads, putting up shelving, building the woodshed and hen-house, and doing the many small things that inevitably demanded their attention.

Now that he had a home for his growing family (Alice had given birth to a baby boy, Cooper, in May 1903), Horace also had a place to conduct surgeries. He soon realized that patients needed somewhere to convalesce. Accordingly, he and Alice used part of their new home as a hospital, taking in thirty-one patients before the hospital itself was completed. Horace wrote:

As soon as we found we would not have the hospital ready for occupation this winter, we at once decided that we must take some of the most needy patients into our own house. So we decided to set aside our sitting room and two bedrooms for hospital purposes for this winter. Before we had been in our house two weeks we had two patients in with us, and we have had two of our rooms occupied by patients nearly ever since. Just now we have three patients with us, two of whom have undergone serious operations and are making good progress in recovery.... We do not mind inconvenience in our home if we find such good results coming from it as this tells us of.

Seventeen of these patients were First Nations. Patient No. 1 was twenty-two-year-old Aleck Morrison from Kispiox. Suffering from rheumatic fever, he was admitted on August 22, 1903, and stayed until October 23. The charge was $31 — sixty-two days at fifty cents a day, a bill that Horace passed on to Loring for the Indian Department to pay. Patients were treated for such ailments as gangrene, pneumonia, ophthalmie, a shattered hand, alcoholism, birth, parturition, dysentery and an axe cut to the foot. Horace also saved the life of a girl who was suffering from the last stages of pneumonia.

Anne Sherwood wrote in a letter of October 1903 that they were using three rooms in Dr. Wrinch's new home for patients until the hospital was ready. There had been seven patients already, she wrote, one white man and the rest First Nations. Three Gitxsan were recuperating in their home at that time, one a child with pneumonia, another a case of compound fracture of the skull and the third with appendicitis. She later wrote, "I cannot tell [you] what a help Dr. Wrinch is to these people by his knowledge of medicine." After relating that Hazelton would be one of the headquarters for the railway operations the following summer, she said she also wished that, "the Gospel had more of a foothold here before the rush that a railroad necessitates. There seems so much evil to cope with."

Horace wrote to his readers in the *Missionary Outlook* about two of his patients. One was an Indian woman from whom he removed an abdominal tumour weighing ten pounds. "She is now sitting up, having made a good recovery, and is brighter than I have ever seen her before. She is the wife of a man on whom we operated about three months ago for appendicitis."

The other patient Horace wrote about was Charles Newell. He

was a miner who lived in Manson Creek with a mining partner, and they hadn't been into town for about three years. At the end of January 1904, an explosive cap Newell was about to set to a dynamite charge suddenly exploded, shattering his fingers. He and his partner knew they had to get medical help from the doctor in Hazelton, 180 miles away. His partner helped him put on his snowshoes and then they set out. The first stage took them twenty miles to their nearest neighbour's camp.

The neighbour, also a miner, dropped everything and walked with them forty miles to the next stage, where someone else took over. At times the snow was five feet deep and the temperature was thirty-five degrees below freezing.

Eighteen days after the accident, Newell and his companions arrived at Horace's door. Although they were exhausted and the shattered hand was painful, the extreme cold had prevented infection from taking hold. Horace operated and did what he could. "We were able to remove portions of the injured members, and the patient is now getting nicely over the effects of the chloroform, and says his hand is quite comfortable already." Newell spent forty-five days at the hospital and was discharged, as the hospital register put it, cured.

Since this was Horace's own home, Newell and his partner took part in the life of the family as soon as they were able. Although they had not seen women or children for three years, they soon became firm friends with Horace's young children. Horace discovered that one of the men was the son of a Presbyterian minister and, bashful at first, soon joined in the family hymn singing around the portable organ. "Both were fond of singing and, although at first they did not join in," Horace wrote "it was not long before they were singing with the rest and asking for favourite tunes when we were having some hymns on Sunday." Music and the children probably played their part in Newell's recovery, and, Horace probably would have hoped, also helped in bringing him and his partner back to God.

By necessity, the only doctor in town is always on call. This often meant saddling the horses or packing a dog sled for days on the trail.

Horace recounted one time in early 1904 when he had to go twenty-five miles downriver to see a woman suffering from internal bleeding. He wrote:

> We were sent for in haste and left at once (10 o'clock in the morning), taking our dog team and riding part of the way. On arriving at 6 p.m., the woman was found to be in a very low condition from internal hemorrhage and from insufficient nourishment since the attack had commenced two weeks before. We told her and her friends that an operation was the only thing to save her life, and that it could not be performed unless they could bring her to our house that she might be under my immediate care. They were also warned that she might not even have strength enough now to stand the journey of twenty-five miles, and that after that there would be doubt if the operation would not be too much. They realized that her only chance lay in coming to us, so next morning they started out. It took them twelve hours to bring her here. Next morning we commenced to give her chloroform for the operation, but found her too weak; in fact, it took about half an hour to restore her breathing. We used building-up treatment for three days, and then got her through the operation successfully. Her recovery was tedious, but at last we had the satisfaction of sending her home to her friends in good spirits and in a fair way towards full strength.

While the Wrinches settled into their new home, Horace continued work on the hospital itself, planning and collecting building materials. It required about sixty-three thousand feet of lumber, besides all the doors, windows, mouldings, which latter, together with hardware and tar paper, had to be ordered and sent up from Vancouver. In early September, the carpenters came back and construction of the hospital began. With the frame up, Horace was hoping that before winter set in the roof could be completed. Then, he wrote, the inside work would be proceeded with in the spring far sooner than outside work could be commenced.

"The undertaking is being pushed" the annual report of the Indian Affairs Department for 1903 said, "with the doctor's indomitable energy." Building went well. The roof was on before winter set in. It also went well financially. "Thus far the work has been accomplished without drawing upon the Society's funds." Sutherland seemed pleased (as well he might), writing to Horace in February of 1904:

> Your report of progress in the matter of the hospital is very gratifying. The negotiations with the authorities seem to have been conducted with great skill. . . . It was a fortunate circumstance that the hospital building was so far advanced before winter set in so as to make it practicable to go on with a good deal of the inside work. . . . When the building is finished, kindly take advantage of the first visit of someone with a good Kodak, so that you may be able to send us a photo for publication.

Horace wrote that they had four carpenters, one plumber and two labourers working on the hospital. He grumbled about the cost of bringing the plumber from Vancouver, paying all his wages and expenses. "It will cost considerably more for putting in the furnace than for the furnace itself and all material connected with it. Even then, however, it will be a great economy in both labour and fuel, and will give far better satisfaction than a number of stoves in a large building. We are getting anxious to have the outside painted and the scaffolding removed so that we may have a picture to send you. I don't think it will be many weeks now before we can do this. It will be a great relief to get into the new building."

Horace's siblings also helped. His brother Alfred came from Ontario to work as a janitor and handyman and stayed for two years. In Ontario, Leonard assisted in the hiring of male staff, his sister Gina posted advertisements and interviewed female staff, and his other sisters, Mary and Agnes, received donations of goods and sent them on to Horace.

By July 1904, the new hospital was almost ready. The carpenters had left and the painting was well along. Horace wrote:

When first planning for the building, we did not include the painting of the inside. We thought that if we got the building up, and with the outside protected by paint, we would have accomplished a good deal, and we were prepared to gaze at the bare board walls and ceiling for a year or two until funds would come in and enable us to paint them. But when we found the carpentering would be finished early in the summer, and so be in good time for paint to dry, and thought, too, of the much greater convenience of painting before the rooms were occupied at all . . . we decided to have it all done before going into it.

Horace spent $300 on this painting and disinfecting, with faith "that the money would come in some way."

The hospital opening was delayed until October, which necessitated the continued use of Horace and Alice's home for the care of patients. "At present," Anne Sherwood wrote, "we have four patients, and one on the way to us. To accommodate this number, the nurses had to give up their room temporarily, and occasionally during the winter we have had to share our room." She recorded the first death. This was caused, she said, by the patient moving too much after surgery, contrary to Dr. Wrinch's strict instructions to keep still. This apparently prompted one Gitxsan Elder to say he was afraid Dr. Wrinch would not take any more Gitxsan patients because one had been disobedient.

Accompanied by Anne Sherwood, Horace went to Vancouver and Victoria in August 1904 to buy equipment and furniture for the hospital and to attend a meeting of the Canadian Medical Association. He was also looking for someone to replace Anne, who in the not too distant future would be returning to Ontario. He came back with Helen Bone, Alice's roommate from Grace Hospital in Toronto, as the new ladies superintendent. Before leaving, Anne furnished one private ward at her own expense. Another was being furnished by a $100 subscription. When they returned they would have been busy getting ready for the opening. Bedsteads, tables, washstands, all had to be made, meaning a busy time for Horace and his helpers.

When Robert Tomlinson, the thirty-four-year-old son of Robert

Tomlinson the missionary, arrived from Meanskinisht with a dislocated bone on September 20, 1904, he was the first patient in the new hospital. In the hospital register, which included those treated at the Wrinch home, he was Patient No. 32. He stayed for eight days. When the hospital was officially opened in October, Tomlinson had already been discharged and the hospital was in full operation.

Whittington came for a visit that October, probably coming for the official opening. He stayed with Horace and Alice in their new home, inspected the hospital and expressed himself as being "very much pleased. It would be difficult to speak too highly of the building and the work being done here."

Horace later summarized the costs. His own home had cost $2,100. The Missions Board had paid for this, but not for the furniture, hardware or supplies. The costs of the hospital and associated buildings were paid by the Missions Board ($1,000), the provincial government ($2,000), the London First Methodist Church Sunday School ($1,000), the Indian Department of the federal government ($2,200), subscriptions and donations ($1,500) and surplus office income (that is, from Horace's medical practice) for four years ($244). In all, the hospital and related buildings had cost a little under $8,000.

Initially the hospital, which could accommodate seventeen patients, had a staff of four: a lady superintendent, two nurses and a caretaker. The main building had two storeys, with a basement and an attic, with room for expansion. Fifty-five feet wide and forty-four feet deep, it was heated by a hot-air furnace using cordwood for fuel and was lit by coal oil lamps. Initially water was brought in by hand-power using a forced pump, but two years later a hot-air engine pump was installed, itself later replaced by an electric pump. Horace even built an ice house, one of the uses for which was to make ice for ice-cream. Visitors, he noted, expressed surprise at finding porcelain-enamelled baths and such fixtures in what they had expected to be a frontier settlement.

Horace drew up a constitution for the hospital and posted rules. Visitors were allowed between 10 a.m. and 9:30 p.m. Spitting inside the hospital and out of the windows was "absolutely prohibited, much to the surprise of the people at first." Smoking was not allowed inside the building and only on the verandas in certain circumstances.

Horace gave tours of the new hospital. One of them was to a Christian chief from Kispiox and his wife, who were astonished most at the furnace with its hot-air registers and foul-air registers and with its concrete chimney running from cellar to roof. It seemed hard for them to believe, Horace wrote, that it would heat the whole building.

The ground floor seemed a large house to them, but when they went upstairs and found another house just as large, and then up another flight into the large open attic, and finally down into the basement where the furnace is, they failed to find words to express their admiration. The idea that seemed uppermost with them was that "there ought to be no more drumming and rattling and dancing over the sick people now that there is such a fine house for them to come to." Even the building itself had, Horace wrote, a strong moral and educating effect.

Horace's son Harold later recalled that as various conveniences became available: "Father always seemed to find out about them and have them installed in the hospital." Horace installed a gas acetylene system, something he perhaps recalled from his work on the community hall in Appleby more than ten years before. This consisted of a generating plant, which was supplied by the Siche Gas Company at a discount for the Hazelton Hospital because it was a mission hospital. (Horace wrote specifically to the Missions Board in Toronto asking them to settle this bill expeditiously because they had given the hospital this discount.) Carbide was mixed with water at a controlled rate, and gas was piped through the hospital and their home. Later, Horace installed a generator to supply electricity to the hospital.

Years before Hazelton had its own service, Horace installed a telephone at the hospital. In his annual report for 1904–1905, he recorded that the hospital had received a donation of $26 towards this telephone. Having come from the urban centre of Toronto, he would, of course, have been familiar with telephones. He would have known how useful it would be to have one at the hospital. The line led to the office of Edward Hicks Beach, a mile and a half away in Hazelton. Hicks Beach was the local stipendiary magistrate, notary public, real estate and insurance agent and later, for a short while, Horace's mining partner.

In June 1905, Alice wrote in one of her few surviving letters that the previous year they had been very crowded, as they no doubt were, in a house with a small family, at least one nurse living with them and several rooms being used as a hospital. Now that the hospital was complete they had more room. The greatest number of patients at any one time so far had been eight. Most of them were First Nations from Kispiox, Kitseguecla, Gitanmaax and the different villages up and down the Skeena, and a few from the interior.

The nurses, Alice wrote, report them as being good patients. The more treatment they get the better they are pleased, but once the orders are carried out there are few suggestions from them as what might add to their comfort. They do not know how to cook for sick people, she said, and few of them, even if they have cows, manage or care to milk them.

She noted that the hospital had received a present of a fine cow from Robert Tomlinson. As the lowest price for a cow was $90, this was a valuable present and the fresh milk was very welcome. The white patients so far that year, she said, had all been men. One had to come seventy miles, and made the journey in three days, travelling on horseback. He made a good recovery. On Sunday mornings, Horace held a service for First Nations patients and any of their friends who were visiting them. The First Nations, she wrote, were "particularly fond of music and can learn tunes very quickly, but do not always succeed as well with the words."

While clearing land for the hospital, Horace was also clearing land for a farm on the hospital site. With patients staying in the hospital for long periods, a reliable food supply was essential. This was not only a necessity for the hospital, however, but also a labour of love and a source of great relaxation for him. It connected him to his years of farming in Halton County and also to his years as a boy on the family farm in Essex. With the first twenty-eight years of his life spent on farms, he was a farmer through and through.

He established the farm, much of it on the land the Gitanmaax had donated for hospital use, tilled the soil, acquired chickens to add to the cow, and laid out vegetable and flower gardens. One of his first steps after clearing the land had been to plant the seeds that his farming friends and supporters in the Epworth League had sent him. He acquired some fruit trees and plants from a nursery in Victoria. He planted four kinds of strawberries, five or six roots each of black-caps and thimbleberries, and three potatoes and some gooseberry slips, all sent by his Ontario friends by mail. All these except the gooseberry slips, he said, did well. Writing to these friends and spon-sors, he outlined how he thought fresh fruit was so beneficial for convalescing patients:

Last summer in our new garden at the hospital we planted a few of quite a number of different kinds of fruit. Perhaps you think that this kind of thing is strange missionary work; but on second thoughts you will see some of the benefits to the Indians. In the first place there is nothing better for maintaining health than fresh fruits in their sea-son; and so if we can show the Indians how to grow these and what to grow we are certainly in the way of bringing benefit to them. And for invalids and convalescing patients, a certain amount of fresh fruit is most beneficial, so that a good variety of home-grown fruit is a great help to us here where but little is grown otherwise, and where it is impossible, either from distance or great expense, to provide them for the patients or ourselves.

Horace acquired a canning machine with which Alice and the staff processed huge quantities of produce from the farm. He supple-mented this with canned goods shipped up from Vancouver. Photo-graphs of the cellars under the hospital show cans of food lining the walls around a billiard table. With the river closed from October to May, this food had to last them all winter. He acquired more Jersey cows for fresh milk to add to the cow Tomlinson had given them. Recuperating patients and pregnant women who had come from far-away places to give birth often helped out, and perhaps relieve their boredom, by shelling peas, washing vegetable produce and doing light chores around the gardens. With eggs, milk and a hospital farm to provide produce in summer and well-canned food in winter, the hospital could well have been the best place in town to eat.

When Horace opened the hospital, he also established a nurses train-ing school. In this, he was perhaps inspired by the nurses training schools at St. Michael's Hospital and Grace Hospital. He was greatly helped by the Women's Missionary Society, which paid the salaries of two, then three and later four nurses. In his annual report for 1908, Horace paid tribute to the nurses: "The whole-souled energy which these young ladies put into their work is the leading factor in the success of the institution. Without such skilled and devoted workers the hospital doors would close."

Nurses usually enrolled every September, and three years later they graduated, fully qualified. They took classes from October to May, studying Clara Week's *Textbook of Nursing*, already a classic and in its third edition. The nurses were also taught anatomy and what was called *materia medica*. In her book, Clara Weeks wrote that, "Nursing is an art, the importance of which can scarcely be over-estimated. It properly includes, as well as the execution of specific orders, the per-sonal care of the patient, attention to the condition of the sick-room, its warmth, cleanliness, and ventilation, the careful observation and reporting of symptoms, and the prevention of contagion."

Annie Lawrence, the first nurse to graduate from the training school, arrived in May 1905 and graduated in August 1908. Until 1922, the hospital set its own examinations and awarded its own diplomas. Presumably the superintendent of the training school and Horace, later assisted by the staff doctor, gave lectures. Laura Moore, who entered the school in 1908 and graduated in 1911, was awarded 88 percent for the theory of nursing, 85 percent for anatomy and physiology and 93 percent for obstetrics. Her student record related that her deportment was "A1" and her health "Fair."

An unidentified nurse described the hospital in a nursing journal, probably in 1906, as a "wooden building, prettily painted green." The same nurse also noted that the nurses had recently taken up cooking and were using the *Boston Cooking-School Cook Book* by Fannie Merritt Farmer. This nurse wrote that "the patients have what are considered in Hazelton real luxuries, fresh eggs, vegetables and milk." Eva MacLean, the wife of the Presbyterian minister, Dan MacLean, who came to town a few years later, told her family in the East to stop sending her recipes that required fresh eggs because she couldn't get any in Hazelton. It was hard, in any event, to keep chickens alive: ravenous dogs roaming free in the town ate them. Horace built a solid stockade to keep his chickens safe, but even he lost a whole hen-yard once.

When Whittington visited Hazelton in the autumn of 1904, it is possible that he brought with him from Victoria the October 9 edition of the *Daily Colonist*. This would have given Horace much food for thought. He would have read the long article on the health insurance schemes that had been in operation in Germany for twenty years. Practically the whole working-class population of nineteen million had health insurance coverage. The scheme, based on compulsory deductions from employee wages and employer contributions, provided free medical attendance and free medicines.

In Germany, they seemed to have solved a problem that had probably been bothering Horace for a while — how to provide health care to those least able to afford it. Health insurance seemed to be working in Germany; it seemed to be financially viable. It was becoming normal. The number of accidents had not increased as employees became careless, as had been feared by many. Could such a scheme work in British Columbia? Over the years such ideas about the financing of public health simmered in Horace's mind.

———

Horace described the hospital site in a letter to his friends in the East, writing that there was a fourteen-acre lot around the hospital enclosed by a neat wire fence and that half of it had been cleared and seeded. He used to watch the pack trains of from forty to seventy mules or horses plodding on the trail to the interior that ran along-side the grounds about two hundred yards away from the buildings. If watching mules was too prosaic, he wrote, you only had to look up to see a range of mountains forty miles away with an immense glacier between the two of them, the whole looking as clear and distinct as if not more than eight or ten miles distant.

A similar view equally distant was to be seen in another direction. A nearer and grander view was presented by the beautiful Hazelton Mountain, "Skeedanden" (he meant Rocher de Boule Mountain) which was going to form the background for the photographs of the hospital to be sent back to the *Missionary Outlook* in Toronto. The mountain was three to five miles distant, but looked very much less. It was so high that in the short winter days one of its peaks kept the sun from shining on the hospital until after eleven o'clock. It pre-sented, he wrote, so many and varied conditions of light and cloud scenes that he hardly ever tired of looking over at it.

For almost fifty years, the mule trains that Horace watched plod-ding past the hospital were the lifeblood of Hazelton. Goods flowed up the river into Hazelton and then, strapped to the sides of mules, flowed out into the hinterland. This flow of goods, determined by Hazelton's physical location as being at the head of river navigation, had given the town its importance. "Hazelton is today probably the greatest pack-train camp in North America," the *Daily Colonist* reported in 1910. "During the summer there is a constant stream of pack-trains leaving with supplies for all parts within two hundred miles on the north, east and south. Over eight hundred horses and mules are used in the business, in which also about a hundred men find employment."

Waiting patiently for the river steamers to be unloaded or goods to be brought out from the warehouses, the mules lined up on Hazelton's Government Street. This ran parallel to the river and close to the riverbank warehouses. Each mule would be loaded with from 200 to 350 pounds of goods. The weight had to be balanced evenly because, as happened occasionally, if the balance was wrong, the mule could topple over and be unable to get up.

After being loaded, the mules would plod in single file back up the hill, with a few yards between each animal, and then on to the little hamlet of Two Mile, half a mile to the east of the hospital. Here the goods were often unpacked, sorted and held for repacking and onward carriage to the telegraph operators, miners, settlers and farmers in the hinterland. Though, as Frank Chettleburgh pointed out, this was also an opportunity for one last drink.

Horace was well-acquainted with Cataline, the legendary packer of the British Columbia interior. Cataline had packed goods to the gold fields of the Fraser Canyon, the Cariboo and Omineca but he now made Hazelton his home and base. During the first twenty years of the century, he was a familiar character around town. His real name was Jean Caux, and he had probably been born in Oloron in Béarn, France, though no one really knew for sure. About his own history, he was at best reticent and at worst deceptive. Legend says he told some people he came from near Catalonia and the name Cataline stuck. Béarnaise, the local dialect of Béarn, was probably his mother tongue, but his speech was made up of some Spanish, some English, some French, some Chinook, with a smattering of First Nations words he had picked up in his packing travels. He abbreviated words of over two syllables. As a result, he was more than a little difficult to understand. "He could speak three languages," someone said of him. "Trouble was, he spoke them all at once."

Cataline was famous for rubbing an amount of whatever he was drinking — rum or whisky — into his hair on the "a little insida, a little outsida" principle. Allegedly, he could not read or write, but he always knew what was owed to him and by whom with great accuracy. With a reputation for reliability and honesty, he treated First Nations with open generosity. When a First Nations band was short of food, he had been known to take in supplies and not worry too much about charging them.

As a consequence, his pack trains did not suffer the shrinkage of animals "going astray" on the trail. Reliability of supplies was absolutely critical to those working in the wilderness. In this, Cataline had no equal. "He was," Sperry Cline wrote, "the best packer British Columbia — and possibly North America — ever produced. He would appear with his mule-train, load up, then at some distant date reach his destination. Nothing stopped him. Storms, rains, fires, insects, the wilderness, he took in his stride. On two occasions most of his animals perished from lack of feed and other hardships. But the supplies got through, once on the backs of Indian women whom he had pressed into service."

Cataline and Sperry Cline were good friends. Cline's own speech had been moulded by his experiences in South Africa and was a mixture of English, Cape Dutch and Swahili. Although few others could understand them when they were conversing, he and Cataline understood each other perfectly.

———

In addition to building the hospital and serving the medical needs of the local communities as a doctor and surgeon — as if this were not enough — Horace was also a missionary. This part of his work was necessarily in a subsidiary capacity, since Pierce, the closest Methodist minister, was less than a dozen miles away. It was, in any event, a heavy load. Sutherland in Toronto was sympathetic. He wrote to Horace with the following advice:

To occupy a field of any considerable extent and fully discharge the duties of both minister and doctor would be manifestly impossible, but in any ordinary medical practice there are opportunities for evangelistic work as good as one could desire, and by occasionally conducting Bible classes, or the like, you can greatly encourage the missionary and strengthen his work. . . . We rely upon your fidelity and good judgment.

Hazelton itself was, on the whole, an Anglican community, having an active minister in Rev. John Field, with his new St. Peter's Church. Horace would, therefore, have confined his missionary work in Hazelton to the hospital, ministering only to those who came there for the Bible classes and hymn singing, as well as to patients.

Horace identified the evils the missionaries had to contend with. In particular, he blamed settlers and others in Hazelton for introducing the First Nations to bad habits. These, he said, were principally drink, immorality, desire for money and Sabbath breaking. They were making it much harder to bring people to Christ. He wrote, "The loose lives of many of the white people in these frontiers make a very bad example for the Indians. And when those very white people will offer them drink and urge them to take it, or hire them to work and then almost compel them to work on the Sunday, it makes it very hard indeed for them to resist the temptations or for us to keep them back."

Horace was a firm believer in temperance. At Pierce's request, he regularly went to Kispiox to give lectures on the evils of alcohol. Hazelton, with its numerous bars, gambling and large number of unattached young men, was a town where liquor flowed freely. Frank Chettleburgh recalled that the Hudson's Bay Company had a warehouse with a liquor supply where all drinks before breakfast were free. It opened when anyone showed up. All drinks, he said, were served from a cup chained to the wall. Hudson's Bay Company rum cost $9 for a two-gallon keg. Until a new policeman with a reforming broom arrived in the autumn of 1909, the bars were open twenty-four hours a day and every day of the week.

—◦◦◦—

While on a tour of the Skeena district in the summer of 1905, Richard McBride, the premier of the province, stopped at Hazelton. Waxing lyrical about the potential of the district, he said the area should be called "New British Columbia," on account of its abundance of natural resources. All that was missing was better transportation. He visited the hospital, one of the first of many dignitaries to do so. "The splendid hospital, lately constructed in Hazelton," the *Daily Colonist* reported him as saying, "must not be overlooked. It is the charge of Dr. Wrench [sic] and a competent staff of nurses. We were shown over the building and grounds."

While in the hospital, the premier paid a bedside visit to J.E. Gobeil, general inspector of the Yukon Telegraph from Ottawa, who, while inspecting a line fifty to sixty miles to the south, had broken his ankle badly (a Pott's fracture) in several places.

The $152 charge for fifty-five days in the hospital stimulated Horace to propose to the Dominion government that it pay the hospital $30 a month for medical attendance on employees working on the telegraph line. Consequently, on May 10 of the following year, 1906, Prime Minister Wilfrid Laurier signed an order-in-council approving such an arrangement. "It is hard to contemplate what might have happened," the Order papers said in referring to Mr. Gobeil's travails, "if the hospital at Hazelton had not been reached for a proper treatment."

With the hospital, farm and nurses training school settling into their rhythms and running well, in the autumn of 1905, Horace and Alice faced a personal crisis that jolted them out of their routines and, for a while, threatened to become tragic.

CHAPTER 5

New York Interlude
1906

ALICE WAS BUSY WITH family matters during the years from 1901 to 1905. When a daughter, Ralphena, was born on June 24, 1905, Alice — she was Patient No. 80 — stayed in hospital until July 7. Horace wrote, tongue in cheek, to his correspondents in Ontario:

Our staff has been recently reinforced by the arrival of a young lady, to be hereafter known as Miss Ralphena Alice Wrinch. We have not yet noticed that she has perceptibly relieved the pressure of work, but we remember that a certain amount of time is required for anyone to become accustomed to a place and to shoulder the appropriate share of care and responsibility, so we will give her all due allowance and hope for remarkable things in the near future. I need hardly add that she has already given evidence of intelligence, not to say genius, of a very high order.

Alongside pride and pleasure in his children, though, Horace had cause for serious concern. Alice was not recovering. She had been re-admitted to the hospital on July 28 with a severe attack of appendicitis and remained there until August 25. Although for a time Horace thought that an immediate operation might be necessary, her health gradually improved. He realized, however, she would need an operation, one that he could not perform, followed by what could well be a long convalescence. (The nature of Alice's ailment is not known, but it could possibly have been complications stemming from appendicitis.) Where would the surgery take place? Vancouver, the logical choice, would be convenient — but what about the children?

They made the decision to go back to Toronto, where Alice would receive the necessary operation. They both had family there who could look after the children and also care for Alice during her convalescence. By the beginning of October, Alice was strong enough to travel. The decision made, they had to act quickly. It was already autumn.

Horace had arranged for Dr. Allison M. Rolls from Chatham, Ontario, to come out to manage the hospital and his practice. He and Alice knew they would be away for the entire winter because once they had left in October, they would not be able to return until navigation on the river re-opened in April or May. With Alice's condition, it was out of the question for them to go over a grease trail to the Nass River and then down to the mouth of the river by boat.

They had to reach the coast before the Skeena River became unnavigable, which it did on October 5. The *Mount Royal* was the last steamer to make the journey downstream to Port Essington, and the Wrinches were probably on board. Tuesday October 10 found "Dr. F.C. Wrench [sic]" and his family from Hazelton staying at the Badminton Hotel, at the corner of Dunsmuir and Howe in Vancouver.

After the two journeys by steamer, first down river and then down the coast, Horace, Alice and the children set out on the third leg of the journey by rail to Toronto. With a seriously ill wife and three children under five — one under six months — this time would have been arduous and fraught with anxiety. Horace would have worried about Alice's health during the journey and how the children would manage the turmoil of being away from the only home they had ever known. In Toronto they would have to stay with relatives they had never met.

And what would happen to all his hard work in Hazelton? Horace had shown Dr. Rolls what was needed, but how competent would he be in running the hospital, the training school and the farm? And would he have the necessary personal and indeed political skills to navigate the delicate balance of relationships between First Nations and the settlers and the many differing factions within each of them? Horace must have wondered what state the hospital would be in when he and Alice both returned — if indeed they did both return.

After the tiring journey of two weeks, they arrived in Ontario. In October 1905, the *Missionary Outlook* published a letter Horace had written from Toronto, no doubt surprising many people who had been picturing him on the Skeena River. The letter read:

> For some little time Mrs. Wrinch and I have been hoping to arrange for a visit to our friends at home. This visit was precipitated some-what by a very serious illness, from which Mrs. Wrinch has not yet fully recovered, and which necessitated our coming out where we could avail ourselves of special advice and treatment.

As far as one can tell, Alice's operation in Toronto went well. Relatives were attentive in caring for her and for the children. Full recovery, though, would take time. As Alice's health improved, Horace wrote, they would be able to spend more time in the East with their friends and families.

Horace was never one to miss an opportunity. Toronto's *Globe* newspaper reported that he had brought with him "to show people here he does not live in a frost-bound region, some fine samples of potatoes, one of which weighs two and one half pounds, and measures eleven inches in length, twelve inches in circumference and twenty-four inches around the longest way."

Back in Hazelton, Dr. Rolls appeared to be managing the hospital and its affairs well. He was also willing to continue the religious services, which pleased Horace. A few weeks after his arrival, Rolls wrote of his first experiences. He said he had heard praise of Dr. Wrinch in Toronto but "when I considered that he engineered the work here practically single-handed and did so much of it himself, I felt that he well deserves all the praise he receives."

He reported also that Miss Bone, the lady superintendent, never had too high a recommendation given her, and Miss Lawrence, a nurse, was all that was to be desired. Miss Tomlinson did excellent work in the kitchen and around the hospital. He also mentioned that Mr. Wrinch — Horace's brother Alfred — was there as assistant and general helper and deserved thanks for leaving his work in Toronto to come out to the hospital. Rolls went on:

The work here is very varied. Sometimes it is medical work, at another an Indian brings around a horse to be treated. Again, a man has a tooth to be filled or something of the kind. . . . Just shortly after I came here I had to go out to attend a patient at a distance. She lived seventeen or eighteen miles away. Word was received at about ten o'clock Sunday morning, and I got there about half-past two. Taking all things into consideration this was excellent time. Being an urgent case I had to stay all night with her. Next morning about 11:00 a.m., I left and, after stopping half-way to treat some patients got home about 6:30 p.m. I felt very stiff for two or three days after my long ride, but it was necessary work and so no complaint was possible.

In Ontario while Alice was recuperating, Horace, not one to sit around doing nothing, spent some of his time on Church matters. At the end of January, for example, he attended the Epworth League Convention in Bowmanville, Ontario, and received praise as one of the missionaries "who are in the thin red line, in the forefront of the battle," and lauded for their work in their arduous fields. He led a devotional service at the convention on the evening of January 24 and the following afternoon gave an address. He also found time to speak at Albert College in Belleville, the school he had left ten years before. He reported to Alice there had been a fair attendance of about sixty. He had spoken for two hours, he wrote, and the audience had kept him for another half hour asking questions.

Horace also spent some of his time in Toronto bringing his medical knowledge up to date by attending the city hospitals. He then decided to take a larger step and travel to New York to enrol in post-graduate training at the New York Post-Graduate School and Hospital. This school, founded by Dr. Roosa in 1882, was one of the oldest and, it implied, the best post-graduate medical school in the United States. "Throughout the world," its 1906 Annual Announcement [Academic Calendar] said, "this is the pioneer Institution of Post-Graduate Medical instruction under one roof, and in this country there was never any systematic instruction by courses in all departments for graduates until they were here organized." The school took evident pride in being an institution at which the students were expected not only to learn but also to engage in hands-on medical treatments.

Although Horace's available time did not permit him to attend for the full term, the school had a system whereby practitioners could purchase a number of tickets for courses of their choosing. Horace chose tickets to study for a period that lasted from the beginning of February until the end of March in 1906.

The fee for three months' instruction was $160, but Horace tackled Dr. Roosa, the president of the school and head of faculty at his office. After resisting the efforts of a secretary who suggested he should to wait and see the president at some uncertain day in the future, Horace went to Roosa's home and sent up his card and a letter of introduction. He had been told that Roosa was some kind of an irascible bear but he obviously found him in one of his gentler moods. He was able to persuade Roosa to lower his fees to $100 on the basis that he was a missionary.

Returning to the school, Horace secured tickets and attended one lecture before one o'clock, thinking he'd had a pretty good morning.

He then attended four more lectures and demonstrations in the afternoon and then another between 8 and 9 in the evening. One of the courses was on diseases of the eye, led by Dr. Roosa, himself a noted eye and ear specialist. Some days Horace had a free ticket and spent the whole day there, picking up plenty of pointers. In a letter to Alice, he wrote, "What I have paid for includes two special courses on operations on 'subs' — one in eye work and one gynaecology. So I think I have plenty of work laid out, don't you? Today I had a splendid lesson on operation for squint, so I am prepared to fix up the cross-eyed posty according to the latest New York cut."

On his first Sunday in New York, wanting to see more of the city and find a good church service, he started exploring. Walking up Fifth Avenue to Midtown in the bright, raw cold of the January day, he found his way first to the Catholic Cathedral. He was impressed with the building and the size of the congregation, but only stayed about fifteen minutes. A little farther he found the Fifth Avenue Presbyterian Church and, seeing that the preacher — Dr. J. Ross Stephenson — was someone he was acquainted with, he went in.

The text of the sermon, a very fine one, he said, was Romans 16:13: Salute Rufus Chosen of the Lord and his Mother and mine. "You can see how a simple analysis of that would suggest many homely thoughts," he wrote to Alice. "The thought of the mother opening her heart to Paul was made very peaceful and tender." After the service, by invitation, he spent the rest of the day with new friends. "Altogether I have had a most pleasant day. Much better than I had expected from first impressions of New York." The only jarring part of the day to him was that he saw men who were busy hauling snow off the streets. To a staunch Sabbath observer, that did not seem right.

Like many an adult student before and since, he found the return to book-studying more trying than he had expected. "I am getting down to steady work now," he wrote, "and am beginning to get into the run of study again. It is really surprising how much I have got out of the way of it. I must not allow myself to lapse so again. In the eye work, to which I have been giving quite a good bit of time, I feel that I have gained some very valuable groundwork and have yet time enough to get quite a lot more."

Dr. Newsom, one of his new friends, introduced him to physicians at other hospitals. Horace was eager to visit them as often as he could because there would be fewer students at their hospitals and, being personally known, he would get a much better chance of close observation. Another connection gave him an entrée into the Presbyterian Hospital, one of the best in the city. The surgeon offered to send him a post card every day announcing the planned operations for that day so that Horace could come and observe. The fittings and equipment of the Presbyterian Hospital obviously impressed him. He wrote that they were exceedingly fine. Marble coated the doors as well as seats for the onlookers, and everything was on a similar costly and substantial basis. What's more, he said, all of it for the poor of New York, and all kept up by voluntary subscriptions.

In addition to studying and watching surgeries, Horace assisted physicians in their daily work. He wrote that he went with one of the professors to a patient in a private house, a brownstone, and assisted him in the operation when the family physician failed to turn up. The professor offered to use him again when he could.

While in New York, Horace lived first at a small hotel but found it expensive and inconvenient. He was paying $1 per day for an indifferent room and had to go to restaurants for all his meals. He tried a good many places and found that it was hard to combine good food and plenty of it for anything less than thirty-five cents a meal. So very soon he moved to Mrs. Purinton's boarding house, one recommended by the school. Conveniently situated at 245 East Nineteenth Street, it was within easy walking distance of the school, which was located at Second Avenue and Twentieth Street. Often, having finished dinner in his lodgings and written his letters, he would walk back to the school for an evening clinic.

At Mrs. Purinton's, he paid $8 a week for a room he shared with another doctor. After one evening's walk two or three miles downtown to a historic old church (Episcopal) for the service, he came back to a delicious dinner. "The swellest since I have been at this boarding house — oysters on the half shell, turkey, cranberry sauce, sweet potatoes, asparagus, stewed onions, ice cream and real strawberries, with raisins."

Most of Horace's time in New York was spent at the school. This was clearly his priority — everything else was secondary. His letters do not show any appreciation of one of the greatest cities in the world at that time. New York in the early 1900s was a melting pot of different peoples: it would have been loud and colourful with Italian, Yiddish, Russian, Spanish and every variety of English. By 1906, the population was about three and a half million. Had Horace wanted to amuse himself in, say, the second week of March 1906, he would have had many opportunities.

He could have gone to the Vaudeville or to see Mr. George Cohan's musical triumph *George Washington Junior*, or he could have travelled to Midtown to see Miss Ethel Barrymore in J.M. Barrie's play *Alice Sit-by-the-Fire* at the Criterion Theatre. More likely, had he wished, he could in all propriety have gone to Carnegie Hall to listen to Mr. Henry Martineau playing Beethoven's *Violin Concerto* with the Philharmonic Society Orchestra, conducted by Mr. Victor Herbert.

He did not mention any visit to, or desire to visit, the Metropolitan Museum of Art. He did not mention the construction of the New York Public Library on Fifth Avenue, still then without its roof. He was not, it seems, interested in Central Park or Brooklyn Bridge. Nor did he express any shock at the Tammany Hall corruption in city government. Horace's letters record nothing of these events. He was more interested in sermons at the churches, his courses at the school and little Ralphena's smiles back in Toronto.

He spent his spare time in the evenings writing, not only to Alice but also to others in Hazelton: Dr. Rolls, Helen Bone, Robert Tomlinson and prospective new staff such as Clara Hollingsworth, soon to be the new matron. His letters show that he was already planning improvements. Everything at the hospital seemed to be going well, but from such a distance it was a great worry. With several mail deliveries every day, he could get a reply by supper time to a letter he had written to someone in New York in the morning and one from Alice in Toronto overnight. Mail from Hazelton took much longer.

During these few months in New York, Horace wrote to Alice almost daily, and she replied just as frequently. Once he noted that he had received a letter from her in the morning's mail and another at noon. "You are indeed putting me in the shade. But I see how it is — they have you in bed and you cannot do anything else so you amuse yourself by writing to me. That is an uncharitable way of putting it, though, is it not? And it would serve me right if you did not write me again for a long time. But then I know you won't be so hard as that." And there was also something rare for him — in writing, anyway — introspection:

February 25th, 1906
My Dear Alice,

I was so glad yesterday to get your card with its assurance that you are feeling really better. It begins to make me feel like old times again. I know I have been irritable and hasty in speech too frequently during the past months but it seems to me I have been under heavy pressure and so allowed myself to be upset by things that I ought not. I believe now that I have been nearer a nervous explosion than I thought. I depended upon a very strong constitution and it has carried me along, but I believe with a somewhat narrow margin at times. And I know that you too have had as much or more to endure than I have, but it looks as if we might be in less troubled waters for a time. I hope so indeed. In the eyes of some perhaps, we looked to be going along smoothly but we know, do we not, that they have been about as heavy as we could very well carry. I know you are taking care of yourself and I assure you I am doing so too. I am working about as much as I can find myself able to take in, but am not by any means over-taxing myself. My time here is almost half gone by, and from the time I return I don't think we need look for much more lengthy periods of separation for some time.

And he was anxious for news about how quickly she was getting better, and a little suspicious that he was not always being told the full truth:

March 9th, 1906
My Dear Alice,

I have been trying to discover from your letter whether you are up and around or still in bed but I am afraid you are purposely avoiding a statement bearing directly on the question. You must please report a little more fully or I shall have to get Miss Aiken to send official reports and I know you will not hear of such a thing as that. I am very glad, though, you are not having much discomfort and hope soon to get the information direct that you are up and around as usual. Do you have any trouble regarding the swelling of the right leg anymore? This extra rest ought to be good for that and you needed it on that account anyway, so perhaps it is as well something occurred to oblige you to give it the rest you needed.

On occasion, Horace went on rather wide-eyed trips to the stores. "Then I took a walk and looked in the shop windows for about three quarters of an hour and got some papers with accounts of the wedding in the White House [of Alice Roosevelt, the President's daughter]. I know that such matters will interest you and the girls." He noted some things he thought he would like to buy, until he saw the price: ". . . don't be looking for much of that character when I come home, for I don't know how to start buying when I see such wonderful decorations and such elaborate stores. Some of these stores are so handsomely fitted out that they look more like wealthy private homes than any kind of public place."

He had to think ahead and plan for his return to Ontario and then on to Hazelton. His calendar was filling up — Central Methodist Sunday School and taking the service at Simpson Avenue, both on March 25, Epworth League Church in Toronto on Monday March 26, London on the following Sunday, then Appleby and Bronte on the 8th, both visits (or services) on the one day. "And the following week would be our last before we started back. We ought to start, should we not, on the 17th or 18th? I thought I would give you these dates so that you could try to make other visiting fall in with them."

Alice suggested drawing up a plan and deciding what they could and couldn't do, recognizing that some of their relatives might be disappointed if they didn't see them. Horace agreed, "I want as far as is possible to consult your wishes in this and will make other things fall in as well as we can." But he was adamant that, with a long and tiring journey ahead of them all, he didn't want Alice tired out by too much travelling and visiting before they even left.

After completing his studies, Horace returned to Toronto. Together, they saw as many of their relatives and friends as they could squeeze into the limited time available and Alice's health would allow. Then, after meeting his commitments to churches and other groups, they travelled back to Hazelton. They took with them Clara Hollingsworth from Picton as the new matron for the hospital. It was the first week of May 1906.

They had a good journey back — the train across the country, a few days seeing friends in Vancouver, the steamer passage up the coast, a day and a half in Port Essington and then up the river by steamer to Hazelton. In Vancouver, he would have heard that the Methodist Annual Conference meeting then taking place in Victoria had declared him "ordained for special purposes." Alice, though by no means fully recovered, was certainly feeling much better. "Mrs. Wrinch," Horace wrote, "is still under instruction that she must take very great care of herself." These, he added, had been crucial times for the family. Even in July, nearly a year after she had become ill, Horace was reporting to Sutherland that Alice "has within the last few weeks been improving greatly and is now on her way to full health." With a recuperating wife, three children under the age of six and the new matron, as well as bales of material for the hospital,

Horace would have been happy when the steamer, tooting its horn, rounded the bend, and at long last Hazelton appeared.

The sight of children running along the bank to greet the steamer and the sound of dogs barking and merchants coming to greet them told them they were home. Flora Martin, a long-time resident, recalled that the arrival of the steamer was always a happy time because it meant contact with the outside world and hearing from friends. "And usually the little boys used to go up on the top of the hill, little native boys, and they would call out 'Steamboat, Steamboat.' And we would listen. Sure enough we would hear the puff. You know you could hear it from miles down the river. Everybody — the whole town — would get their coats and fly down to the wharf, you know, to see the boat coming in."

Some years later, Wiggs O'Neil remembered the dogs at such a time joining in the welcome. "Even the dogs got excited," he wrote, "and lined up along the river-bank. Everybody, both Indian and white, joined them at the landing and when the captain blew his whistle at the big cottonwood tree on the point, everyone cheered. The dogs, not to be outdone, sat on their hind ends, opened their mouths to the sky and howled their heads off."

Horace and Alice walked down the gangplank, recognizing friends and acquaintances in the crowd. Dr. Rolls had brought a wagon to take Alice, the children and their luggage back up to their home on the hospital grounds. Horace and Rolls, though, decided to walk. On the way back through town, Rolls told Horace what had been happening during his seven-month absence. He would have given Horace the full story of George MacKenzie and his harrowing ordeal in the wilderness.

MacKenzie, a veteran prospector, suffering from scurvy, had survived an epic journey in a temperature of minus sixty-five degrees, but somehow, thanks to First Nations trappers, he had managed to reach the safety of the hospital. Apart from a few amputated toes, he would recover. Rolls may also have told Horace about the new hotel and bar at Two Mile that Constable Kirby and other respectable people in town were not at all happy about.

Once home, Leonard and Cooper jumped off the wagon and ran ahead, seeking out familiar people and places. Alice noted happily that their home had been freshly cleaned and dusted. Water was boiling on the stove for tea. The smell of fresh bread filled the kitchen. How nice it was to be back! Rolls invited them to the hospital for dinner with the staff and nurses.

Soon there would be farewells to make. Horace's brother Alfred and Helen Bone were returning to Ontario. Rolls was going to Port Simpson to allow Dr. Kergin to take a holiday. Clara Hollingsworth would settle into her job. Routines of medical practice and of the hospital would once again take control of their lives. Horace knew he would have much to do on the farm since Rolls, with all his now-proven medical and administrative virtues, was not a farmer.

A few weeks after they had settled in, Hazelton was shaken by one of the most famous murders and subsequent manhunts in British Columbia's history. This murder, moreover, was committed on Horace's own land.

CHAPTER 6

Murder, Missionaries and Medicine
1906–1908

"ABOUT 9 O'CLOCK in the morning of the day in question," Horace testified at the trial, "I received a telephone message that Alex MacIntosh's body was lying on the trail between the hospital and Two Mile. I went out and found the body lying near the fence of the hay field. . . . I examined the body superficially. Life was extinct. I knew MacIntosh. It was his body. I found a wound in the chest, on the left side about two inches from the middle line, about an inch below the collar-bone." It was June 19, 1906.

The corpse was lying — splayed-out, coatless. Horace noticed the dirty rag wrapped around a superficial knife-wound to the little finger of the corpse's right hand. He also observed that MacIntosh had received a bullet in the back of his spine that had travelled up through the base of the heart. Examining the wounds, Horace deduced that the shot had been fired upwards, as if by a man lying or kneeling on the ground. This was no accidental killing, he thought. This was deliberate murder.

Because the Gitxsan were matrilineal (that is, deriving their status from their mother), MacIntosh, with a Scottish father and Gitxsan mother, was Gitxsan. He was a worker from the river steamers, with a reputation for both strength and temper. He was so strong, it was said he could lift a hundred-pound sack with each arm. His temper had led him into trouble on numerous occasions. He had a bad reputation and was sometimes in trouble with the law for selling liquor to the Gitxsan. He also knew how to handle mules and horses, and that made him invaluable as a packer with the pack trains.

Constable James Kirby soon arrived on the scene. After he had surveyed the murder site and Horace had finished his examination, Kirby directed that the body be taken to the lock-up in town to await a post-mortem. Ironically, MacIntosh had only been released from that same lock-up the day before, having been serving a three-month sentence for supplying Gitxsan with liquor.

He had been released early to ride with the Barrett packtrain, then assembling at Two Mile. Kirby then decided to go to the hotel. There he looked around at the topsy-turvy scene at the bar. There was ample evidence of drunkenness and of a fight. After interrogating some of the people still there, he quickly decided who the murderer was.

The suspect's English name was Johnson, but he preferred to use the name by which he is known to history: Simon Gunanoot. A Gitxsan from Kispiox, Gunanoot had already had one brush with the law. The police (perhaps Kirby) once had kicked in his door at midnight, suspecting, wrongly, that he was operating an illegal still and selling home-brewed alcohol. Gunanoot, furious at this indignity, had threatened to shoot anyone who did that again.

About thirty-one years old, a strong and proud man, Gunanoot was a good businessman, with an excellent head for figures. He owned the general store in Kispiox — which was where Horace had come to know him — and was doing well in his business. In his store that day, he had stock worth $3,500, all paid for. He used to go to

Vancouver and, allegedly, on occasion to Seattle and San Francisco to sell marten, fox, lynx and beaver furs, thus cutting out the middlemen at the Hudson's Bay Company. When he was away from home, his wife Sarah looked after the store.

Gunanoot owned land in the Bear Lake country, as well as a farm of approximately a hundred acres at Anlaw on the south side of the Skeena River, towards Hazelton. On this farm he kept between eighteen and forty-eight pack-train horses, with which he occasionally ran supplies out to miners and telegraph operators. Although generally well-liked and well-respected by Gitxsan and residents of Hazelton alike, some packers resented the fact that he, a Gitxsan, was doing so well. True, there were also some who thought he drank too much. He had recently returned from a long hunting and trapping trip. Known to be an excellent shot, he preferred to shoot his prey in the spine just below the neck.

On the day before the murder, Gunanoot and his family had gone to his farm at Anlaw to see if the hay needed cutting. When he decided to go to Hagwilget to buy some fresh fish, he was not expecting trouble. But trouble found him. Along the way he stopped for a drink at the "disreputable caravanserai" at the Two Mile Hotel. This was close to where pack-train owners assembled their teams, including the Barrett and Charleson pack train that was getting ready to leave the next day. The bar was a place where drink could be bought and women rented. The licence had been granted to the hotel over Kirby's objections, when Horace, a magistrate and a member of the licensing authority, had been away in New York.

This particular night had been rowdy. Packers, leaving with the pack train the following morning, were drinking and preparing themselves for the long days on the trail. The inebriated manager of the bar, James Cameron, sank to the floor, asking MacIntosh to take over serving the liquor, which MacIntosh did, liberally. Gunanoot and MacIntosh argued. Although some witnesses said he was in a drunken rage, others said that, while he had certainly been drinking, Gunanoot did not appear to be wildly drunk. In his book *Trapline*

Outlaw, David Ricardo Williams suggests that Gunanoot could have been upset with MacIntosh for helping himself to free drinks. The talk at the time, though, reported by Loring and by Pinkerton's men searching for him later, was that MacIntosh had boasted that he had been sexually intimate with Gunanoot's wife. This part of the story remains murky. Words, insults and fists flew. Gunanoot went for MacIntosh, who pulled out his knife and cut Gunanoot's face. Gunanoot then used his own knife and cut MacIntosh's hand. The manager of Charley Barrett's pack train heard the row and entered the bar, looking for MacIntosh. He managed to separate the fighting men and made them shake hands, which they did, though unwillingly.

Described by witnesses as having been bested in the fight, Gunanoot left in a rage, swearing, according to some witnesses, to return with a gun and kill MacIntosh. Other witnesses testified he said only that he would return and "fix" MacIntosh. One witness later said he saw Gunanoot riding hard back to his farm at Anlaw, lashing out furiously at him with the spare bridle in his hand. Another said that Peter Himadan, Gunanoot's brother-in-law, had gone to collect their rifles. Meanwhile, MacIntosh was helping to round up the horses for the pack train. When MacIntosh complained of a sore and bleeding hand, he was told to go to the hospital and get it looked at. On the trail, which ran over Horace's land, someone shot him dead.

Horace, his examination of MacIntosh's body completed, had packed up and, after looking in at the Two Mile Hotel, had returned to the hospital, his plans for the day utterly disarranged. There he collected the instruments he would need for the post-mortem later that day. Then, at about one, his telephone rang again. Another body had been found.

Already cold by now, this one was lying on the trail to Kispiox, close to the junction with the Salmon River trail. It was Max LeClair. The person who found this body had dragged it to one side of the trail and placed a handkerchief over his face. This news was taken to Kirby, who was trying to assemble a posse. He asked Edward Hicks Beach, the coroner and magistrate, to telephone Dr. Wrinch and tell him about the second body. Residents of Hazelton, by now buzzing with the news, were becoming agitated at the thought of a double-murderer on the loose.

Horace's plans changed again. He saddled his horse and was examining the second body when Kirby arrived with Hicks Beach. Once again Horace knew the victim, later testifying, "Life was extinct. I knew Max LeClair and recognized the body as his. . . . I moved the branches and saw that blood had been oozing freely from the nose, and seeing no wound on the head, I turned the body till I could see the back. I saw a round blood stain in the middle of the vest. . . . I pulled up the vest and found a bullet hole in the back."

The entry wound was at the point where the fifth rib on the right side attaches to the body. From the way the bullet had travelled up through the body, Horace again concluded that the shooter had been low down and firing upwards.

LeClair's role in the affair is still unclear. He had not been in town for very long. How had he got mixed up in all this? He had not even been at the Two Mile Hotel that evening and might not have known either Gunanoot or MacIntosh. There has been much speculation but no clarity about why he was shot. Had LeClair known who had shot MacIntosh and therefore, as a witness, had to die? Had the murderer mistaken LeClair for a policeman coming after him?

More likely, LeClair had met the still-angry Gunanoot — if he was indeed the murderer of MacIntosh — got into an argument with him and taunted him for having been bested in a fight. This taunt to an angry man could have precipitated the second murder.

What evidence there was pointed to Gunanoot having shot both men. Certainly Kirby had no doubt at the time. Not sure whether he had a mass murderer to deal with or not, he continued looking for his posse. With many residents out of town prospecting, this took some time, but eventually he found enough men and had them sworn in. In a scene reminiscent of a movie from the Old West, Kirby then rode out of town with the posse to search for the murderer.

Kirby, though, had a problem. Gunanoot was popular and respected. People had sympathy for him: many thought MacIntosh had it coming. Some of the help given to Kirby, therefore, was less than helpful. The first time he and the posse came to Gunanoot's farm at Anlaw, he found that three of Gunanoot's horses had been shot and one killed with a pickaxe.

He came back a couple of days later, and, after placing his posse strategically around the farm, rushed the house. The house was now guarded by dogs blocking the entrances. These he had shot. Gunanoot was not there, though there was evidence that he had been in the house recently.

Kirby noticed a man walking on the other side of the river and thought he recognized Gunanoot. Barney Mulvaney and others in the posse said it wasn't him but rather someone who resembled him. Kirby later came to believe that Mulvaney had deliberately let Gunanoot through the cordon and had advised him how to get away. (Many years later, Kirby's belief that it had been Gunanoot on the riverbank was confirmed.)

Kirby took Gunanoot's father, Nahgan, into custody, partly for helping his son escape and partly as bait to entice Gunanoot into a trap. He was confined in a cabin next to the police station in Hazelton because the lock-up was being used as a morgue for the murder victims. Allowed out to go to the outhouse, Nahgun managed to escape with some ease.

Gunanoot slipped away into the forest. With him went his parents, his wife Sarah, their two children, another child she had had with a previous partner, as well as his brother-in-law Peter Himadan and his wife. Himadan's role in the murders remains unclear to this day.

Gunanoot's escape led to a massive and fruitless manhunt that subsided only when the police realized they had no chance whatsoever of catching him. At first, though, there was much excitement, and the police put great effort into the search. They offered a reward of $500, later raising it to $2,000.

After some initial bungling, they continued the search with special constables, with irregulars and finally with Pinkerton's Detective

Agency, whose agents, disguised as prospectors, sent in detailed reports of their travels and conversations during 1909 and 1910. Some bounty hunters set out full of confidence and returned empty-handed.

Some search parties, it was suggested, were using public money to finance their prospecting trips into the mountains. Several never left the bars of Port Essington. For a time, the authorities thought Gunanoot and Himadan had died in the harsh winter of 1907. "Peter and Simon Believed to Have Perished," headlines in local newspapers said. But they hadn't. After a couple of years of fruitless searching, the police gave up the active hunt.

The community gave remarkably little assistance to the police. No one stepped forward to claim the reward. Gunanoot was certainly in communication with Gitxsan friends in Hazelton and Kispiox. They undoubtedly warned him of any plans to send out search parties. Rumour at the time, reported on by Pinkerton's agents, held that Rev. W. Pearce, the Methodist minister at Kispiox, was a friend of Gunanoot, and had acted as a go-between for his friends in the district, sending him supplies and information. If you needed to get a letter or a message to Gunanoot, the rumours said, give it to Pearce. Few settlers or businessmen, it seemed, wanted to see him caught.

In the autumn of 1909, when the Pinkerton's men were coincidentally in Hazelton, Horace treated Gunanoot's children at the hospital, not telling the police until March of the following year. The authorities then angrily admonished him for this, saying it had been his duty to report the fact at the time so that they could have followed the children to their father. Horace, perhaps a little too innocently, said he had not thought of that.

He may well have had conflicting loyalties. On the one hand, he was a magistrate and a pillar of the establishment in town, and it would certainly have been his duty to turn Gunanoot in or help the police catch him. On the other, like so many, he sympathized with him and wished him no harm. He would, moreover, have been aware that if he had turned Gunanoot in or had given his location away, he would have made enemies among the Gitxsan. They would have seen this as betrayal.

The police authorities would have been even more unhappy with Horace if they had learned of his involvement in an incident in December 1912. Rev. William Lee, who was then the Methodist missionary in Kispiox, told the following story to Rev. Chas. R. Sing, a fellow Methodist minister. Sing retold it in a letter to the *Victoria Times Colonist* in 1945. A version had appeared in the newspapers in 1912 but had omitted Horace's part in it.

Before the murders, Gunanoot had been a shareholder in the co-operative that ran the sawmill at Kispiox. Lee managed its finances. Sing related that a man had come to Lee, saying that Gunanoot, whom Lee did not know, was in the village and wanted to claim his share of some funds owing him relating to the sawmill. Lee confirmed the amount and told the man to ask Gunanoot to come in himself that evening to claim it.

When the man had left, Lee hurriedly went to consult Horace at Hazelton. Sing said that Horace was regarded as being "father confessor to all Indians." He wrote that Horace's first thought was to report the matter to the police at once. This would have been his clear duty. He was, after all, a magistrate. The police could then have gone to Kispiox and arrested Gunanoot when he came back to collect his money. Horace, however, thought the matter over and decided against it. He told Lee to try to persuade Gunanoot to give himself up and to tell him that he would be treated fairly.

When the man — who of course was Gunanoot himself — came to see Lee that evening, he was heavily armed with two revolvers and with two belts of shells around his waist. He also had a friend with him. After giving him the money owing, Lee passed on Horace's advice and assurances. Gunanoot at first agreed to give himself up, but his friend then spoke to him in Gitxsan. At which point Gunanoot changed his mind. When Lee asked him why, Gunanoot said, in perfect English, "I hear the climate is not good at Westminster." (The prison — and scaffold — were both at New Westminster.) This could have been the best chance the police had of catching him.

Confident of his safety, Gunanoot likely slipped into Kispiox and Hazelton more often than is known. Constance Cox, Hankin's daughter, told the story that she was walking on a trail one day when Gunanoot stepped out of the bush in front of her. His wife was ill. Could she obtain some medicine from the hospital for her? She did. From his sources, James Maitland-Dougall, the chief constable in Hazelton since September 1909, received information about when Gunanoot had been in town — always afterwards, never before.

On March 22, 1910, for example, he recorded in his diary that he had learned that Simon had come into town a while before, got drunk and was looking for trouble, threatening to kill the first white man he came across. Another time, he came into town and asked a couple of newcomers, white men, whether the government was still looking for him.

On August 13th, Maitland-Dougall noted that on the evening of the 8th, Gunanoot had met a Gitxsan on the road between Glen Vowell and Hazelton. On August 23rd, he noted that Charley Sterritt, whom he called a friend of Gunanoot and met with him often, said he was trying to persuade him to give himself up. There is even a report that Gunanoot came into town to watch the new moving pictures being shown. Others present at the show would probably have recognized him but would almost certainly have maintained the conspiracy of silence.

Gunanoot evaded all attempts at capturing him. No one ever gave him away. He was never caught.

———

The increase in population in the district inevitably meant more work for Horace's medical practice. This, in addition to his contract work for the Department of Indian Affairs and responsibilities as a provincial health officer, kept him busy. In October 1907, for example, after a passenger arrived on the steamer *Hazelton* suffering from measles, he had to fumigate the stateroom and take special precautions to prevent the contagion from spreading. The hospital was also becoming busier. The annual report for the year that ended in March 1907 records that Horace had performed forty surgeries and that the hospital was treating the sick in record numbers.

When Horace was in New York, he had already been thinking about upgrading the water and gas systems at the hospital. He was hoping to obtain money from the federal government in Ottawa to cover the costs. The materials themselves, he reckoned, would cost $1,200 and on top of that he would have to pay for them to be transported from Vancouver to the mouth of the Skeena and then upriver by steamer. Vancouver newspapers reported in July 1906 that the steamer *Camosun* was taking five tons of plumbing and other supplies up the coast to the hospital, together with a plumber to install all the material.

Once it was installed, Horace was able to make hot and cold water available throughout the building. Aware of the fire risk, he also set up taps in each hallway with sufficient lengths of hose to reach the farthest parts of the building. "We now have 'almost' all the modern conveniences," he wrote in the hospital annual report for 1906–1907.

Improvement of the facilities became a constant pre-occupation. In planning the hospital, Horace had allowed for additions. By the spring of 1907, he already had designs and plans for extensions of twelve feet by thirty-seven feet below and twelve by thirty-one feet above. These would, he said, be fitted with large windows on hinges that could be closed tight in storms and left with three sides open entirely in more clement weather.

His plan was to have open-air wards there for tubercular patients. "It is next to impossible," he wrote, "to do them much good unless they can be the greater part of their time in the open air." The third storey was also completed to provide more living space for the nurses and the matron, who lived there until a new residence was built for them in 1925.

One day in July 1906, Mrs. H. MacArthur, the wife of one of the owners of the mine down river at Lorne Creek, was talking with her husband, who was operating the nozzle of a monitor at the hydraulic claim. She slipped and fell into the sluice box. The enormous rush of water carried her down the full length of the sluice some three hundred yards, and she shot out onto the dump several feet below. "Fortunately the steamer *Mount Royal* happened to be at the landing and Mrs. MacArthur was taken to Hazelton where she was placed in the hospital and is recovering nicely under Dr. Wrinch's care," reported the *Daily Colonist* in Victoria. She had a double-fractured fibula, though, and had been badly shaken up. She stayed in the hospital for over two months, which cost her $156.

Mrs. MacArthur had been lucky the *Mount Royal* had been at the riverbank. Many times Horace was called away to an emergency in the mountains or up the river valleys. "An accident happens," he wrote, "or someone is taken seriously ill, sixty or perhaps a hundred miles from here. A telegram comes for the doctor to hasten to the spot." And so, of course, he went. One can imagine him setting out on horseback with perhaps a helper — the going rate was $2 a day — and a couple of horses, with bedroll, food and medical supplies. Alice might, perhaps, have packed a bag for him with spare clothes and some food, bacon and beans being the standard trail food.

Horace was an early riser — it was his farming background. Someone knocking on his door at four o'clock one May morning, though, could only mean a medical emergency. He was needed urgently up the Bulkley Valley. Thirty miles south of Moricetown (Witset/Lach-al-sap), a tree had fallen on Thomas Michell, a twenty-one-year-old Wet'suwet'en survey worker. He had a broken skull and could be dying. An hour after receiving the news, after hastily putting his surgical bag together and preparing the horses for the trail, Horace was on his way.

Riding towards the rising sun, he had to go slowly at first but then with the increasing light he would have been able to pick up speed. Four hours later, he reached Moricetown. The men carrying Michell to Moricetown had not arrived there yet. Horace rode on for another ten miles until he met them. Michell had a badly fractured skull but was still alive. Horace knew he had to operate then and there. Watched by a ring of Wet'suwet'en workers and family who had come from Moricetown, he dressed the wound and removed a bone pressing on the man's brain.

Then — there really was no alternative — he arranged for a relay of bearers to take Michell to the hospital. By changing the bearers at every stage, the party was able to maintain an even speed. As they passed through his home village of Moricetown, they picked up fresh bearers. They arrived at the hospital later that evening after what for Horace would have been a ride of over seventy miles.

After their arrival at the hospital, Horace gave Michell further treatment. His friends watched, and when it was time for the still-sluggish patient to eat, they shouted in his ear to wake him up. "He'll get up some day soon," Horace said, "and be ready for the woods again." Recovered, Michell was discharged after eleven days in hospital. The cost, which Horace passed on to Loring for payment, was $15. In the patient register, Horace noted laconically, "A very severe injury, almost resulting in death."

In September 1907, Horace recounted another emergency. He had been called at 7:30 in the evening to attend a case of what turned out to be acute appendicitis ninety miles downriver. He spent the night, he wrote, looking for a canoe and crew to take him there. With Helen Bone as nurse, he started out at six in the morning. By nine that evening, Horace had removed the infected appendix, and the patient, G. Graham, had started to improve.

Leaving Helen to look after Graham, Horace came back upriver by canoe, taking four days to return to Hazelton. On another occasion he had to apologize to the readers of the *Missionary Bulletin* for not having written sooner. He had, he wrote, just picked up his pen when "an emergency call, for a hundred mile horseback journey to attend a broken limb, made everything else stand aside, and it was within a few hours of a full week before I was home again."

In another case, Horace wrote:

An urgent call came for me to attend two men severely injured by dynamite at a place about ninety miles away. I went to them and found them in such critical condition that it was four days more before we could begin the trip with them to the hospital. We brought them here in a lumber wagon, with four horses to drag it over "places," not roads, that no Ontario farmer would think it could be driven over at all. I had gone out to them on horseback in a day and a half, but it took four tiresome days to bring the patients in. It was the only thing to be done, however. They both made good recovery, as far as recovery was possible. They had received the charge full in their eyes. One man recovered good use of one eye. The other poor fellow will have to depend upon others for sight for the rest of his days. His was one of the saddest cases I have known in a long time.

With Horace's medical workload growing so quickly, it was becoming increasingly clear that he needed an assistant. Someone had to take charge of the hospital while he was away on calls. The coming railway with its crowds of workers, as well as increased mining activity, inevitably meant more medical emergencies and hospital admissions than could be handled by one doctor alone. This, he argued, more than justified the employment of Dr. Albert Henderson Wallace as his assistant.

Dr. Wallace arrived at the hospital when Horace was away for over a week on an extended medical call in the mountains. Before having met his new colleague or settling in, Wallace had to admit "more patients . . . to the hospital than during any similar period of its history." He must have wondered what he had got himself into. "Not long after," Horace wrote:

A telegram came stating that one of our Indians, out hunting about two hundred miles north of here, had been severely injured in an encounter with a grizzly, and asking that one of us meet him on his way in. That took Dr. Wallace away ten days. He was able, by a little operative treatment, to give him some relief in the meantime. Later a more extensive operation was performed in the hospital and the patient is now back among his friends again, grateful for the hospital and doctors to whom he owed his life.

With the growth in fees from the growing non-Indigenous population — miners, railway workers and settlers — the hospital was able to survive financially without the annual grant from the Missions Board. Accordingly, in the autumn of 1906, Horace wrote to his friends in Ontario that the hospital would experiment in doing without their grant. He would, however, still welcome donations from them. In March of the following year, he wrote:

> The response to our appeal last year was so generous that Miss Bone, our superintendent, has not come to me yet with any list of shortage. We are not making definite requests this year, but I may say that these things are always wearing out, of course, and need replenishing from time to time. Anything in the line of bedding and linen of the various sorts will be appreciated all the time. About mid-summer we have goods shipped from Toronto. Miss Wrinch, 9, Rowanwood Avenue, will gladly enclose with these goods anything sent to her for us.

At this time Horace's sisters, Mary and Agnes, were living at this address and would have sent donations on to the hospital.

That spring, Horace wrote that, despite the thermometer having at one point reached fifty-three degrees below zero (Fahrenheit), they actually had had a "beautiful winter." Strangely enough, he said, he had no frostbite cases to treat during that time. The dry air meant they had treated few cases of pneumonia or lung troubles, other than the consumption (tuberculosis) that was always with them, and almost no rheumatism. Fevers such as measles, typhoid, diphtheria and scarlet fever, he wrote, were almost unknown. He had seen only one case each of measles and typhoid since he had arrived. He feared, though, that *la grippe* (the flu) that was reportedly in Vancouver could reach them soon.

———

Horace reported on the havoc that the Skeena River played with the river steamers in those years. The *Mount Royal*, which had been built in 1902, was one of the biggest and most luxurious. One hundred-and-thirty-eight-feet long and twenty-eight-feet wide, it had, reportedly, stateroom space for a hundred — twenty-five staterooms with four beds each — and cabin room space for two hundred passengers. Empty, it could sail in eighteen inches of water. In 1907, the *Mount Royal* was spectacularly and tragically wrecked coming through the Kitselas Canyon.

After it had hit some rocks, the captain ordered all passengers off the ship, including a young lady working at the hospital, while six of the officers and crew attempted to tie the steamer to the rocks to enable them to repair the damage. A surging current suddenly overturned the ship, drowning all six officers and crew. This disaster had not only taken these lives and destroyed the mail but also caused several thousands of dollars of damage to the cargo.

Writing late in 1907, Horace noted that the year had been a tragic one. There had been six accidents of canoes and steamers on the river and fifteen lives had been lost. One steamer had become a total wreck the previous November and two of the three that had started the season were also wrecks. A third had been disabled and was, according to Horace, "stranded on a gravel bar with about twenty-seven feet of her bottom torn up." He added:

> It is exceedingly doubtful if we shall see another steamer trip to Hazelton this fall. And what makes it more serious is the fact that even now there is a serious shortage in the visible supply of foodstuffs for our proper population. . . . You will agree that it is small wonder that we wax enthusiastic over the coming of the railway into this northern country. It will revolutionize things in a short time, and will make us independent of this old river, whose reputation grows rapidly worse year by year.

The wrecking of so many steamers so close to the end of the navigation season had serious implications for Hazelton. Horace wrote that there would probably be some food shortages during the coming season as a result of the loss of provisions. Providentially — and thanking Providence was no mere figure of speech for him — he thought the hospital had enough supplies to last until spring. He reported that he had made a practice of buying most of the hospital's needs wholesale and having them sent in well before the end of the season. Doing so had relieved the situation as far as actual living was concerned.

One of the steamers on its last trip had brought groceries and the biggest drug orders. He said, however, he would be short of carbide for lighting. Some few others things in furniture, hardware, paints and some drugs that were on their way up would probably have to winter at Port Essington or be returned to shippers. But on the whole, he said, the hospital was much more favourably situated than many others in the community.

The Victoria newspapers melodramatically reported that "Famine prices prevail in Northern District owing to the inability to get in supplies." Although Hazelton ran out of cigars, tobacco, beer and whisky — hardship enough for some — Horace played down reports of looming famine. The winter of 1907–1908, nevertheless, was a hard one for many residents. All the stores in Hazelton were short of supplies to tide the community over until spring. Horace was one of the proponents of the railway because, by making supplies more reliable, it would make life in Hazelton safer.

———

Horace loved his farm and his garden. Many years later, Harold recalled that his father

> . . . was a very good horticulturalist. He put up a good farm around the hospital so that they could be self-sufficient in a thirty-bed hospital for all winter. . . . No pigs, though; he drew the line there, for some reason. He had two or three horses for transportation, and chickens. Although, the chickens were difficult to keep because the Indian dogs were very ravenous — if that is the right word if they're eating chickens. Two or three times they cleaned out the hen-house and ate all the chickens, and he had to send to Vancouver for another batch.

For Horace, the hospital garden and grounds were not merely to grow food for the hospital community. They were more even than for his own relaxation and pleasure. They were, he said, also to provide a beautiful place so that patients would find an environment that would be conducive to their speedy recovery.

In the winter of 1906, Horace experimented with sowing winter wheat to see if it would grow so far north. A friend in Manitoba had sent him some samples of Turkey Red and White Clawson seeds. He sowed these in the autumn and even after the exceptionally hard winter, with a heavy snow cover, the seeds survived and by early May the wheat was over a foot high.

In November 1907, the *Vancouver World* reported that "a record yield of wheat, which is probably unrivaled throughout the province" had been grown on the hospital farm. Three kinds of wheat had been grown, at a rate of no less 90, 87 and 75 bushels per acre. The straw in one case, it reported, was six feet high. A correspondent of the *Daily Colonist* visited Hazelton in the summer of 1907. Very much taken with the garden and farm, he described the hospital as being one of the first institutions in the North. He wrote:

The head officer is Dr. Wrinch, a splendid man for the position, being not only an excellent practitioner with a wide knowledge of conditions in the north, but also a man of marked executive ability. . . . The hospital has a splendid garden and in this Dr. Wrinch is making the first experiments in horticulture to be carried on in the country. So far his efforts have been crowned with the greatest success and the results, although at present by no means complete, go to show that almost anything can be grown in the country. The doctor shows with pride a splendid strawberry bed which stood the frosts of the past winter and from which your correspondent had the pleasure of picking some luscious berries. In addition to this, he has cultivated currants, such as have been grown nowhere else in British Columbia, the fruit having attained the size of small grapes. Oats, barley and fall wheat have been ripened, and the doctor is now experimenting with larger fruit.

With a contract with the Department of Indian Affairs to provide medical services for the local First Nations, Horace was able to serve the Gitxsan and Wet'suwet'en, both in his medical practice and in the hospital. Although paternalistic, Horace had high regard and great sympathy for both nations. "My own opinion," he wrote in February 1912 to Rev. A.C. Farrell at the Missions Board in Toronto, "if I may express it, is that Indian character does not differ so much from that of the noble Anglo-Saxon as much as some would like to believe. And wherein it does differ, we may sometimes have to look to our laurels that we do not appear in the second place."

This letter was written to bring attention to an act of generosity by the Gitxsan of Kitseguecla, who had collected money to pay for the hospital treatment of Rev. Edgar, a First Nations missionary. "To me," Horace wrote, "it is difficult to conceive of a more loyal and appreciative action than this. The band of Indians is less than a hundred and none of them have any means ahead. [That is, money to provide for the future.]"

Horace had few illusions about the unqualified benefits of European civilization for the First Nations. In October 1905, a journalist from the *Vancouver Province* had caught up with him in Vancouver, calling him Dr. Wrench (a common mistake), and asked him about the First Nations in the Hazelton District. "There were a certain number who had learned cleanliness from the white men," it reported him as saying, "but most of them had only learned drunkenness. The Skeena River Indians have received more harm than good from the white men." They are, he said, "an easy prey for the white man's diseases. No less than four fifths of the deaths around Hazelton are caused by consumption [tuberculosis], which the Indians say was unknown among them before the white men came."

Harold Wrinch recalled his father being able to speak both Gitxsan and Wet'suwet'en languages well enough to converse. "I think he adapted himself pretty well," he said. "He never had trouble to my knowledge speaking with any of them. Chinook, yes, that would be one of them, one of the languages he could speak." (Chinook jargon was an easily learned trade language composed of words from Chinook, French and English as well as other languages).

Horace had taken an early interest in the Gitxsan fisheries. In the autumn of 1904, he had prepared a plan for the fisheries on the Skeena and sent it to the Indian Superintendent in Vancouver, A.W. Vowell, who sent it on to Ottawa. Horace recognized the hardship the Gitxsan were experiencing as a result of the enforcement of fishery laws.

In 1906, federal fisheries officers had been taking down Gitxsan fishing weirs and fining those who resisted. In one case, eight Gitxsan had been sentenced to prison, convicted of theft, illegal fishing and resisting arrest. They were, fortunately, almost immediately pardoned. Horace could see that this dispute might have caused serious complications if a final settlement had not been reached. Sounding very modern in his comments, he wrote in a letter published in the *Missionary Bulletin*:

The special grievance at present is that salmon canning is so extensively carried on at the mouths of our rivers, that the fish are getting scarce, and laws have to be made to protect them. These laws restrict the manner of catching the salmon by the Indians as they take them for their own subsistence up here in the interior. . . . But we all know that these laws favoring large corporations are only made that corporations may make a little bigger dividend for their shareholders. What do the great corporations care if a few hundred Indians away in the interior of the northern part of British Columbia suffer on account of it. Then when these Indians refuse to obey, warrants are issued for their arrest for disobeying the laws made by the enlightened and highly civilized white man, and the poor Indians must be compelled to feel the power of the law. And so at the expense of much public money the Governments must send in extra force to compel these people to obey laws made solely in the interests of these avaricious corporations. One cannot wonder that the Indians sometimes ask us if there is one law for the white man and another for Indians. You can imagine too how much more difficult it is to teach the liberality of Christianity to a people when the laws which we are expected to teach them to uphold and obey are anything but liberal. I could, if I gave vent to my feelings, write in much stronger terms, but it might not be to any good purpose.

———~/\/\~———

The clash between Gitxsan and non-Indigenous culture led, inevitably, to a clash between Gitxsan traditional medicine and modern medicine. Traditional medicine was part of the belief system of the Gitxsan. The weakening of it could have been felt as the loss of an integral part of their culture and submission to an alien and all-powerful otherness.

The two systems, traditional and modern, existed in parallel, with competition between the scientifically trained doctors and the Gitxsan shamans or halayts. These halayts, gifted with special powers, were central to the spiritual life of the Gitxsan. They connected the living and natural worlds with the spiritual world. Many missionaries and others in settler communities, though, dismissed the halayts as witch doctors, frauds and conjurors, and tried hard to reduce their influence.

This tension between the two medical cultures lasted through all the years Horace was in Hazelton. On the one hand was the lore and practice of traditional Gitxsan medicine: on the other, the modern knowledge and scientific techniques of Trinity Medical College, Grace Hospital and the New York Post-Graduate Medical School. A power struggle was to be expected. Each side thought its methods were effective; each reached for the ascendency of its medical treatments; and each brought its own knowledge, spirituality and beliefs to the matter. Trained doctors, being medical men of their times and imbued with assumptions of superiority, did not believe in such Gitxsan remedies as bone-setting, drumming and rattling, healing herbs and natural cures. Showing little willingness to learn about traditional medicine, they inevitably ignored the opportunity to study the purported effectiveness of its remedies.

In 1998, a Gitxsan-Wet'suwet'en–sponsored study looked at Gitxsan herbal healing practices and described Gitxsan medicine:

> Reflecting beliefs about the harmonious interaction of people and the land and the balance of natural forces, the fundamental Gitxsan approach to health is holistic and preventative. When problems arose in pre-contact times, healing was handled by various specialists. Halayts [spiritual healers], herbal healers, bone setters and mid-wives all participated in the maintenance of health and prevention and treatment of disease. Extensive use was made of plant products as medicines. In the past sixty years with the influence of the missionaries and modern Canadian life, the halayt, bonesetters and midwives have largely disappeared. However, traditional herbal remedies have continued to be employed.

A Gitxsan with arthritis or a skin ulcer may, the study noted, have used the sliced root of yellow pond lily as a salve. Dried leaves of the soapberry, steeped in water as a tea, were used as a diuretic and to treat bladder infections. Pitch from the lodgepole pine, subalpine fir or white spruce, collectively called *skyen* in Gitxsan, was used to heal all types of wounds. Red elderberry was used as an emetic. Cow parsnip or Indian rhubarb was used as a poultice. Indian hellebore, known as '*mulgwasx*, was used for spiritual purification and also to remove bad spirits.

Devil's club was also a widely used plant, being collected in the autumn, preferably after the first snowfall. The Gitxsan stripped the bark off and used it as a poultice to heal wounds, rheumatism, respiratory ailments and stomach ulcers. Devil's club was also used as a chewing substance for general health, and hunters used it to purify themselves before hunting and to bring them luck. Bathing in devil's club was reported to remove human scent, which would obviously have been useful for a hunter.

A doctor of the 1890s, trained in a Western medical school and with a grounding in science and rationalism, would not have had much understanding of, or patience with, such traditional remedies. Many descriptions of the methods of halayts sound patronizing and dismissive today. Dr. Alfred Bolton, the missionary doctor on the coast, for example, described the Tsimshian medicine in 1896 in his *Medical Work Among the Natives*. His comments could be applied equally well to the attitudes of many, perhaps most, missionaries towards First Nations medical practices:

> As long as any tribe remains in heathenism, witchcraft and jugglery continue. I have heard the medicine-man's rattle clash over a fevered subject of *la grippe*, and have seen an old hag blowing and sucking with unearthly sounds while pressing her lips close to the skin over different parts of the body in a case of pulmonary haemorrhage. . . . As physician, I am brought into contact with the sick and dying, who are impressionable to Gospel truths; as missionary, I am constantly consulted by natives in trouble or in search of spiritual light; as Justice of the Peace, I deal with criminals and settle disputes, and perhaps repress illegal traffic in intoxicants; and since becoming conversant with the Tsimshian language and dialects, and the Chinook jargon, which is of some moment in teaching and leading a people who can read so little, I have opportunities as a preacher.

This then was the medical missionary's ideal. Helping to cure the body would help to cure the soul.

As long as he was living in Hazelton, Horace and the halayts competed to heal the bodies of the Gitxsan and, at a deeper level, their souls. As Horace tried to bring them to his God, the halayts, too, tried to keep them in their traditional beliefs. Horace was a doctor of his times. He laboured hard, and sincerely, to bring anaesthetics and God to the Gitxsan. Being a medical missionary, he endeavoured to prove his medicine effective and thus reduce the power of the halayts, who, in turn, did what they could to reduce his credibility. Horace once wrote of his suspicion that halayts were sending people they knew to be dying to the hospital so that they could attribute the death to his ineffective treatment. When Horace saw Christian progress being made and a soul saved for eternal life, he rejoiced. On the occasion of the conversion of a halayt he would have been — and was — happy, proud, relieved and grateful. In 1903, he recounted one incident when dealing with a First Nations patient:

> Just before administering the anaesthetic to a patient this week we had a very serious talk with him and were glad to find out he was in a most repentant condition. He had formerly been a Christian, but for some two years had been gradually falling back, and had even told some that he did not believe there was anything in Christianity. But when this attack came on, it brought him back to himself and he began to pray again. He promised us that it was his full purpose if raised up again to turn his back upon his godless friends, and strive with all his power to live the better life. He believes, as we suggested, that God had sent this sickness to give him a warning and to bring him back.

Horace's sympathy for the Gitxsan did not prevent him, though, from occasionally being exasperated by the attitude of some to medical treatment. In a letter in the *Missionary Outlook*, he wrote:

> At the root of the high rate of mortality among the Indians is the insidious enemy, tuberculosis. These people cannot understand the necessity for months of treatment for what looks like a very simple ailment, perhaps a slight cough, or a little stiffness in a joint, or a few enlarged glands, or a small abscess not at all painful — these and other of the early manifestations often seem most trifling, and when we tell them that it is necessary to encase the joint in plaster, or put some apparatus on the back, and that treatment must be continued for six months or a year, or, perhaps longer, they at once conclude they will not send the child to hospital (for it is usually a child) for such protracted treatment, for such a little thing. They ask for medicine and think that a bottle or two of medicine should ensure a cure.

While Gitxsan and Wet'suwet'en did come to the hospital in great numbers, Horace's medicine did not always prevail. Although written reports are scarce, there were instances where modern medicine was said not to have worked. An article in the *Daily Colonist* as late as 1931 was headed, "Indian Proves His Magic More Potent Than That of White." While not naming Horace, the article noted that a Gitxsan woman from Kispiox had been unsuccessfully treated by the nearest doctor.

Reportedly, a halayt called Billy Williams, dressed in bearskin, had then cured her of the intense pain in her knee. The halayt had blown smoke into the knee and sung healing songs. He took a good spirit from his own body and placed it on the woman's head. Then he told her she would get better. She did, the paper said, in less than a week.

The two systems of medicine ran in parallel tracks, and the edges between them were often jagged. The settlers' experience of Gitxsan medicine was often only of the outer signs and symbols of it — the herbal remedies, the regalia, the rattles and the drums. Not unnaturally, the Gitxsan, well aware of their prejudices, would have been reluctant to let them see their system in operation.

Over time, the use of some aspects of traditional medicine declined. Some Gitxsan medical practices, such as herbal and plant remedies, have survived longer than others. Loring had written in the 1890s that drumming and rattling were things of the past. They were not. Dr. Geddes Large, the son of Horace's old friend from Trinity Medical College, Richard Large, came to Hazelton Hospital in 1924 for two years. He recalled that the annual potlatch at Hagwilget that year was perhaps the last. He also recounted that drumming and rattling over patients was still common. Horace's son Harold, who was born in 1911 and who grew up in Hazelton, recalled the drumming:

Medicine men drummed and treated sick natives. Often the patient would die while he was being treated instead of being brought to the hospital where he might have been saved. Well, they drummed over sick people. Our house was well into the hospital property and the lower end was probably half a mile away from our house. Many nights there would be drumming for a sick patient. It came from a native house on the edge of the property. I heard it night after night. That's when I lay in bed, so that it was clearly audible from our house. I mean it was nothing. You just heard it and never thought much about it. I am sure it was of concern to Father because he always wondered if this was going to continue until the patient died or whether the patient was going to survive.

Whatever Horace thought about the drumming at the edge of the hospital compound, he took comfort from his progress. In 1907, with perhaps more than a touch of wishful thinking, he wrote, "Our work is settling down to an established basis with the Indians. They have not the old superstitious fear of our medicine or our methods. Nor do they look so much for miraculous results from medicine or treatment. On the other hand, they resort much less than they did to witchcraft methods of doctoring."

———∿∿∿———

In 1908, the residents of Hazelton finally had their own newspaper. Joe Coyle, an entrepreneur from the Bulkley Valley, published the first edition of the *Omineca Herald* in July. No longer did residents have to rely for their news on snippets from the telegraph, passed around by word of mouth, or on the *Daily Colonist* arriving from Victoria after a long journey up the coast.

The *Herald* brought news from the outside world once a week: from the tragedy of approximately 150,000 deaths in Italy after an earthquake in December to more personal items, such as the birth of a son to Dr. and Mrs. Wrinch, or the wedding in London of young Mr. Winston Churchill. It also published news of local interest: from useful information about the canoes going downriver to who in town was ill; from who was buying land to who would be awarded the contract for carriage of the winter mails. Its four or five pages contained local news in short paragraphs, then a number of editorials, advertisements and always a large number of mining and real estate notices.

It published with varying fidelity the names of those arriving and leaving Hazelton by river steamer and canoe. That September 1908, no doubt to the relief of many but perhaps to the chagrin of Horace, it announced that the steamer *Distributor*, on its penultimate voyage of the season, had brought up the winter supply of 105 barrels of beer for one of the hotels. The *Herald* gathered all the local news and passed it on to its readers, providing a detailed picture of small town life at that time.

—∿—

With an innovative mind, Horace was always seeking new solutions to old problems and better ways of doing things — new buildings, new equipment and machinery, new processes, and, commencing in 1907, an unusual way of raising money for the hospital.

Examining the *Herald* on the morning of October 31, 1908, a reader would have seen on the front page two notices from Horace. One informed readers that the supply of vaccines in the hospital was running out and there would not be a new supply until the next spring. The second item was about the hospital ticket scheme. "A hospital ticket," this item read, "is a form of insurance against illness and accident which the person of ordinary means can scarcely afford to be without."

It was accompanied by an advertisement that appeared in almost every edition of the *Herald* for the next three decades that ran as follows: "The Hazelton Hospital issues tickets for any period from one month upward at $1 per month in advance. This rate includes office consultations and medicines, as well as all costs while in the hospital. Tickets obtainable in Hazelton from E.C. Stephenson and E.H. Hicks Beach; in Aldermere from the Rev. F.L. Stephenson or at the Hospital from the Medical Superintendent."

Some years later, the *Herald* reported: "When you carry a hospital ticket you do not have to worry about a hospital and doctor's bill when you get better." Half the subscription went to the doctor and half to the hospital. Apart from an increase to $1.50 per month in

1920, the scheme did not change. This then was a basic form of health insurance.

The correspondent of the *Daily Colonist* who visited the hospital in 1907 wrote that the hospital ticket scheme that had lately been put into effect was proving to be extremely popular and had been taken advantage of by "nearly all those having business in the wilds." Horace may even have had some form of this scheme in place much earlier than 1907. When Robert Tomlinson was admitted as the first patient in the new hospital in 1904, he paid by using a hospital ticket. A year or so later, in April 1906, A.W. Corner paid for treatment for a skin condition with a ticket.

There are other indications of how this health insurance scheme worked. In the hospital annual report for 1910, Horace said that $236 had been raised from the sale of these tickets, slightly more than the $227 from donations. Hospital records show that, between the first ticket used in 1904 and the outbreak of war in August 1914, approximately a hundred patients had paid for treatment at the hospital by using tickets. This number does not include those who paid for a ticket but never had cause to use it. Nor does it include those who merely went to the doctor for medical advice.

The basic principle was neither new nor complicated. The concept of a person paying a sum of money into a common pool and then being entitled to a benefit if a specified event occurs can be traced back over 2,000 years. The Greeks created guilds called benevolent societies that paid out funeral and care benefits to the families of dead members. A century before Christ, the Roman general Gaius Marius reportedly persuaded soldiers to pool some of their wages to pay for the funerals of dead comrades. This led to the Roman collegia, which were societies or guilds, one of which was the Collegium Dianae et Antinoi, a society founded in AD 133 to pay for members' funeral costs.

The practice of making a regular payment into a fund to finance medical benefits when needed later divided into two streams. The first was the payment into a pool, the primary benefit of which was to pay medical and burial expenses of members. This developed through the medieval trade and craft guilds, and later, as social and employment relationships in Europe changed, into friendly societies. (The second, not relevant for this discussion, was the commercialization that led to the insurance company business.) By 1900, a large number of friendly societies had been flourishing in Britain for over 200 years. In the nineteenth and early twentieth centuries, they were the premier working-class self-help organizations.

In Britain in 1835, it has been estimated that perhaps as many as one million of a population of about 5.5 million adult working males were enrolled in such organizations. By 1910, the number had risen to between nine and ten million.

Some societies were huge; others were very small. Some were even confined to a single village. Others supplied only one form of benefit, while others paid more extensive benefits. Many different types of organizations set them up, including medical benefit societies and trade unions. These societies were also seen as ways to reinforce values and build communities. Many of the friendly societies paid for hospital beds and supported their local hospitals.

There were also other models. One common arrangement was the one whereby an employer contracted with a doctor for the supply of medical services for his employees, deducting a monthly amount, usually $1, from their wages.

There were several drawbacks to the friendly society model for financing medical services. Some funds were managed badly, negligently or fraudulently, with consequent financial loss. Sometimes managers miscalculated, and the society ran out of money. The schemes were also subject to the whims and winds of economic depression and epidemics that disarranged the actuarial models. Furthermore, friendly societies only benefitted those who paid the premiums. The poor, the elderly, the sick and the unemployed were often without the wherewithal to pay those premiums and so were without health benefits. In an attempt to remedy these problems, governments in the United Kingdom and in Canada enacted legislation to regulate friendly society management.

Friendly societies came to British Columbia with European

settlers in the mid-nineteenth century. When the Hudson's Bay Company, for example, brought miners from Britain to Nanaimo in the 1850s and 1860s to work in the coal mines, the miners brought friendly societies with them. As in England, many of these societies had exotic names like the Ancient Order of Foresters and the Independent Order of Odd Fellows, the latter of which in Britain had 4,000 branches. To reduce fraud and mismanagement, in March 1871 the colonial government in Victoria enacted legislation to regulate them and give them legal status.

When Horace started his hospital ticket scheme in Hazelton, he was being practical but not groundbreaking. It is clearly within the same tradition as the friendly society: a member of a club, by whatever name it was called — collegium, trade guild, or friendly society — paid a monthly fee and in return received a benefit should a specified event happen.

In both Canada and the United States, the ticket scheme had been used as a largely unrecognized way to finance small hospitals. Such schemes had also been used before in British Columbia. Although the records seem scarce, some community hospitals found them a useful way to raise much-needed money. In the *Fort Steele Prospector* in 1899, Ruth Fulsom, matron of the Victoria Diamond Jubilee Hospital, drew everyone's attention to its hospital scheme whereby a person could pay $1 a month and then be entitled to medical benefits. Dr. Kergin also set up a hospital ticket scheme at the Methodist Hospital at Port Simpson, although it did not last long there.

The Presbyterian-supported St. Andrew's Hospital in Atlin, a mining town near the Yukon border, had a scheme that was probably similar to the one at Hazelton. In December 1905, an editorial in the *Atlin Claim* described the perilous state of the hospital finances. The Presbyterians had announced — probably to the shock and dismay of the whole community — that the hospital should stand on its own feet financially and that they were withdrawing their financial support. The only solution, the editorial said, would be for more people in the community to subscribe for hospital tickets.

Helen Bone, Alice's roommate in her nursing days at Grace Hospital, was one of the two nurses at St. Andrew's Hospital. When she came to the Hazelton hospital as lady superintendent, she would likely have shared with Horace her experience of how the ticket system had worked in practice at Atlin.

Subscribers for tickets also became patrons of the hospital. Patrons formed a hospital community and were entitled to attend the annual meetings and other hospital events. Here they were kept informed about hospital finances, what problems it faced, and what successes it had. The staff gave them cake and refreshments, and after the meetings musical members presented a concert.

In the same way as many friendly societies bound communities together, the ticket scheme of the Hazelton Hospital and its patrons helped maintain community support for the hospital. Well-managed and long-running, it became an essential element in the hospital's success. Although neither unique nor revolutionary in larger world medical history, the Hazelton Hospital ticket scheme had a long, quiet and honourable history.

———

As 1908 moved into 1909, Horace and Alice settled into now-familiar routines. Change, though, was coming. Dog-sled travel, four mails each winter, pack trains and posses riding out of town in a cloud of dust to catch a suspected murderer would soon be memories of a frontier past. Talk of a railroad and questions about the location of a new town were becoming louder and more strident. As new mineral finds were made and as new technologies were being developed, the pace of mining was also picking up. New stores were opening. People travelling to Vancouver returned with stories of automobiles and even of machines that could fly. The town did not have electricity yet, but sooner or later it would come. Dr. Wrinch up the hill at the hospital was talking about the need for an X-ray machine and of the need to install his own electricity supply. Hazelton was growing up.

CHAPTER 7

Community, Cars and the Coming of the Railroad 1908–1913

HAZELTON HAD CHANGED considerably since Horace and Alice had arrived in the autumn of 1900, but perhaps not enough for Horace. Despite having set up a hospital, a training school, and a farm, he lamented that he had not accomplished as much as he had hoped.

When he arrived, he wrote in a 1909 letter to the *Missionary Bulletin*, Hazelton had consisted of Loring's Indian office, a post office, John Field's new Episcopal church and mission house, the Indian School and three stores, the business of which was almost entirely in catering to First Nations and miners. Some mining was being done in the summer months at points from one hundred and fifty to two hundred miles to the east, and all their supplies had to be forwarded through Hazelton. Several Hudson's Bay Company trading posts, ranging from sixty to four hundred miles away, also received their supplies via Hazelton. Brought there by steamer, they were then taken farther by pack train over trails, by schooner on the interior lakes, or by canoe up the rivers. The previous year, some supplies for the hospital shipped from the East had taken a year to arrive. Some took two years from the time of shipment to delivery at interior posts.

By 1909, though, Hazelton had become a thriving townsite, with three or four times the volume of trade being done as before, with three hotels, a government land office, in which five or six men were kept busy recording land, mineral and other rights, a telegraph office, a weekly paper (the *Omineca Herald*) with a good printing office, schools for both white and Gitxsan children, a tailor, a blacksmith's shop, a restaurant, real-estate offices, large warehouses, a watchmaker, a bakery, a barber shop, a superintendent of police with a staff of four constables, and a hospital that could accommodate about twenty patients.

Horace reported on the changes that the prospect of a railway was causing. He would have remembered the debates about the railway along the Skeena that he had watched from the visitors' gallery in the Legislature in Victoria a few years earlier. Now it actually seemed to be coming. Contracts had been let for construction of the section of the railway that would pass Hazelton. (But where would the station be?) The sub-contractors were building up supplies to enable them to make a start at the more difficult portions of rock work before winter set in. There were now seven steamers on the river, five of which were employed solely in supplying the railway camps.

Everyone, it seemed, was anxious for the railway to arrive. Settlers, miners and railway workers were flooding into the district. With the best of the agricultural land being nearly all taken, farming was growing fast. New "strikes" by miners were being reported all the time. The passage of the river steamers to Hazelton was too precarious, though, and too expensive to be a reliable means of communication and transport for the business that was trying to develop.

The influx of single men working on the railways and groups of hopeful or disappointed miners pumped oxygen into the fires in the saloons. Frank Chettleburgh, who arrived about the same time as a new reforming police chief, was one who told tales of a wild town. He arrived in Hazelton in 1909 to open up a coal mine and stayed for many years. Years later, he recalled that Hazelton, despite the presence of such clergy as the kind and cheerful Irishman, Rev. John Field, and such professional medical men as Dr. Wrinch, was still a Wild West town.

Sometimes as many as 150 pack horses and mules crowded the streets near the warehouses on the riverbank. Packers from the mule trains took themselves up to the hotel at Two Mile, where, outside the town and reserve limits, liquor flowed freely. At one time as many as twenty-two girls entertained the packers there, he said, giving them memories for long days on the trails. Railway workers and other men from the district also enjoyed the hotel's amenities. There was, Chettleburgh said, "a regular taxi-service backwards and forwards from Hazelton."

The Hazelton Hotel, with its regular games of poker, faro and blackjack, was the wildest of the three hotels in Hazelton — the other hotels being the Ingenika and the Omineca. When prohibition was introduced in British Columbia in 1917, Chettleburgh bought all the wines and spirits that the Hudson's Bay Company were no longer allowed to sell, which kept him going, he said, for a long time.

Selling alcohol to the First Nations was illegal. The *Herald* was full of reports from the police courts of fines being imposed on violators. In 1908, for example, a white man, Herman by name, was given six months in the "skookum house" (jail) for selling whisky to a Gitxsan, who thereupon became rip-roaringly drunk all around the town. Many (including Loring, who was also a magistrate) suspected that Richard Sargent, one of the storekeepers and liquor sellers in town, knew more than he let on about how the First Nations got their liquor. It was becoming time to clean Hazelton up.

James Maitland-Dougall arrived as the new chief constable at 3:30 p.m. on August 27, 1909. He set about improving law and order at once. Enforcing the liquor laws strictly, he gave severe warnings to offending establishments and imposed new rules. He obtained permission to build a new jail, for a cost not to exceed $3,000. During that October, the existing jail was host to eleven prisoners and Maitland-Dougall had collected $265 in fines, fees and forfeitures. Pinkerton's Agent No. 28 — although unnamed in all the reports, he was probably W.T. Bennett (he was one of two, the other being No. 6) — searching for Gunanoot in the summer of 1909 soon reported: "The saloons which previously kept open all night and Sundays, are now closed promptly at 12 midnight, and not open at all on Sundays. It is noticeable too that Indians who during the summer bought whiskey by the bottle at the two saloons are not able now to buy it. Tonight three different Indians endeavoured to buy some whiskey at the Hazelton saloon, but were refused. John, the bar-tender, told me that . . . they were not taking any chance of arrest." Maitland-Dougall soon recorded in his diary that he had given instructions that all gambling must stop.

On October 29, 1909, Maitland-Dougall also noted that, since he was under the impression that the three hotels in Hazelton were paying too small a license fee, he had counted the population. The 154 inhabitants he recorded justified him, he wrote, in raising the half-yearly fee on the hotels from $37.50 to $62.

With the growth of mercantile business and mining, and with the approach of the railway, came the need for a bank. The nearest one was the Royal Bank, which had opened in 1907 in Port Essington, about 180 miles away. With the river being closed by ice for about five months every year, the lack of a bank in Hazelton caused great inconvenience for local businesses. Bank notes circulated until the denominations became illegible. They also became filthy and, allegedly, carriers of disease. There was actually a shortage of legal tender.

Mrs. V. Simms, who had been a young girl in Hazelton, many years later recalled those days. "Everything was paid for in gold dust," she said. "And we used to sew the pokes [small bags] up for Dad." She remembered also that some of the stores, like the Hudson's Bay Company and Cunningham's, issued their own tokens and that she didn't see much real money. "Just in small amounts until latterly, of course, when the country began to wake up." Letters were written to the Union Bank asking for a branch to be opened in Hazelton. In June 1910, representatives from the Bank came to town and reported that, unable to find space to rent, they were securing a lot from Dr. Wrinch and would build a bank. Meanwhile, they said, they were setting up a temporary branch.

Hazelton indeed was "waking up," as Mrs. Simms had said, to the twentieth century. The Galena Club, a new social club, with a pool and billiard parlour, offered members the latest newspapers and magazines, brought upriver as far as possible by steamer and then packed in. The Assembly Club held a masquerade dance in February 1910. No dancers, it pronounced, would be allowed onto the floor before eleven if they were not in costume. Practically the whole town attended. Richard Sargent was floor manager and "performed his duties in the able manner that might be expected of him."

The Omineca Photographic Company opened a shop across the street from the *Herald*'s office and advertised for sale excellent post-card views of the town and its environs. Bobbie Reed started to build a skating rink for hockey matches. By 1913, there were serious dis-cussions about the introduction of electricity for both house and street lighting. A telephone system, initially with seventy-five sub-scribers, was proposed, but not set up at that time. Advertisements appeared in the *Herald* for Remington Typewriters, for dry-cleaning and pressing services at the Hazelton Pantorium and for fresh oysters at the Hazelton Bakery. In August 1912, the *Herald* carried an adver-tisement for an "auto stage" to carry up to eight passengers three times a day from Hazelton across the river to the new town there that had been named New Hazelton.

—∾∾—

Horace and Alice had their hands full raising Leonard, Cooper and Ralphena, who in 1908 were seven, five and three, respectively. Alice had recovered sufficiently to have another baby, Arthur, who was born later that year. Their youngest son Harold would arrive in August 1911. In what must have been idyllic surroundings, the children grew up on the hospital grounds, playing with the children of Fred Goddard, the caretaker and gardener, and with the Gitxsan children around the hospital. They walked to school in Hazelton through the Gitxsan cemetery on the bluff. All of them took their share in the many jobs around the house and garden.

Summer days would have been enlivened by the fairs and fêtes held on the hospital grounds. There were many fundraising events. The ladies of Hazelton organized an ice cream social, for example, on an August evening in 1909, with proceeds going to hospital funds. The Hazelton band provided the entertainment, and there were games, sports and speeches. Despite rain, the event was a great success and raised over $120.

The Dominion Day festivities on the hospital grounds on July 1, 1910, were also held in showery weather but were nonetheless considered very successful. There were games of baseball, races and a prize for the woman present who had given birth to the most children. Horace and Alice entered their son Arthur in the contest for the best-looking baby under three. Sad to relate, though, he did not win the first, or even the second, prize out of a field of five.

Horace celebrated Guy Fawkes Night on November 5, 1911, with a party on the hospital grounds for about twenty-five young people. They gathered around a huge bonfire he had prepared for them and enjoyed themselves toasting apples on sticks. Afterwards there were games in the house.

Alice was occupied with home, family and community service. Even in those days when parents allowed their children to manage their own free time — especially on a safe hospital compound — she would have had her hands full with their growing family. In the years between 1901, when she was already over thirty, and 1911, she had given birth to five children. She had also been seriously ill for a year. Nevertheless, she looked after the household and garden, placed fresh flowers in the hospital in summer and canned produce from the garden and farm for the winter. She was, it is clear, as fired with religious zeal as Horace. With her training as a teacher and a nurse, with her experience, albeit short-lived, of acting as superintendent of Grace Hospital, and with the self-confidence from speaking at Methodist rallies in Ontario, she was in her own way a strong community leader.

In their 2006 book *Good Intentions Gone Awry*, Jan Hare and Jean Barman note the importance of missionaries' wives and lamented the lack of information about them. In writing their book about Emma, the wife of Thomas Crosby, the missionary on the coast for many years, they were fortunate to have the letters Emma wrote to her mother in Ontario. Almost no letters from Alice have survived. Horace's letters to the *Missionary Outlook* as well as newspaper reports in the *Herald* contain few references to her specific activities.

Horace himself was by now firmly established as one of the leaders in the community. In the years after he had first moved to Hazelton, he had been busy practicing medicine and building the hospital. He and Alice had been in the East for approximately seven months when Alice had been ill. In February 1908, the provincial government promoted him to be a health officer for the province. In the years between their return from Toronto in the spring of 1906 and the start of the First World War in 1914, he took an ever-increasing part in Hazelton activities.

Many years later, Mary Wrinch, Horace's artist sister in Toronto, wrote to her niece Ralphena, "I know how awfully difficult it is to relax. We Wrinches are 'blessed' or 'cursed' with too much passion for 'doing things' and it is the hardest thing in the world to curb it. I can, to a great extent get over it and am learning to loaf about too well perforce — but you are so much younger — proportionately, more eager to get going." Horace had this passion to a great degree.

Even though it was becoming clearer that the coming of the railway meant that New Hazelton, the town established south of the river, would be the railway town, Hazelton was still thriving and acquiring more clubs and associations — all signs of a maturing community. Horace seems to have been involved with most of them. His position in the community was such, it seems, that every worthy organization wanted to have him as an officer or benefactor in order to give it status and respectability. The inhabitants may have told each other that if Dr. Wrinch were involved, it must be a proper organization to support.

Horace was on the executive of the Hazelton Rifle Association, which had a membership of over thirty. There is no record, though, of his ever having gone hunting or indeed having remained on the executive for very long. The annual Thanksgiving Day "shoot-out" at the rifle range in 1910 was pronounced a great success. Horace participated in the second class, but, while shooting respectably, didn't shoot well enough for any prize. An athletic association was formed in 1911, and a subscription was organized to which, along with many others, he made a $15 contribution. He allowed the association to build a skating rink on the lake on the hospital property and encouraged everyone to skate there.

The Hazelton Overseas Club was formed in 1911 for the purpose of celebrating different national holidays and historic gatherings. Horace was appointed its second vice-president. In October 1911, he was elected as one of three fire wardens for the town, along with William Larkworthy and A.C. Aldous. Taking the risk of fire very seriously, the wardens then decided to enforce the regulations and announced they would be inspecting all buildings in town to ensure compliance.

In addition to all these commitments, he was drawn into politics. In August 1911, he was elected as a vice-president of the recently founded Hazelton Liberal Association, although at this time he does not appear to have been noticeably active. In 1912, after a service in St. Peter's Anglican Church, a branch of the Canadian Bible Society was set up, with Rev. John Field for the Anglicans as president and Horace for the Methodists as treasurer.

When in October 1911 the Hazelton Club was formed for literary, debating and social purposes, Horace was elected vice-president. "It is expected," the *Herald* said, "that many profitable evenings will be spent this winter by Hazelton's young people." The club had an inauspicious start. "Woman is the Intellectual Equal of Man" was the motion set for the first meeting, ruffling many feathers. The *Omineca Miner* — the new newspaper in Hazelton and rival to the *Herald* — reported:

> Taking umbrage at the implication that there might be any doubt as to their equality with the sterner sex, the militant suffragettes of the town took action to demonstrate their intellectual capacity. To the number of fourteen, they invaded the hall, wearing streamers with the inscription "Woman's Rights," and evinced their determination to sit out the debate. The unfortunates who had been slated to take the negative side refused to proceed in the face of the formidable fourteen. The debate was abandoned.

That seems to have ended the Hazelton Club.

In 1909, Horace became a member of the American Hospital Association and retained his membership for several decades. He was one of two members from British Columbia, the other being Dr. Kergin, his colleague at the Port Simpson hospital. The Association's 1908 convention had been held in Toronto, and this had perhaps inspired Horace to join. Every year the Association published a report which included the speeches given at the convention. At the convention in Toronto, for example, Miss Alline gave a talk on "The Inspection of Nurse Training Schools" and Dr. McClure gave a talk on the "Problems of Small Hospitals."

For Horace, the importance of this membership meant that he was in touch with all the latest developments in hospital management and surgery. It also meant that he had almost a decade of experience with its organization, limitations and benefits when he helped establish a similar organization in British Columbia at the end of the First World War. Meanwhile, the Association's journals and reports landing in his mailbox gave him information about new medical procedures and practices. Isolation was a problem; this was an important way for him to stay up-to-date.

To oversee administration of the hospital, Horace set up a hospital board. One purpose was to create a bond between the hospital and the local community. The public and ticket holders could then see — often with brutal frankness — how the operation was run and how healthy its finances were. The provincial government appointed one member to the board and the patrons of the hospital appointed another. The medical superintendent, lady superintendent and Indian Agent were members ex officio.

Each year, usually in January, the board reported the year's activities to its patrons at a well-attended and well-reported meeting. Normally, as medical superintendent, Horace would deliver the report. These annual meetings were convivial affairs becoming, along with Dominion Days and, later, Hospital Days, part of the regular social life of the town. The auxiliary and ladies of the hospital staff were always there and served refreshments.

At the annual meeting in 1909, every chair in the hospital dining room was occupied. After C.F. Morrison had been elected as chairman, Horace summarized the main points of the report which had already been printed in full in the *Herald*. "Another cow is needed," he said, "for which pasturage is required." More significantly, he also reported the important statistics. "At the beginning of 1908," he stated, "we had six patients in the hospital and during the year we admitted 103. We had fifty-six medical cases, forty-seven surgeries and six obstetrical cases." Sixty-nine of the patients had been First Nations and the others had been non-native. Of all these, only four had died. "The average length of stay," he went on, "had been almost twenty-eight days. First Nations had received 2,371 days of treatment and non-natives 533 days."

He also reported on staff changes. Dr. C.G. MacLean had replaced

Dr. Wallace, who had left to open a practice in Telkwa. Clara Hollingsworth, the matron Horace and Alice had brought back from Ontario with them, had returned there to get married. Miss Broughton had taken her place. They had now replaced the handmade wooden beds, he said, with modern iron hospital beds. They had not done much work to the fabric of the building during the previous year except for painting the new extension.

They had, however, cleared eleven more acres on the hospital site, part of which they ploughed and made ready for spring planting, and part of which they had planted with sixty-two fruit trees. "Besides the aspect of simple utility, the hospital grounds and surroundings are being beautified," he reported. "We are trying to develop to the highest degree the natural advantages of the situation so that our patients shall find an environment most conducive to their speedy recovery."

He listed the donations received, which included salmon, eggs, blankets, clothing for patients and a clock. Some patients had trouble paying their medical bills and paid in kind. Horace's youngest son, Harold, recalled later that some mornings the family would discover on their porch gifts of food or tools, baskets, spoons and other artwork from Gitxsan who had been unable to find cash to pay outstanding bills. Over the years, Horace accumulated a large number of such objects in this way. Stopping at the hospital for tea and an inspection of his collection became part of the tour of Hazelton for distinguished visitors.

The hospital itself, filling an obvious need, was thriving. The *Herald* reported in July 1909 that there were at that time twenty-two patients in the hospital, the largest number since it had been built. The 1910 New Year's Day edition of the *Herald* devoted most of one full page to describing it. The volume of work, it noted, had about trebled in the five years since the hospital had been operational. "Its nearest neighbouring hospitals have been distant approximately as follows: to the west, 160 miles, north 400 miles, east 600 to 800 miles, south 550 miles."

Even, however, with the per diem per patient payments from the provincial government and the Indian Department, hospital finances were never strong. Horace never expected there to be a profit. It was a community hospital and financial support from that community was always necessary to keep it solvent.

The annual report for 1911 noted that there had been a "decided increase in all departments." Admissions during the year had increased to 257. The staff had increased and the number of patients had increased. In one two-week period in the autumn, four patients were operated on for appendicitis. In 1908, the average length of stay had been approximately twenty-eight days whereas in 1911, a year in which the hospital had provided 5,777 days of treatment, the average stay had dropped to twenty-three days.

More buildings were going up on the site, including a five-room cottage for the caretaker, Fred Goddard, formerly a policeman in London. The 1911 report also highlighted the further needs of the hospital. These included the increasing need for an X-ray machine, something to which Horace was now turning his mind. An editorial in the *Miner* reported, "To his skill as a practitioner, Dr. Wrinch adds a large measure of executive ability, as evidenced by the fact that, since the building of the hospital, it has not been necessary to make an appeal to the general public for funds." This would soon change.

That the hospital was appreciated was evident. R.O. Jennings, the superintendent of roads for the district, in a letter to the *Herald*, wrote that he had been in the hospital for ten days with an acute attack of muscular rheumatism and was grateful to Dr. Wrinch and the staff for their unremitting care and attention. "One would not expect," he wrote, "to find in a frontier place like this an institution so well-equipped with all the modern conveniences that the Hazelton Hospital has. I cannot find words loud enough to sing the praises of Dr. Wrinch, his assistant and staff, who are all laboring to maintain the hospital in its high state of efficiency. . . . Through the fact of its existence, it makes possible for men to bring their families into this country who would otherwise be compelled to leave them outside."

Despite Mr. Jennings's praise, improvements were becoming necessary. The hospital had an urgent need for an X-ray machine if it was going to stay up-to-date and provide medical services. "The quiet, simple life that has heretofore held sway in our little shut-in community is about to be rudely disturbed," Horace had written to Dr. Sutherland in 1910. "In anticipation of the opening of the country by the GTP [Grand Trunk Pacific] Railway, for the past few years, settlers have been taking up and improving the land so as to be ready with the produce [farm products] for the railway builders and for the many others who will accompany and succeed them."

The demand was growing: the hospital had to be capable of dealing with it. "We ought to have had it [the X-ray machine] long ago, but had not the wherewithal. But with all the dangerous work that will now be going on around us, it would be almost criminal not to have it."

There were, however, two problems. First, the hospital did not have the electricity to provide power for an X-ray machine, and, second, the hospital did not have the money to pay for it.

Without electricity (which the town of Hazelton did not have, nor would have for many years), there could be no X-ray machine at the hospital. A reliable supply of electricity, therefore, had to come first. Horace wrote that he had hoped the development of the railroad would stimulate some enterprising state or private enterprise to build a dam or plant, but since that hadn't happened, he realized the hospital would have to generate its own power. "It seems impossible to operate it at all conveniently or economically," he reiterated in the annual report, "without having some kind of power plant in connection with the hospital itself."

The hospital had by now nearly outgrown the capacity of its water supply and gas plant. The need for greater capacity was becoming increasingly obvious. In making the case for improvements, Horace said that it should be possible to get a single engine to supply the necessary power, fuelled either by gasoline or oil. It would operate a pump to raise about 750 gallons per hour, and also run a motor that would charge storage batteries during the day sufficient to run electric lights at night. It could be so arranged that if necessary the motor could operate the lights directly instead of through storage batteries. Furthermore, it would be able to operate the X-ray whenever required. This scheme, Horace argued, appeared to be the most feasible of any yet presented.

How to pay for all this? Horace had already applied to the Missions Board for $1,500 to pay for the extensions completed during the previous year. In 1911, he wrote to William Manson, the local member in the provincial legislature, and in replying to Manson's inquiries about the hospital, he explained:

> Personally I have no interest (financial) in the Hazelton Hospital. I am simply the employee of the Methodist Church in the position of Medical Superintendent and Acting Secretary of the hospital. There have never been any profits from the Hazelton Hospital nor, as I understand it to be, are there ever likely to be any. . . . If any profit is accrued, I suppose they would belong to the Methodist Church, but I expect you personally understand enough about the management of hospitals to have an idea of how remote a possibility there is of any such contingency. . . . The Hazelton Hospital does as valuable and disinterested work for the general public as any hospital in British Columbia. Up to the present it has not been a very heavy tax upon the resources of the province. For several years, while our annual expenditure was running from $5,000 to $7,000, we were only receiving from $350 to $600 from the provincial treasury, yet our doors were kept open to the general public in compliance with the Hospital Act.

The provincial secretary, to whom Manson passed Horace's request for $1,000, sent a cheque for $500. After graciously thanking the provincial secretary, Horace expressed disappointment that the full amount requested had not been granted and warned that it might be necessary to come back to the Province for more assistance later. "This," he told patrons of the hospital more bluntly, "had left us nothing with which to pay the cost of further necessary improvements." To put this in context, the summary financial statements showed that, with some bills unpaid and some to collect, at the end of 1911, the hospital had $335 cash in hand. Income for the year had been $13,771, whereas expenditures had been $13,828.

The problems were clear. Solving them would take an appeal to both the community and governmental authorities, research into the most appropriate type of machine, buying and installing it, and training those who would operate it. This, without any other such X-ray machine or experienced operators in the North, would not be easy.

———

Articles in American motoring journals in 1910 were reporting that it was impossible to tour the Hazelton district by automobile. This publicity was not welcome to Hazelton's city fathers, who wanted to open up the district for settlers and to encourage motorists and tourists to visit. Consequently, they eagerly supported the proposal of a contest for the first automobile to reach Hazelton from the South. A prize was offered to the first automobile driver to reach Hazelton from any one of a list of named cities — Seattle, Vancouver and Victoria included.

The published rules of the contest stated that, apart from ferries traversing under one mile and apart from the necessary ferry for any competitor from Vancouver Island, the entire journey had to be made under the automobile's own power. The *Daily Colonist* declared that this would be "a point farther north than any motor car has ever yet penetrated under its own power." (This might have been true for North America because automobiles would have been taken into Alaska by ship and therefore did not get there under their own power.)

Why Hazelton? The Pacific Highway Association was an enthusiastic group of motorists whose aim was to improve the road system. To that end the membership was "bent on securing one magnificent highway through the coast states, and extending north to the limits of civilization in British Columbia, and south to the Panama Canal."

Hazelton was chosen as the northern terminus. The Victoria jewellers Challoner & Mitchell, through the Pacific Highway Association, put up a handsome gold medal trophy for the winner.

The trouble was that the story about the bad roads around Hazelton was largely true. The roads were awful. There were some wagon tracks, to be sure, but few roads. Anyone who had been to Vancouver would have been familiar with automobiles, but there would still have been many in the Hazelton district who would not have seen one before.

Two automobiles, though, were brought to Hazelton in 1911, probably upriver by steamer. In a 1911 version of a pub crawl, drinkers had driven from the bars in Hazelton up the hill past the hospital to the bar at Two Mile. "At both places were profitable dispensaries of hard drinks for soft intellects," Brab Hoops, a Bulkley Valley pioneer, remembered many years later. "When you got tired of the booze in one place you just jumped into a car along with other gentlemen of convivial dispositions and motored to the other. The ride and jolts sobered you up and probably emptied you out, so you could start all over again."

The absence of roads made longer journeys practically impossible. There was, moreover, one stretch of rough track between Hazelton and Quesnel, more of a mule-train path than a road, which no one really knew much about. Many thought the planned journey couldn't be done, and later did not believe it had been.

P.E. Sands, the president of a Studebaker agency in Seattle, was the only one who took up the challenge. He set out from Seattle for the 1,200-mile journey on August 28, 1911, in a Flanders 20 Studebaker, which had cost $800 and which was fitted with a thirty-gallon auxiliary gas tank, a set of spare tires, two rifles, 200 feet of rope and camping gear. A photographer — this was one of the conditions — went along to record the journey.

With his two companions, D.F. Batchelor and W.T. Curtis, Sands drove north from Seattle. They had problems crossing the Snoqualmie Pass in Washington State, where they had to build a track to get through. They had problems crossing the border at Oroville, where they had to promise Canadian customs they would take the car out of the province after the journey. They had problems with rain. And they had problems finding the way north from Kamloops. But they persevered. Sands himself seemed irrepressible. "One of the finest roads I ever saw," he wrote of the Cariboo trail north of Ashcroft. In Quesnel, he said, people who had never seen a car before came out and stared.

By September 9, however, the drive became more difficult. The forest was becoming impenetrable. They had to cut down trees to get through. The track was difficult to find and, at best, a muddy path. They hired a First Nations guide to help them find the way. At one point the car turned over, but they managed to set it back up and carried on. It took them twelve days to get through from Quesnel to Aldermere, where they had a fine reception complete with chicken, steak and champagne.

"The Flanders No. 20 Automobile," the *Herald* said, "arrived in Hazelton Wednesday evening at 9:40 o'clock, it being the first automobile to come into this town over an all land route from Seattle or any other point." Forewarned by the telegraph, a crowd had gathered. It was October 4, 1911. "The Flanders No. 20 accomplished the impossible and came over a road, or at least over a country, that no other vehicle ever travelled and some parts of it even horses have not been over." The brave explorers arrived in Hazelton to a warm, almost rapturous, welcome. The Studebaker account of the journey said:

> When the muffled beat of the busy little motor made itself heard, a cheer went up which showed the travelers that their task had ended and their hardships had been appreciated. Escorted by cheering men and women, dogs barking and the whole village in violent eruption, the Flanders 20 made her way to the hotel, where across the portal stretched a great canvas sign inscribed with the word "Bravo."

The following afternoon they re-created the arrival for the photographers. That evening the town fêted their arrival with a banquet at the Hazelton Hotel.

Before dinner, Horace, who presided, stood and quietened the crowd while he could still command their attention. In his speech and toast to King George and President Taft, he described the purpose of the expedition and congratulated Sands and his party on their accomplishment. "I feel sure," he said with the rhetorical flourish the occasion demanded, "that Seattle will be glad to receive the party back after their trip into a civilized country where everyone was prosperous and where there was lots of room for the investment of millions of dollars."

There were more speeches, songs and toasts, and later there was a lively dance. "Without doubt it was the biggest success of any similar affair ever held in this town," the *Herald* proclaimed. "The banquet hall was very nicely decorated with bunting and flags, while tires off the Flanders 20 were hung around the walls and decked with flowers. . . . The wine list was perfect and the service excellent." The Studebaker account stated that "Sands chronicled in his log the fact that sixty persons were present who consumed seventy-three bottles of champagne, as well as other liquid refreshment, and then adjourned to the bar of the hotel."

That should perhaps have read fifty-nine persons, because Horace not only did not drink alcohol but also disapproved of the drinking of it: he knew the damage it could do to human health. One wonders how he reconciled those bottles of champagne with his conscience. Perhaps, being pragmatic, he accepted the inevitable. The party had the predictable consequences. "Spent day recovering from the banquet," Sands wrote. "So did everyone else in Hazelton. Some haven't recovered yet." The *Herald* was eloquent in its praises. "Mr. P. Sands of Seattle and his friends" it said, "are heroes and they deserve all the credit that can possibly be bestowed on them."

A journey through almost-impossible terrain by an automobile entirely under its own power was a great feat. A marvel! Sands and his companions were intrepid pioneers! Heroes indeed! But was it all true? Some had doubts. An old prospector, Bob Montgomery, who had a criminal record and served time in prison, alleged that he had met them on the track and had seen mules carrying automobile parts.

160 / Service on the Skeena

Could it be that they had not in fact driven all the way but had paid a mule packer to help them? If true, the rules of the contest had not been followed and the prize should be forfeited. The question hung in the air: could they have cheated?

Montgomery thought so and, arriving in Hazelton before they did, went to the notary public, Edward Hicks Beach, to swear an affidavit to that effect. Then nothing more was heard of the matter. That weekend the usually indigent Montgomery was suddenly flush with money and started paying off his many debts. Alvin Kingsley, for one, doubted the official story, writing later that Montgomery had repaid him some of the money owed him. Montgomery, he wrote, had also shown him a roll of four $200 bills, and had given him a knowing wink about where it had come from. Kingsley believed money had changed hands, and the affidavit had been quietly lost.

True or not, Sands and his friends probably need not have worried that they would forfeit the prize. One story was that the Hazelton city fathers knew very well what had happened and were not going to make a fuss. Sands, it is alleged, confessed during the banquet that he had indeed disassembled the car and brought it over the difficult parts by mule. After all, the notary, Hicks Beach, was one of those city fathers and probably knew the truth. Perhaps they believed that Montgomery had made the whole story up and had merely tried to blackmail Sands. More likely, with all that champagne, they were having far too much of a good time at the banquet to worry about it.

Everyone seemed happy. Everyone had achieved their objectives. Sands had publicity for the Studebaker and his auto dealership, as well as the trophy. Hazelton was in the news and had photographs of the car in town to show it had completed the journey. Bob Montgomery had his money, and Kingsley got his money back. The city fathers had wanted to promote the accessibility of Hazelton. They probably saw no need to let a small thing like an observant prospector spoil the story.

Although Horace appears to have become less of a missionary and more of a doctor, hospital administrator and community leader as time went on, he was still deeply committed to his faith. In 1908, he was a lay representative at the Methodist Conference in Vancouver. In 1910, he was ordained as a Methodist minister in "full connexion."

He preached in St. Peter's Anglican Church in Hazelton on Hospital Sunday in 1911. This was an annual service to keep the hospital in the forefront of the community. He relished the opportunity of discussing its work. There was always a risk that a smoothly running hospital could fade from peoples' minds; this, for an institution that depended on public support and funding, would not have been helpful. In his address, Horace expressed the view that hospitals should engage in more social work:

> A patient in a poor home is taken to the hospital where he is temporarily cured and then sent back to his home where the conditions of that home are so often the cause of the trouble, and it is only a short time until the patient is at the hospital again. The new plan is to treat the whole family by improving the conditions of the home and thus removing the chief cause of the trouble. . . . This social branch of hospital work could be worked to advantage in some cases in this country should the people so desire it.

New plans, hospital social work, helping the poor, preventative medicine — here we see Horace at work.

Seeing the devastation that alcohol caused to the social fabric, Horace had always advocated temperance. Had he not, when farming in Halton County, been a member of the Sons of Temperance? The Methodist mission at Kispiox set aside one Sunday each year to discuss the evils of alcohol, and Horace was usually a speaker. On Temperance Sunday in 1909, for example, he spoke of the dangers of alcohol and took along with him illustrated charts that showed the effects of this firewater on the human system. On one such Sunday he brought in a bowl of alcohol and set fire to it, showing his startled listeners what alcohol could do to their insides. After what Pierce called his splendid talk, many of those present came forward to renew their pledge to give up liquor.

Horace went to Vancouver to attend the Methodist conference again in 1912. While there he spoke to the delegates about the hospital and the service it was supplying to the community. Two months later, Methodists from the whole Skeena district came to Hazelton for their annual meeting, with Rev. George Raley from Port Simpson presiding. Horace represented Hazelton and was chosen as a representative to yet another provincial conference. The delegates toured the hospital and went to see the Methodist mission at Kispiox. The Board of Trade treated them to a public reception in town, where "vocal and instrumental music and choice refreshments rounded out the pleasant occasion."

In 1911, a Presbyterian minister, Donald MacLean, and his wife Eva, arrived in Hazelton. Since Hazelton was so crowded, they lived on the bench above the town in a canvas tent erected over a wooden foundation and with low walls. The MacLeans were an unconventional couple. He was a qualified veterinarian and developed a good practice tending to the horses of the district, as a result of which he was known as "Doc." Among his skills was an ability to tame wild horses, something he had learned on ranches in Alberta. Another — and this would come in useful later — was that he was an excellent shot with a Colt revolver and a Lee Enfield rifle. He quickly set up the Presbyterian Club in rooms rented from Horace above the Up-To-Date drugstore to foster reading and writing.

MacLean's lively wife, Eva, was a modern young lady who saw nothing wrong in being friendly with the prostitutes in town and who compared the illegal but still practised potlatch, with its extravagant gifts, to Christmas. She was sympathetic to Gitxsan customs and once attended a potlatch, incurring a censorious lecture from one of the Tomlinson daughters. An excellent musician, Eva played the organ in church and on occasion incurred the displeasure of some of the more straitlaced inhabitants by playing a piano at dances. Respectable people in the Hazeltons did not, perhaps, approve of the MacLeans.

During these years the Methodist, Presbyterian and Congregational churches were moving closer together. Not only was a formal merger being discussed but also the ministers in the Hazelton district were working ever more harmoniously. In early 1912, the Presbyterians of Hazelton voted unanimously for merger. The following April, MacLean for the Presbyterians and Horace for the Methodists entered into an arrangement whereby a Methodist service would be held in the Presbyterian Hall in the evening of the first Sunday of each month, and Horace would no longer take so many services at the hospital. This was later changed to every Sunday.

They held a joint reception and party with the Anglicans at Thanksgiving. Horace took the chair and "added considerably to the success of the evening." He didn't sing, as did a number of the ladies, but he did give a reading. Afterwards the young people had a dance that lasted several hours. So quickly were the Methodist and Presbyterian churches coming together that, when MacLean had to go to Vancouver for eye treatment in 1913, Horace took his Sunday morning service in the new Presbyterian Church.

Horace would have read the *Miner* on the morning of August 10, 1912, with special interest. It reported that in the United Kingdom the National Insurance Scheme, introduced by Chancellor of the Exchequer David Lloyd George, was now legally in effect.

Horace was aware that a number of European states had much earlier developed various forms of publicly funded health insurance. Saxony and Prussia had set up state health programs as early as 1854, some of them being compulsory for certain classes of workers. Clearly, public health was not an entirely new idea. As early as 1694, Dr. Hugh Chamberlen had presented a proposal to the English Parliament recommending a form of state health insurance with a tax on people to pay for the provision of medical benefits to those who needed it.

Daniel Defoe also argued for it, as did John Bellers, who set out proposals for what was almost a national health service in the early eighteenth century. Nevertheless, the reforms of Chancellor Bismarck in Germany in 1883 and the reforms of Chancellor of the Exchequer Lloyd George in 1911 were the first major national programs. Much of the framework of state-supported social welfare is based on their achievements.

Lloyd George's legislation in the United Kingdom was the first wave of similar legislation in the English-speaking world. This, the first step in the emergence of the modern welfare state, shifted an outlook from a system that appeared to be designed to encourage moral reform of the recipient to the acceptance of the principle that the State has a responsibility for the health of its citizens. The First World War subdued — but did not stop — discussion of the Lloyd George reforms and whether they should be adopted in Canada.

Horace had always taken an interest in how people should pay for medical services. Although Hazelton was isolated and far from the centre of the debate, he was able to follow it in the journals and newspapers. As has been seen, his interest had led him to set up the basic insurance of the ticket system at the Hazelton hospital in 1907. Could reforms similar to the British and German schemes work in British Columbia? And if not, why not? Wasn't the health of its citizens something that a progressive society should be prepared to pay for? These were probably questions that stayed with Horace through the next decade and led him to take action after the First World War.

—⚬⚬⚬—

The railway arrived. No one doubted that it would come through the Hazelton district. People had been talking about it for well over a decade. Everyone knew it would change everything, in good ways and bad. On the bad side, it would mean the end of an era, the end of a time where everyone in the community knew each other, the end indeed of Hazelton's *raison d'être* as the jumping-off point for supplies into the hinterland. The Gitxsan and the Wet'suwet'en rightly feared the railway would lead to the loss of more land and to a deeper disturbance of their way of life. The physical landscape would change as bridges and tunnels were built, and as engines shunted and whistles boomed around the valleys.

On the good side, it would mean opening up Hazelton to the outside world and giving its residents ready access to the coast and to Vancouver. It would mean an end to the threat of famine (or higher prices for supplies) should the river steamers be wrecked as had happened in 1907. A railway could bring mining machinery in, and take the ore out, leading to greater prosperity. Subject to winter storms and flooding on the rail tracks, Horace would be able to get medical supplies from Vancouver as often as required and not, as hitherto, four times every winter.

Everyone also knew the railway would run south of the Skeena and Bulkley rivers. Hazelton, as the *Herald* pointed out, "is not on the railway line and [there is] no chance that it ever will be. It is pretty well covered with buildings and at the rate building is going ahead at the present time there will be no vacant ground in a short time." Many believed that the town would die altogether, and so made plans to move to a new town south of the river.

In 1903, the Grand Trunk Pacific Railway, with concessions from Prime Minister Laurier's government as an inducement, had been incorporated to build the railway from Winnipeg to the West Coast. This stemmed from the government's desire to link the prairie provinces to a Pacific port along a northern route. After much debate and intrigue, Kaien Island near Port Essington was selected as the western terminus. A competition to find a name was held, and the new port was then named Prince Rupert. Soon the district started filling with contractors and surveyors. A party of forty Grand Trunk Pacific men, surveying the route for the railway line, was in Hazelton in the autumn of 1908. Cutting it fine and leaving Hazelton in November after the river had closed to steamers, the men returned to Prince Rupert by canoe.

Construction commenced. Steel rails moved out from Winnipeg

in the East and from Prince Rupert in the West. The difficulty of building the route from Prince Rupert up the Skeena to Hazelton may well be imagined: the manufacture and transport of explosives; the establishment of camps every two miles; the problems of supplying the workers with food and water; the challenges of attracting and keeping workers and dealing with all the consequences of having such a work force; the necessity of building many bridges (the first being from Prince Rupert to the mainland) and the pressing need to have medical assistance along the lines. Steamers were built to bring logs, rails and other supplies up to the railhead. Gunpowder blasted tunnels and routes through rock. Workers were hired, fed, worked, injured, paid and discharged.

Per mile, the stretch of line between Prince Rupert and Hazelton was one of the most expensive railway lines built in North America. The basic outline of the story does not, though, tell of the broken bones and dynamite-blasted limbs, the sweat and anxieties, and the hopes, fears and expectations these roads of steel generated.

From very early on, Horace understood the impact of the looming population growth. He saw that the hospital must be prepared to deal with a corresponding increase in the demand for medical services. Given the sad inevitability of injuries, he also saw it as an opportunity for revenue for the hospital. As early as June 1908, he wrote to Sutherland at the Missions Board in Toronto:

> In railway construction, I am told that the companies always prefer to use hospitals already in operation in reasonable proximity to their work, rather than erect and equip their own. It will certainly be to our advantage in every way to take in all such work as we can. It will extend our "sphere of influence" and will also enable us to keep more assistance in the hospital and make it easier for us all to work thoroughly and effectively. A little more work would enable us to have a medical assistant resident at the hospital. That would greatly lighten my own responsibility in relation to surgical work. Supervising the anesthetic and performing the operation is really more than one person is justified in attempting except under circumstances that render

it impossible to do otherwise. However, when it has to be done, and of course here there is no alternative, we find, as in other things, help is "given according to the need."

Horace also saw an opportunity to sell the land owned by the Methodist Church on Mission Point. Would not the Grand Trunk Pacific jump at the chance of buying it as a place to land supplies, build a bridge and expand its townsite to the river? Thomas Crosby, who had pre-empted the land for the church many years previously, was quick to write to Rev. Sutherland in Toronto in 1909 that the land on Mission Point would be an ideal townsite for the Grand Trunk Pacific. Horace was in charge of leasing this land, mainly to farmers.

Receiving offers from would-be purchasers, Horace wanted to sell the land in 1910 and 1911. This was in part because he was making enemies in Hazelton among people who were aggrieved he did not rent it to them. And in part it was also because the prospect of the coming the railway and the uncertainty about the location of the new townsite was raising land prices throughout the area. Once the decision about the townsite was made, all other land prices would be sure to collapse.

Since the railway would not cross the land on Mission Point but run only adjacent to it and approximately 800 feet higher, Horace came to the conclusion that the Grand Trunk Pacific would not in fact want to use the land there for its townsite. It made sense to him, therefore, to take advantage of the artificially high prices and sell. The Missions Board in Toronto, nevertheless, politely turned down his recommendations and dithered regarding what to do.

Horace made enemies in town because he refused to lease land on Mission Point if he thought it would be used for the sale of liquor, for gambling or for a house of "ill-fame." Accordingly, he turned down offers from the hotel keepers in town who, trying to take advantage of what they saw as the inevitable increase in business resulting from the Grand Trunk Pacific supply steamers, wanted to open hotels and saloons there.

For much of 1909 and 1910, Horace was in negotiations with J.W. Stewart of Foley, Welch and Stewart, the principal contractors for the railway, to lease part of the land to the Grand Trunk Pacific for use as an unloading point for supplies. Caught in the middle of discussions among existing tenant farmers on Mission Point, Stewart for the contractors and the Missions Board in Toronto (which saw no need to hurry or even seemingly to make decisions), Horace was not able conclude a deal. Stewart and the contractors then gave up and settled on a site a few miles downstream.

Horace was gratified, though, to learn that the contractors were as much in favour of the no-sin clauses as he was. They wanted sober workers. Horace was able to lease part of the land for two years to Burns Meat, which drove herds of two or three hundred head of cattle at a time up from the South. They set up a meat-processing and cold-storage plant on Mission Point to feed the railway workers.

Although the Grand Trunk Pacific did have a number of staff doctors of varying abilities of its own, it appointed Horace as its district surgeon, and a contract was signed whereby all railway patients would be treated at the Hazelton Hospital instead of going to Prince Rupert, "which will be better," the *Herald* said, "for all concerned."

As might be expected, the *Herald* and *Miner* followed the progress of the railroad carefully. By July 1909, the western railhead had reached fifty miles east of Prince Rupert. The Grand Trunk Pacific then called for tenders for the 140 miles of track from below the Kitselas Canyon, past Hazelton and on up the Bulkley Valley to Aldermere. Mile by mile, bridge by bridge, tunnel by tunnel, the rails came closer to Hazelton. After the railway lines had passed Kitselas Canyon, travellers were able to take a train from the coast to Skeena Crossing (Kitseguecla) and then by steamer up the remaining stretch of river to Hazelton.

The first four passenger cars that pulled out of Prince Rupert for Hazelton in June of 1912 were so full that there was standing room only. The passengers would have had a strange sensation not only of the telescoping of time but also of the ending of an era. The Skeena

River, which had been such a terror and challenge to steamers, when seen from the train was a pleasant, fast flowing but otherwise calm river, with merely an eddy or two to disturb its placid surface. The long, wide valleys of trees and pastures above the riverbanks could be seen for the first time.

The City of God, Meanskinisht, (about to be renamed Cedarvale) that so many had heard of but few had visited, was seen to be a pretty village with a quaint church. The totem poles along the river at Kitwanga flashed by too quickly. The perilous journey of days up the Skeena had become a few comfortable hours of watching the scenery. Nothing would ever be the same again.

A prolonged and acrimonious dispute between local promoters and the Grand Trunk Pacific led to there being two new towns and two railway stations. In the end, New Hazelton would be the principal townsite, partly because so many people and businesses had already moved there from Old Hazelton and partly because the new bridge across the Hagwilget Canyon that fed into it was already under construction. The Grand Trunk Pacific was clearly faced with a *fait accompli*.

In August 1912, the *Miner* noted that the rails would soon reach South Hazelton, the town that the Grand Trunk Pacific was promoting. "The whistle of the locomotive," it reported, "is now a familiar sound in Hazelton." The steel tracks arrived in South Hazelton and then moved on to New Hazelton a week later. By September, the Grand Trunk Pacific was advertising a through service to Vancouver in fifty-seven hours, with the train leaving South Hazelton at 10:30 a.m. on Thursdays and Sundays. The Thursday train connected at the coast with the SS *Prince Rupert*, which arrived in Vancouver at 7 p.m. on Saturday. A traveller could now check bags all the way to Vancouver. The change would have been akin to suddenly being able to fly from Vancouver to, say, Toronto, after many years of only being able to take the train or drive there.

Railway construction carried on eastwards to join with the line coming out from Winnipeg. As far as the residents of Hazelton were concerned, though, the completion of the railway from New Hazelton to Fort George in the East was not noteworthy. They already had what they wanted — the line to the coast and thus easy passage to Vancouver. The last spike in the line from Prince Rupert to Winnipeg was driven in at 2:30 on April 6, 1914. The point was near Mile 273, about two miles east of Fort Fraser. About twenty officials from Winnipeg arrived by special train. The *Fort George Herald* reported that, although no public announcement had been made, about 1,500 people had congregated there.

The track-laying gangs had left a mile open for a speed contest between the men laying from the east and the men laying from the west. Both teams started at the same time, but it was soon clear that the team from the east had more system and arrived at the spot fourteen minutes before the other team. When they met, a large Union Jack was run up the centre post. The last nine iron spikes were driven in, the photographs were taken, and the dignitaries climbed back into the train for the journey to Prince Rupert.

For people of the Hazeltons, the arrival of the railway ended the steamboat era. The "Last Steamer Has Gone Below," the *Herald* reported on September 13, 1912, saying:

> On Tuesday the *Inlander* whistled for the last time in the northern waters and pulled away from her old berth and started downstream for Port Essington at a good clip. . . . It was just noon hour when the steamer whistled and in a couple of minutes the lines were cast and the boat started down while a number of citizens stood on the shore and waved a last farewell to the captain and his crew. With the departure of the *Inlander* ends the transportation on the Skeena River as far north as Hazelton.

The main headline on the front page that day, however, was not of the ending of an era — that was already history — but of the fact that the Harris Mines would start packing ore out as soon as the Grand Trunk Pacific got a railcar to New Hazelton. The steamers, no longer needed, were moved to other rivers. The *Inlander*, the last of them, was left to rot on a beach at Port Essington.

As Horace had foreseen, Old Hazelton, confined by the river on one side and the Gitxsan reserve on the others, had no room to grow in either land area or population. It did, however, grow in liveliness as mining boomed. More miners, settlers, farmers and railway employees arrived. As the railway linked Hazelton to the modern world, people settled down, formed clubs, started sports associations, acquired land, farmed, and bought and sold mineral claims.

With the coming of the railway, the isolation and the tight sense of community that isolation brings came to an end. Old Hazelton's population increased to 200 and kept rising. The town was so full that new residents like the MacLeans had to rent homes and even live in tents in the Gitxsan reserve on the bench above the town.

The arrival of the railway was a turning point between old and new. Before the railway arrived, there had been mule trains, travel by canoes, river steamers, and prospectors with spades, gold pans and the standard trail food of bacon and beans. Horace had travelled on horseback or by dog-sled to patients in outlying villages. After, there were automobiles, roads, telephone exchanges, electricity and easy railway access to the coast. Soon, Horace would buy a business, acquire his own automobile and become a leading mining entrepreneur.

CHAPTER 8

Mining, X-rays and Daylight Robbery 1912–1914

ONE DAY IN JUNE 1912, Roy Ridsdale and Billy Gore rode along the trail past the hospital, and then followed it down below the Gitxsan cemetery bluff and on into Hazelton. After two weeks prospecting in the Owen Lake district to the south, they and their horses were tired and dirty. The men were looking forward to hitting the bars and blackjack tables in the Hazelton Hotel, but first they wanted to get their ore samples assayed. A prospector named Jim Holland had been in the Owen Lake area not long before and had returned with a few odd rocks to show around town. Thinking Holland might have stumbled on a promising mining prospect, Ridsdale and Gore had gone to check. They had found the ore they were looking for in a narrow canyon down which a creek ran into Owen Lake. At present, the site could be reached only on horseback, but a six-mile track would put it conveniently near the river and only twenty miles from the railway.

In town, excited to see what the first discovery of the season brought in, a crowd of miners quickly gathered. Experienced ones among them turned the rocks over in their hands, quickly realizing that the samples showed great promise. One of them was so enthusiastic that he offered to buy an option on the five claims that had been staked even before Austin, the assayer, had delivered his report. They were too late. Ridsdale and Gore already had three partners, two of them being the Hicks Beachs, father and son, and the third being Horace. The partners had in all probability financed the prospectors' speculative expedition.

Horace had a restless, entrepreneurial side to his nature. In Ontario he had managed a family farming business — buying, selling, taking care of the accounts, always looking for practical ways to reduce expenses and increase income. He brought this expertise with him when he came to Hazelton. Christianity in those days apparently had little against honest endeavour and energetic entrepreneurship.

In fact he was buying land almost as soon as he arrived, the first, as far as is known, was the district lot next to the hospital that he acquired in 1902. This, being almost adjacent to Two Mile Creek, was perhaps insurance in case he could not find water on the hospital site itself. After the site had been acquired and he had found water, he quickly sold one half of his land there.

Most of his life he was buying and selling land. He bought several lots in Old Hazelton, including the triangle lot and its neighbour. Between 1903 and 1923, the Crown awarded him thirteen Crown grants, and it awarded two to Alice. The government had granted most of the river valley land not already in First Nations reserves to incoming settlers. This land, settlers knew, was plentiful and cheap. First Nations protested, but were on the whole ignored.

Reporting in January 1914 on the state of mining in Hazelton, the *Herald* included Horace in the list of men who "with their capital and mining experience, or their energy and their brains, have battled undauntedly against a combination of odds, opposition and vicissitudes rarely visited upon even the famous "hard luck" camps of Bret Harte and Mark Twain." It paid tribute to the owners and operators of the various mining properties who had steadily forged ahead in spite of the slow arrival of the railway, excessive freight charges, bad roads and uncertainty of labour. Horace may have smiled at the hyperbole, but what would he have thought about being described as a mining financier? For one thing, it was probably true.

After his death, one obituary said that he was "part and parcel of everything that went to make up Hazelton and development of the district, and there were a great many during the mining boom of thirty years ago to know his open generosity in the matter of 'grubstakes.'" (A grubstaker is one who supplies material or food to a prospector in exchange for part of any profit from the venture.) This suggests that he was a soft touch not only for every organization for the public good, but also for money-short prospectors and grubstakers.

This though was only part of the story. As early as 1904, Loring wrote that he was not yet able to repay a loan Horace had made to him in connection with a mining venture. Horace was not immune from the infectiousness of mining in Hazelton in the years before the First World War. Few were. It seemed that everyone of any consequence in town — Sargent, Loring, Kirby, Chettleburgh and Larkworthy among them — was in some way active in mining or mining investment.

Mining had been the main business of Hazelton since the days of the Omineca gold rush in the late 1860s and early 1870s. The steamers up the river, the storehouses, the mule trains taking goods to miners in the hinterland — they all fed this business. In the early days of the twentieth century, mining activity increased and rose into an excited buzz known, to many as the Hazelton mining boom. In 1910, in a banner headline, the *Herald* described the district as "Canada's Land of Opportunity" and went on: "Within this district is a wealth and diversity of natural resources scarcely to be equalled anywhere else in the world. Farm lands, coal, precious and useful metal in the mountains, timber and placer gold are all here. . . . The Northern Interior of British Columbia spells opportunity to the man who is dissatisfied with his present condition in life."

Both the *Herald* and the *Miner* fizzed with news of mining exploration. Almost every edition of these newspapers carried reports of new strikes, new claims and excited prospectors coming back into town after weeks or months in the mountains with rock to be assayed for gold, galena, coal, copper or lead. The front page of a March 1913 edition of the *Herald*, for example, contained eight headlined items, four of them on mining.

It proclaimed with excitement such dramatic events as "New Strike at Silver Standard," "Butte and Rocher de Boule Copper Company Will Start" and "Another Big Strike Made at Rocher de Boule Mine." As it turned out, there was enough metal to excite everyone and to tempt those who could invest, but not enough, except in a few cases, to sustain viable industries. The Hazelton mining boom was lively but short-lived.

In August 1913, a group of investors met to discuss the formation of an association to be called the New Hazelton District Mine Owners' Association. The stated intention was to bring capital and mining men into the district to develop various mines of promise. At the meeting, Horace was appointed vice-president. Others on the executive included C.H. Sawle, the publisher of the *Herald*, which explains some of the excitement on the front pages.

The next month, "at the most enthusiastic meeting ever held in New Hazelton," the Association met again. "From the opening of the proceedings to the end, the greatest harmony prevailed and enthusiasm was roused to a high pitch." The aim of the Association, now restated rather grandly, was "to develop all the resources of the northern interior of British Columbia through its mineral resources." Horace was re-elected to the same position at the first annual meeting, held in October. The committee met early the following year in the offices of the *Herald*, and agreed to publish a brochure on the mining prospects of the district.

Like so much of life in the Hazeltons, the nature of mining was changing, and the new railway had much to do with it. The image of the lonely prospector with his shaggy horse and gold pan, his heavy moustache, suspenders and floppy hat is a familiar one from the Canadian North. The Upper Skeena was well travelled by such people. Prospectors returning from the Omineca Gold Rush in the early 1870s and settling at the Forks, where the Skeena and Bulkley rivers met, had helped establish the community there. They panned for gold in such creeks as Lorne, Chimdedash, Fiddler and Kleanza.

By the time the railway arrived, however, the prospector of this picture was becoming a figure from the past. He was still around — the *Herald* over the years contained many obituaries of old-timers from the gold rush days — but they became increasingly part of the romance rather than of the business of mining. Even placer mining had changed and had become more industrial. Miners were tunnelling deeper and using larger, more efficient machines.

A railway would be able to bring the bigger machinery that was becoming necessary to work the mines, as well as men with new ideas about mining and more capital to invest. The ore was there. The people were coming to explore and mine it. What was needed urgently was efficient transportation to bring the machinery into the district and to take the ore out. This had to be the railroad, and when it arrived in 1912, the already energetic mining in the district exploded in the short-lived Hazelton mining boom.

There were several main mining areas around Hazelton. One was down the Skeena at Lorne Creek near the Kitselas Canyon, where Mrs. MacArthur had the misfortune to fall into the sluice chute. The first claims here had been filed as early as 1893. There were gold and copper in the rocks, enough to entice and tease but, after the first few happy years of gold extraction, not enough to enrich. Now it was barely enough to justify further significant investment.

Another area was in the mountains around Hazelton. On Nine Mile Mountain, to the east, were forty to fifty claims and several mines, including the Silver Cup and the American Boy Mine. There were also mines on Four Mile Mountain, Hudson's Bay Mountain and Groundhog Mountain. The Rocher de Boule Mine, one of the two on this mountain, was brought into production in 1911. This mine in time had its own hydroelectric plant and an aerial tramway to bring the ore to the railway at a place called Tramville.

Horace was involved in at least three mines: the first was an investment in the property at Owen Lake, the second was an association with the Harris brothers in the American Boy Mine, and the third appears to have been some claims on Rocher de Boule. Like many a prospector and investor before and since, he does not appear to have made much money from his mining ventures.

Billy Gore, who had brought the ore samples back into town from Owen Lake, sold his interest to Horace, who then had the largest share. The claim was thereafter called the Wrinch property. Despite being a copper property, it was called the Silver Queen Mine. Soon the site boasted a Wrinch Creek and a deep and narrow Wrinch Canyon. In October, highly encouraging returns were being reported for the assays of general samples from the tunnels at the property. By November, they were making great headway and finding "yellow copper coming in good."

The Silver Queen Mine, however, never amounted to much in the years that Horace held the claims. Every few years he and his partners were able to interest someone into looking into developing it, but nothing much by way of profit seemed to result. Duke Harris, a professional miner, went to Owen Lake in May 1916 to have a look, and came back reporting that the low-grade copper there was indeed worth developing.

In 1916 and again in 1923, Horace and his partners tried to capitalize on their investment. "The Federal Mining and Smelting Co.," the *Herald* said, "have taken options on two groups of prospects in the Owen Lake district that are owned by Dr. H.C. Wrinch and Jim Cole, Houston." They tried again in 1929. "The Silver Queen group, owned by H.C. Wrinch," the Annual Report of the Minister of Mines said, "is described in the reports for 1916, 1923 and 1924. No work, apart from cleaning out tunnels, has been done on this property since 1924. F.H. Taylor organized the Owen Lake Mining and Development Company in 1928 and worked the mine for a while."

One particular cut in a tunnel in the mine was "referred to by mine management as the 'Wrinch System.'" In 1928, reports indicated that the significant ore bodies at Owen Lake could only be developed with the investment of over $200,000. Horace was now well out of his league. That year, the granted options were exercised. Horace had sold his interests, but Wrinch Creek, Wrinch Canyon and the Wrinch vein system remain.

Horace was in another mining venture with the four Harris brothers — W.S. (Duke), Al, Edgar and Hugh. Between the 1860s and the 1890s, the family had lived at Nelson in Halton County, Ontario. Since they were Methodists, it is at least possible they had known Horace or Alice there. After mining in Nelson and in the Atlin Gold Rush near the Yukon border, they came to Hazelton and leased a farm opposite the hospital, where they were among Horace's closest neighbours.

The Harris brothers — the newspapers called them the Harris Boys — were associated with some of the most famous mines around Hazelton. They owned seven claims in the American Boy Mine on Nine Mile Mountain, actually turning down an offer of $110,000 for them in 1911. Keeping these claims for themselves, they started a company to develop them called, appropriately, Harris Mines Limited. (One of their claims was felicitously named Ore-Or-No-Go.) Doubtless needing more capital, they offered the public an opportunity to purchase shares in Harris Mines at fifteen cents each. The American Boy group is "right in every particular to make a big mine," an advertisement soliciting investment said. "In short, it is Hazelton's banner prospect."

Horace became the president and a director of Harris Mines. The Harris brothers had mining, not bureaucracy, in their blood. While they were out in the mountains prospecting or actually mining, they would have needed someone back in town to look after their interests and to offer to the world a respectable, stable, reassuring face. Who better than Horace? At the annual shareholders' meeting at the end of October 1912, Horace was re-elected president and a director.

In a pitch to raise more money for development, the Harris brothers reported on progress so far. The *Herald* (Sawle, the editor, was probably also an investor) had no doubts. "One thing is certain," it editorialized, "the people who put their money into the Harris Mines Ltd. will get full value." The Harris brothers, who were also directors, unashamedly promoted their project, "The directorate of the Harris Mines are men whose integrity and knowledge of practical mining is unquestioned and you will get an honest and capable administration, every dollar being put where it will give you the best run for your money."

After describing in detail the veins and the shipment plans, they asked for more money, "firmly believing that we can make you some money before the summer is over. . . . It is only reasonable to suppose that you can at least double the price of your shares this year."

The mines produced ore and promised more. The Harris Boys, however, knew when to sell in order to recoup their own investment. In May 1922, control of the Harris Mines Limited was sold to British capitalists presumably for a tidy sum. It isn't clear when Horace ceased to be the president and a director, but it is unlikely that mighty capitalist investors would have wanted the local doctor looking after their interests in the district.

Horace did own a number of other claims. A short note in the *Herald* in May 1919 said that "Dr. Wrinch and Vic Procter are getting assessment work done on their claims between Golden Wonder and Hazelton View." These claims were on Rocher de Boule Mountain. Horace was also granted another claim, the Mandon M.C., on the western slope of Rocher de Boule in 1923, but that claim later reverted to the Crown.

When the First World War came in August 1914, British Columbia's economy sagged, and the pace of mining activity slowed. The fall in the price of copper and other metals inhibited the mining industry, especially in those marginal areas such as Hazelton, where the cost of taking ore to refineries and on to buyers became too high. The unreasonably high freight rates that the Grand Trunk Pacific decided to charge put additional financial pressure on the mines' balance sheets. The mine on Rocher de Boule suspended production in 1917. More mines closed in 1918.

The shortage of shipping during the war raised the costs further. With many miners joining the army, labour became harder to find. Much of the investment from the United States dried up. Furthermore, the provincial government cut appropriations for public works in order to provide social assistance to the unemployed and underfed in Vancouver.

Mining did carry on — the metals and minerals were needed as resources for the war — but it all became much quieter. The reporting of mining also slowed down and became less excited. The front pages of the *Herald* and *Miner* that used to throb with stories about mining were now full of stories about the progress of the war. After the war, the energy seems to have gone out of the Hazelton mining boom. Local newspapers ran stories of sports and news from the growing towns of Terrace and Smithers. Many of the mines never did become commercially successful and closed. The New Hazelton District Mine Owners' Association was heard of no more and perhaps merged into the Board of Trade.

—√√√—

The Grand Trunk Pacific provided quick access to the coast for residents, farmers and miners. It also established stations along the line and important ones at divisional points, some of which grew into large towns. One of these was Smithers, named after its chairman, Sir Alfred Smithers. The townsite there, put on the market in 1913, was located on a swampy lot at the base of Hudson's Bay Mountain. Wiggs O'Neill was given the contract to clear and drain it. Terrace, to the west of Hazelton, was a small settlement of a few houses and a store, having been laid out as a townsite in 1910.

With the growing population came the need for more medical services in the Bulkley Valley. In the summer of 1911, Dr. Wallace had moved to Telkwa and possibly may have opened a small hospital there. The demand clearly was becoming almost too much for the Hazelton Hospital to meet. In December 1913, the hospital treated the largest number of patients it had ever treated in one month. It was so busy in the winter of 1913 that Horace had to telegram for another nurse. "Records broken at the Hospital," the *Herald* announced in February.

Yet Horace and the staff somehow found time to produce an in-house journal — the *Hazelton Hospital Herald*. Since this was not heard of again, perhaps it did not last long, but it does show the energy in the hospital that, in addition to the demanding medical work, the staff could even think of publishing a journal.

Horace noted in the hospital annual report for 1912 that the 290 patients admitted during the year had been provided with 6,484 days of treatment. Two hundred and fifty of these patients had been, as the hospital register put it, cured. The average mortality rate at the hospital, Horace wrote with noticeable pride, compared very favourably with other hospitals. For the previous five years, it had been 5.5 percent, which he compared with the 6.2 percent rate for a large city hospital.

An increase in mortality in 1912, he noted, was largely attributable to accidents in the mining and railroad business. Of the nineteen patients who had died at the hospital in 1912, eight had died within forty-eight hours of admission and four more within a week. Most of these, he said, had been almost beyond hope when they were admitted; all that could be done for them was to make their last days comfortable.

There were always staff changes, of course. Helen Bone, lady superintendent for seven years, had returned to Ontario in June 1911 and was replaced for a time by Miss Tomlinson. May Hogan arrived the following year to take over as lady superintendent, and she remained at the hospital in various capacities for the next twenty-five years. Dr. MacLean left the hospital to open a practice in Smithers. Dr. Stone, who had succeeded MacLean as assistant physician, left in early 1914 and Dr. A.F. MacAuley came to replace him.

Student nurses came, learned their profession and graduated. Gertrude Martin, for example, graduated in May 1913. After the usual celebration in the Wrinch home with her friends and colleagues, Rev. John Field presented her with a bouquet of lilacs. She then returned to her native province of Prince Edward Island. At the time of the annual meeting in 1914, the nurses in training under the watchful eye of May Hogan, were Margaret Crawford, Winifred Soale, Annie Sisko, Eva Martin and Hester Wilson.

The hospital farm prospered. In the spring of 1914, Horace allowed H.E. Walker, the government agricultural representative for the northern part of the province, to use several acres on the hospital grounds for experimental purposes. Walker, wanting to assist local farmers in farming practices, planted a number of crops, including alfalfa, oats and field peas. "As a result of the experiments," the *Herald* reported, "Dr. Wrinch is quite an enthusiastic advocate of farming in this vicinity."

Horace, it said, had been conducting farming experiments with wheat on his own account, noting in July that it was growing well and already had full and mature heads. Horace said he had sent some to the Ontario Agricultural College at Guelph, which was also experimenting with it. "A trip to the hospital farm is a treat and an education," the *Herald* continued. "Mrs. Wrinch is just as enthusiastic over the farming as is the doctor and personally superintends many departments of the work."

—⁓—

Horace had announced in 1910 that he would be constructing a two-storey building, which became known as the Wrinch Building, on one of his pieces of land in Hazelton. He used part as his office in town and part he rented out. The first service of the Methodist Church in Hazelton was held there in 1912 when the Rev. R.W. Lee, then the missionary at Kispiox, came down to take the service. A number of other associations, including the local Masons, also used the Wrinch Building for their meetings. It was here that the

Rev. MacLean had established the Presbyterian Club when he first arrived in town in 1911.

A pioneer businessman and druggist in the district, J. Mason Adams, took over the ground floor of the Wrinch Building and established a drugstore and stationery business. This was the Adams Drugstore, sometimes advertised as the Kodak Drugstore. Horace, in what today might be called vertical integration, decided to buy the drugstore, together with all its stock-in-trade. On November 1, 1912, Horace and Adams, who then moved to Telkwa (and later to Smithers) to open a drugstore there, signed the agreements.

Leaving the existing manager, A.V. Johnstone, in charge, Horace renamed the business the Up-To-Date Drug Store. At about the same time, he opened a second drugstore with the same name in New Hazelton. "Everything to be had in the drug line. Finest selection of chocolates, candies, stationery and magazines," its advertisements in the *Miner* said. "We carry a large stock of Kodak goods, cameras, films, papers, etc. Developing and printing a specialty." Horace gave a job there to his nephew Hubert Wrinch, when he came to visit in 1913.

Fire almost destroyed the drugstore in Old Hazelton more than once. As with so many towns of that era, fire was a constant hazard. Over the years, many of the old buildings burned down, were rebuilt and then sometimes burned down again. In 1910, someone knocked over a lamp in the reading room of the Hazelton Hotel at about two in the morning, and the whole building was soon engulfed in flames. Three of the guests and employees had to jump for their lives from upper-storey windows. Except for a couple of barrels of whisky that were rolled out into the snow, everything was lost. Maitland-Dougall, the police chief, who was up all night, had to remove all four prisoners from the jail next door in case the fire spread.

Soon after, a much-needed Hazelton Fire Department was set up and the organizers asked for subscriptions. To this Horace donated $25. In September 1912, an early-morning fire destroyed two Hudson's Bay Company warehouses and one belonging to Broughton &

McNeil. After the fire had been spotted and the alarm raised at three in the morning, the fire department and other volunteers formed a bucket brigade in time to save adjoining buildings.

In December, fire destroyed the Hudson's Bay Company's store itself together with about $40,000 worth of goods. This fire also burned the old logbooks that went back to when the store first opened. Horace was well aware of the fire risk to the hospital. As early as 1907, he was reporting that there were hose pipes on each floor. "The danger of fire," he had written, "is still further lessened by using Siche gas [acetylene] instead of lamp and coal-oil."

With Hazelton growing and with transportation becoming easier, politicians came through town more frequently. Premier McBride, making his third visit to Hazelton, together with his Attorney General, William Bowser, came to speak to the Hazelton Board of Trade in 1912. "Sir Richard McBride, and his distinguished colleague, the Attorney General of the province, have seen," the *Miner* said, "Hazelton and the Skeena Valley in the dawn of a great period of development." In the provincial election that March, the Tory William Manson competed with the Liberal Alex Manson in the Skeena riding, with William winning the seat. McBride won the election and remained premier.

In April 1914, Harlan Brewster, the Liberal party leader, John Oliver, and T.D. ("Duff") Pattullo, a rising young politician from Prince Rupert, were in town speaking to a local Liberal party meeting. The *Miner*, a Tory newspaper, reported haughtily that the attendance at this meeting was low and devoid of all enthusiasm. All these men, except the Mansons, later became premiers of the province. Oliver, Pattullo and Alex Manson were to play a significant part in Horace's own future as a politician. Now in his late forties, Horace was becoming one of Hazelton's old-timers, and a foray into politics was probably the last thing he could have seen for himself.

One by one the pioneers were moving away or dying. Captain Bonser died. He had been a captain of steamboats on the Skeena since 1892, just after the first successful run upriver to Hazelton. His death would have put a bookend to the steamboat era. The Hicks Beach family left town and went to live in the South. In late 1913, Robert Tomlinson, who many years before had set up the City of God at Meanskinisht and from whom Horace had purchased the lumber to build the hospital, sickened and died. Horace had gone downriver to help, but there was nothing he could do. Tomlinson's son, also Robert Tomlinson, the first patient in the hospital, and later to work at the hospital, had remarried in August 1913 and returned with his bride to take over the mission at Kispiox.

———

Horace all the while was planning for improvements to the hospital. Even before the Missions Board had approved the acquisition of the X-ray machine, he had begun campaigning for funds so as to show community support for the upgrade. In a letter sent to patrons and other friends of the Hazelton Hospital at the end of January 1913, Horace asked for money, "believing you to be a friend of Hazelton Hospital and that you take pride in it and desire to see it kept — as it always has been — fully up to the requirements of the district."

He was looking for $2,420 in donations, the rest to come from government and mission sources. "Will you," he asked innocently, "confirm our belief that this is your attitude?" He outlined the hospital's needs: $1,000 was needed for the X-ray apparatus and power plant, $800 for linoleum in the wards, $600 for renovation and painting of the inside walls, $30 for three adjustable bedframes, $30 for two fracture beds, $45 for one air mattress, $45 for an invalid's wheelchair and $70 for improving the sterilizing plant.

In April 1913, Horace took his family to Ocean Park, in Santa Monica, California, for a two-month holiday. They spent much of their time enjoying the beaches and sunshine. On one day, they all took the Electric Railway Trolley to the famous Cawston Ostrich Farm in Pasadena, where the children went riding on the ostriches.

Horace's time in California was not, though, merely a vacation.

He wanted to study X-ray machines: how they were used, what their requirements were and what information he needed to make an informed purchase decision. While in California, his ever-inquiring farmer's mind also noted the damage done by frost to orange orchards. When he returned to Hazelton, he was quoted in the *Herald* as saying that California was a fine place to go for a holiday, but he preferred the Hazelton district and believed that the miner or agriculturalist who used his time and knowledge to advantage would make quite as much money in Hazelton as anywhere on the continent.

Following his return and having his report on the X-ray machine, the power plant and the now-projected cost of $4,500 in front of them, the hospital board made the decision to launch a public canvass for funds. Horace said he would be making a personal canvass, which presumably meant he would be knocking on doors. To free him up for this, Horace asked Dr. MacLean to take over his responsibilities at the hospital. The community stepped up to the challenge of raising the money for the machine that Horace wanted to have installed before winter. "Dr. Wrinch," the *Miner* reported, "is confident that the response will be prompt and liberal."

By October, it noted that "Dr. Wrinch, who is making a personal canvass, is meeting with gratifying success." It was recommended that it would "greatly aid Dr. Wrinch, if intending subscribers indicate to him the amount they intend to subscribe, without waiting for him to call upon them." Horace himself was the largest contributor, with a donation of $100.

The residents of the Hazeltons did respond generously. The listing in the *Herald* of the names of contributors, reading like a who's who of Hazelton, together with the amount they each gave, probably helped. By the end of the second week, the sum of $750 had been raised. A fund-raising concert was held in the Presbyterian Hall in September. Local thespians gave an amateur performance of *The Hat Box*. Every seat was filled for this comedy, which raised over $120. In the concert that followed the performance, Miss Hogan played a piano solo and accompanied the quartet made up of Miss Adams,

Miss Grist, G. Milburn and — Horace. "Encores," the *Miner* reported, "were frequent."

With the money coming in well, Horace raised his sights to include an ambulance. He also stated that, contrary to some rumours being put about, the fee for the use of the X-ray would be nominal, $5 or $10 depending on the size of the sheet used. Contributors to the fund, he said, would get their first treatment free.

In September 1913, Horace wrote to the provincial government again, this time asking for $1,500, "which is less than one-third of the estimated amount required." His letter continued:

> The need of this new equipment is most urgent. With a railway running through our district, a large number of mines being opened up, extensive road construction going on, and the various other industries incidental to a developing country being started, and all bringing in increased population, it is imperative that the hospital be brought more up-to-date if it is to maintain the place of usefulness it has hitherto occupied, and which we venture to believe has been as much a matter of satisfaction to you and other members of our government as to ourselves who have been recipients of its benefits.

At the same time, he wrote a personal letter to Dr. H.E. Young, the provincial secretary. He noted that the hospital had "more than once been subject to unfair criticism, when patients have passed out of our hands to where they could get X-ray examination and on the other hand it works a hardship on patients to have to send them to Vancouver for treatment. It is too far." The government, still not convinced, was afraid that it would be putting money into the hospital, and then the Methodist Church would sell the land, sell the hospital and take all the benefit of provincial generosity.

The local members of the legislature, Manson and Cox, together with the provincial minister of lands, visited the hospital to make a personal investigation. Satisfied, they recommended payment. The provincial government was still hesitant. What was the federal government contributing? it asked. How much had been raised locally?

If Horace was frustrated by this prevarication, he did not show it in print. He calmly replied that the federal government had agreed to contribute $1,500 and local donors had given over $3,000. Finally satisfied, the provincial government consented to the request and sent a cheque for $1,500.

By January 1914, Horace knew he had enough money, not only for the X-ray machine but also for the ambulance. The total cost would be almost $7,000 (nearly as much as the hospital itself had cost a mere ten years before), and this amount had been almost fully subscribed. So successful had the campaign been that he could afford a bigger and better machine than he had originally proposed.

The only X-ray machine in the North, it was the most modern there was, being identical to new ones being installed at the Mayo Clinic in Rochester, Minnesota. Contracts were awarded. Kelley-Koett from Covington, Kentucky, and Canadian Fairbanks-Morse would be installing the power plant. "Next year," the *Herald* said with evident pride and laudable hyperbole, "the report will be from the most up-to-date hospital in the country." It would also be from a hospital in a country at war.

Progress at the hospital in these months before the war was considerable. The new ambulance — essentially a two-horse stagecoach converted to take stretchers and costing $1,700 — arrived and was put into service. The new electrical lighting and power plant was installed. Electricity also proved extremely useful in powering the electric saw that cut the many cords of wood used in the hospital kitchen and laundry, thereby saving many hours of manual labour. The pump, with its capacity of 720 gallons an hour, was working well and, best of all, the new X-ray machine, "which is of the most modern pattern" would be installed within the next week or so. The future looked calm and assured.

—∿—

With all the mining activity in the district, it was useful that there were now reliable banks, both in Hazelton and New Hazelton. The cash circulating in the economy stimulated growth. The Union Bank branch on Pugsley Street in New Hazelton was a log building, with bars separating the cashiers from customers and with a strong box to keep the cash. It seemed safe enough to meet local needs.

C.J. (Jock) McQueen, a nineteen-year-old vacation relief cashier, and Ray Fenton, the ledger-keeper, stepped out for their evening meal in New Hazelton on November 7, 1913. When, at about six o'clock, they came back into the bank for their shift, they found themselves staring at the wrong end of several revolvers. Masked robbers had hacked their way into the bank through a back-bedroom window. McQueen tried to put up a fight but was shot in the face by one of the robbers, who then forced Fenton to unlock the strong box. As soon as the robbers had left, Fenton gave the alarm by firing his revolver into the air. The robbers, though, had by then disappeared into the bush with about $16,000.

Horace was quickly on the scene and gave medical help to the injured McQueen, while others gave chase to the robbers. The police eventually arrived and tracked them on to Rocher de Boule Mountain, where they found their camp but not them. A hunt was started. A few days later, in the general nervousness in the community, a deputized tracker with a police party shot dead an innocent person he thought was behaving suspiciously. A coroner's jury later found two trackers culpable of homicide, but the Crown did not prosecute and they were set free. McQueen seems to have survived.

In February 1914, the *Miner* reported that, even though the surgeons in Vancouver had decided not to remove the .38 bullet from his skull, McQueen had returned to work as a bank clerk. Later that year, he mysteriously disappeared, and his friends were worried that the bullet had affected his mind. Newspapers speculated that he had been murdered by one of the robbers whom he had recognized in Vancouver. One later account, though, states that he enlisted in the army and survived the war with a superficial wound.

On the morning of April 7, 1914, it happened again. Seven heavily armed men tried to rob the Union Bank in New Hazelton. Fenton was there for his second robbery, along with Bishop, the teller, for his first. "They [the robbers] came in the private entrance of the bank and into the interior," Bishop later testified. "They came round with guns pulled and calling out, 'Hands up.' The man who was leading them pointed the gun at me and told me to put up my hands and called out 'money, money.'"

The robbers tried to get Bishop to open the new safe that Tatchell, the manager, had installed after the previous robbery. Two people, however, were required to open it. One of the two, Tatchell himself, was out. The robbers' threats increased. They picked up whatever cash they could find, including about $250 of mutilated bills that Bishop had been painstakingly repairing, $1,100 from the cage and about $375 from Albert Gaslin, the assistant postmaster, who had been in the bank depositing cash at the time.

Fenton ran back into the bedroom to get his gun. "I just had time to get the gun from under my pillow, turned round and pulled the trigger, and pulled the door to, and thinking I should get shot through the door, I slid on to the floor and put my feet up against the bed. He made several feeble attempts to open the door. . . . I heard them threatening Mr. Bishop. I heard several shots in the office and they seemed to be giving him a pretty rough time altogether. . . . I just got scratched — hit by one of the shots."

At about the same time, Tatchell, on his way back to the bank, rounded a corner and found himself looking at a surprised robber, armed with a rifle, who was meant to be keeping a lookout. Recovering his wits before the robber recovered his, Tatchell ran and raised the alarm at Rev. Donald (Dan) MacLean's house and then at the Lynch store, where someone telephoned the police.

The citizens of New Hazelton, believing, with good reason, that the robbers might harm Bishop and Fenton, weren't going to wait for the police to arrive. They went for their guns. Unluckily for the robbers, there were two good shots among them: Ben Smith, known as Arizona Smith, in whose hotel at least five of the robbers had stayed a few nights before, and the Presbyterian minister, Dan MacLean. His wife, Eva, later wrote:

Dan tossed his .44 Colt six-shooter to Barrie [Tatchell] and seized his Lee Enfield army rifle from the wall where it hung. Before more than a few seconds had elapsed they were running back down the street. Dropping flat on the ground behind the ore pile, they turned their guns on the bank doorway where a man with a rifle was clearing the streets with a hail of bullets.

MacLean had taken his firing position behind a couple of large rocks of galena ore that had been placed together as an advertisement outside the mining broker's office. This gave him a clear view of the bank, ninety to a hundred yards away. MacLean later testified:

I saw a man, or just about half of him, standing in the bank door holding a rifle, a man with a mask on his face. . . . I ordered him to come out and put his hands up. I thought I had too easy a chance to shoot him. I wanted to give him a chance. He raised his gun and fired. I just had time to duck behind the ore pile to avoid the shot. A piece of the ore I was hiding behind was blown off and a shower of splinters flew over my head, two or three inches over my head. . . . I just had time to get down. Then I fired back at this man and he returned it, and about this time Mr. Smith slipped up behind me and began firing too.

With other citizens who joined them in the gunfight, they kept the robbers pinned inside the bank.

"We were shooting back and forth there six or seven times," Ben Smith testified. "Every time he showed up in the door [of the bank] with a rifle, I shot at him and he jumped back. When they came out of the bank, they all came out in a bunch. . . . I emptied my rifle and hollered for more shells."

The robbers tried a Butch Cassidy–style escape from the bank, coming out firing and running fast for the bush. "They left the bank," Bishop testified, "and as they left they fired their guns at us." In the two-minute gunfight, in which over 200 shots were fired, two of the robbers were killed, one was fatally wounded, dying later in hospital, and three of the others were hurt, two by bullets and one by running into a tree-branch. These three men and a fourth escaped into the nearby woods.

Horace and Dr. Stone were soon on the scene tending to Fenton, who had been grazed by a bullet, and to one badly wounded robber. Citizens followed the robbers into the woods, capturing three of them. The one that got away, Dzachodt Bckuzaroff, escaped with more than $1,000. People speculated that he had changed clothes and taken the next train out of town.

Thus ended one of the few shoot-outs in the old Canadian West. The gang members were all Russians. The three who had survived and been captured were quickly tried and each sentenced to twenty years in prison, after which they were deported. The *Herald* reported that the bullets the gang were using had been "split and notched" to cause maximum damage. The grateful Union Bank held a grand banquet to thank the citizens for the assistance they had given and presented a purse with $100 to each of Tatchell, Bishop and Fenton.

A curious footnote to this story intrigued everyone. Two of the robbers had been wounded and taken to the hospital, one so badly that he died a week or so later. While he and the robber who did survive were being treated in hospital, two Russians arrived in New Hazelton by train. They took the stagecoach (perhaps auto-stage) to the hospital, where they showed up using homemade crutches and asking for medical help. After an examination that found nothing wrong with them, they left, appearing not to be in need of crutches any more. Who were they? What had they wanted? Could it be, the citizens of Hazelton asked each other, that they had been planning to rescue the robbers from the hospital? This mystery was never solved.

———

The First World War came to most people in Hazelton like a hail-storm from a clear blue sky. There was surprise, and anxious questioning about where it had come from and how it had been allowed to happen. Although there had been warning signs for some years, no one had really paid much attention. In 1912, for example, there had been reports of a possible Anglo-German war, averted as always, and of a sinister military organization in Servia (Serbia) called, somewhat melodramatically, the "Black Hand." Archdukes in brightly-coloured uniforms with old-world feathers on their helmets seemed to be from some comic opera, somehow a different dimension from life on the frontier. Then one of them was assassinated in Sarajevo.

At the beginning of August 1914, alarm bells about the situation in Europe began to ring loudly. On August 1, the *Miner* reported that the "Great Powers [are] on the Verge of War." Russia, it said, was mobilizing its forces. Martial law had been declared in Germany. Austria had formally declared war on Servia. Could it really be true that Europe was about to plunge into strife? "In Great Britain," the *Miner* went on, "there is a feeling of confidence but no great excitement. It is generally hoped that mediation will be accepted by the belligerent nations before other powers become embroiled."

Such hopes were unfounded. By the time of the next issue, August 7, the war between the European nations had broken out. King George had signed the official papers and issued a statement to his overseas dominions expressing his confidence that the Empire would stand united, calm and resolute. The first men of the Canadian militia were ordered to report for duty at Halifax to relieve the 63rd Rifles and the 66th Fusiliers, who had been ordered for defence duty elsewhere. Assuring everyone that the army would absolutely be a volunteer force, the government issued orders for a Canadian Division numbering 21,000 men.

Few people at the picnic in the hospital pasture that week would have understood what it was all about. Led — or misled — by the newspapers, they blamed the evil Kaiser and believed it would end soon. A minor spat in a distant land, no more. Europe was, after all, far away and far distant from the experience of many residents. Even fewer would have expected the war to last for four years and lead to huge casualties that would affect Hazelton deeply.

Two hundred attended the hospital picnic that week, which was described by the *Miner* as "the most successful affair of its kind ever held here." Dr. and Mrs. Wrinch were given credit for organizing yet another enjoyable social event with, as the *Herald* said, their usual skill. Everyone had a good time and enjoyed the sports. Cooper came second in the boys' race for those under twelve. Horace and Arthur came second in the wheelbarrow race. Notwithstanding that Leonard played in the ball game between the old town and the new town, the new town won. "New Hazelton captured the banner and felt proud," the *Herald* said. "It will hang in that most public place, the *Herald* office. This office is a sort of shrine for all valuable souvenirs."

In the races, the *Herald* went on, when any contestant held back and did not enter, "Dr. Wrinch propelled the laggard into the arena. Men who had not run for years, unless to a fire, sprinted like colts." Soon, many of them would be volunteering to join the army and running in less bucolic pastures. No one in Hazelton would have had any idea of what was about to sweep over them.

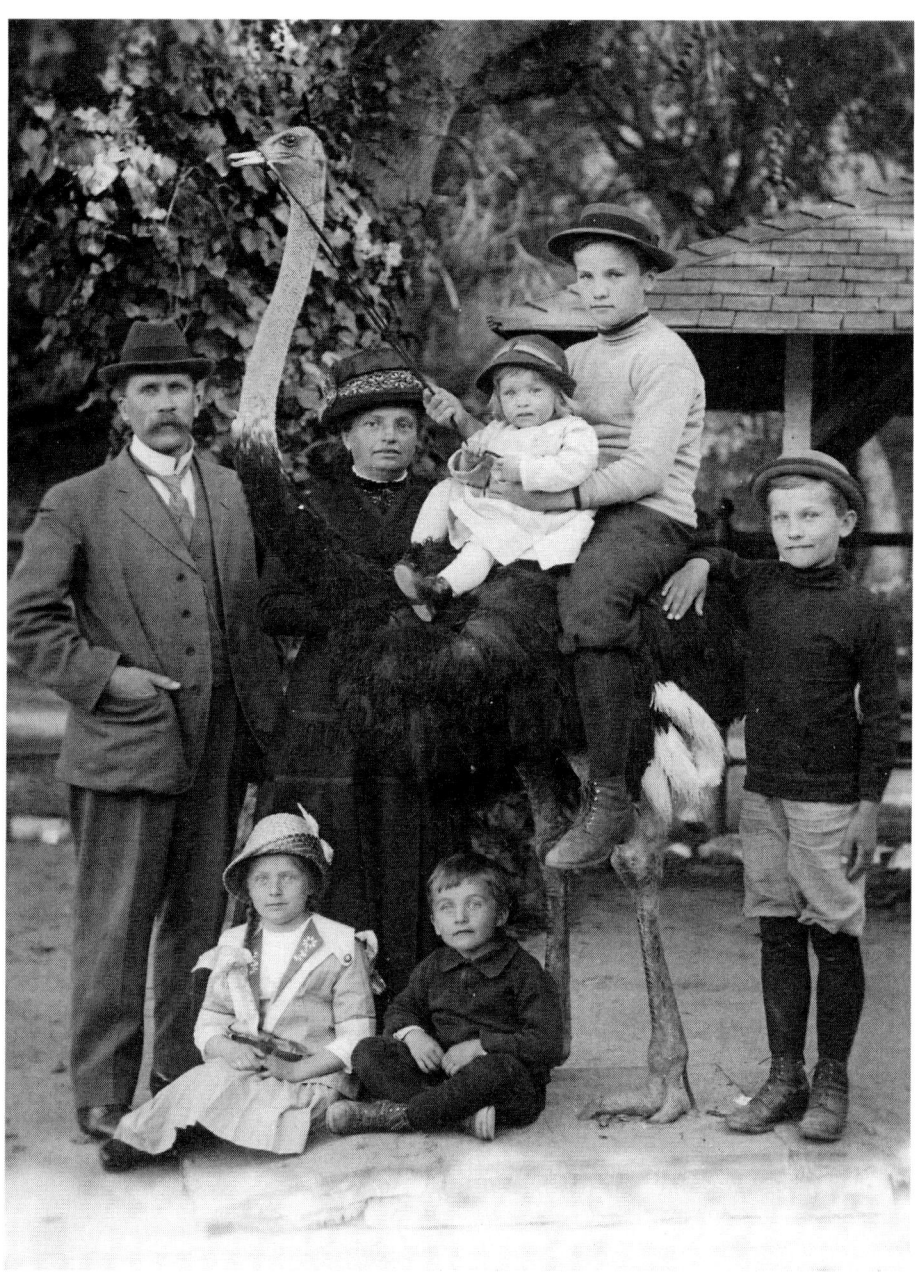

The Wrinch family at the Cawston Ostrich Farm in Pasadena, California, in 1913. Leonard on the ostrich is holding Harold. Ralphena and Arthur sit on the ground. Cooper is standing.

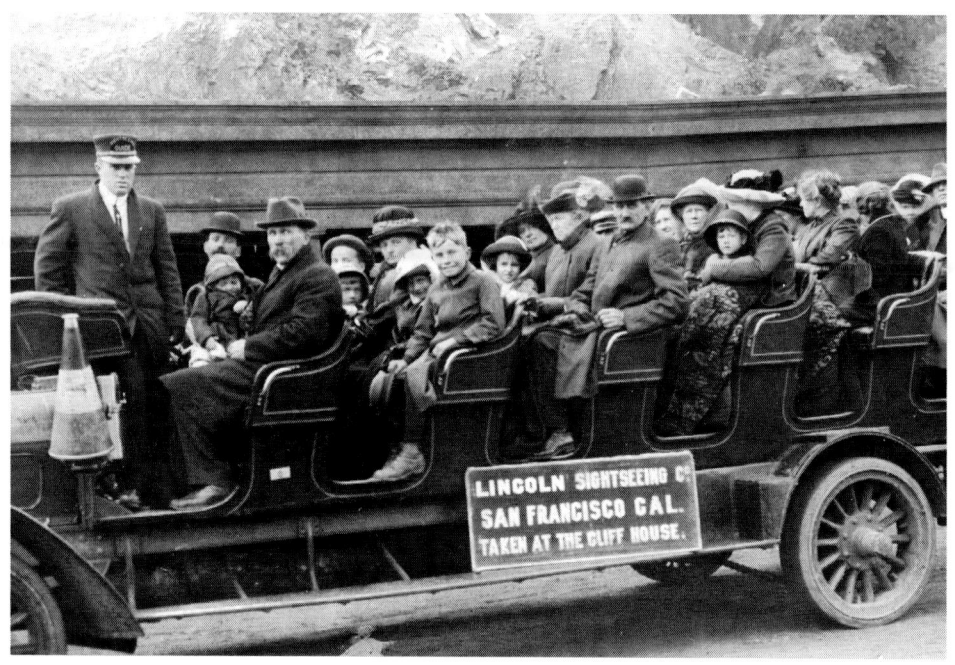

The Wrinch family, in front two rows, sightseeing in California in 1913.

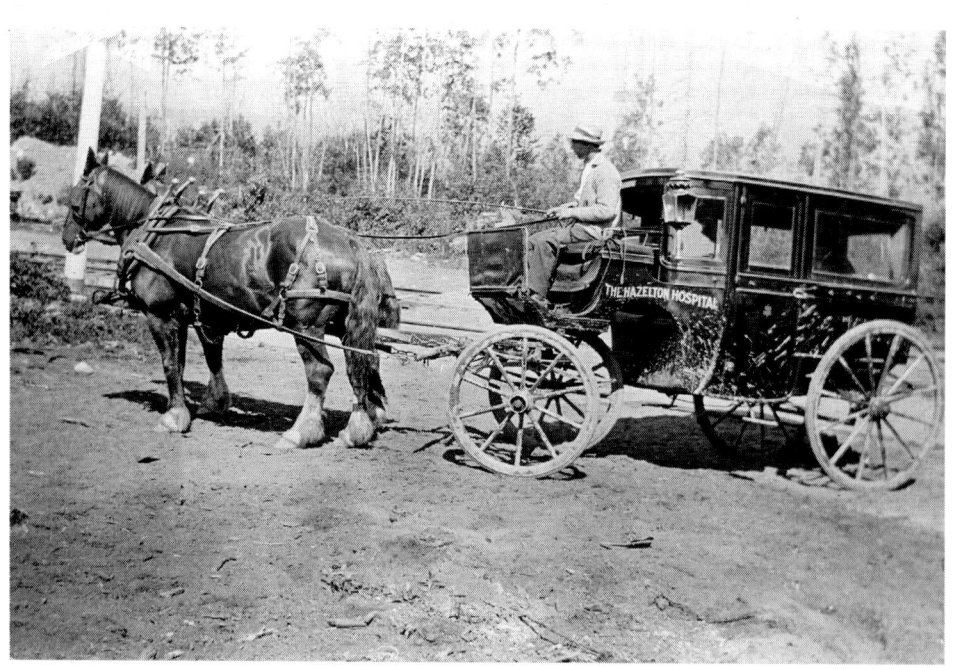

The Hazelton Hospital ambulance.

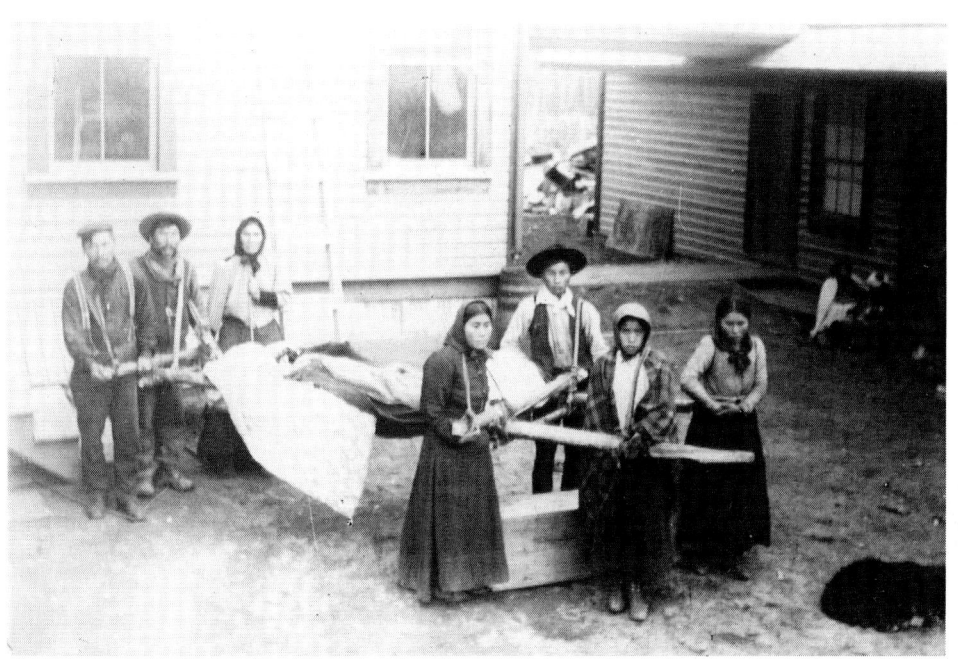

First Nations stretcher party.

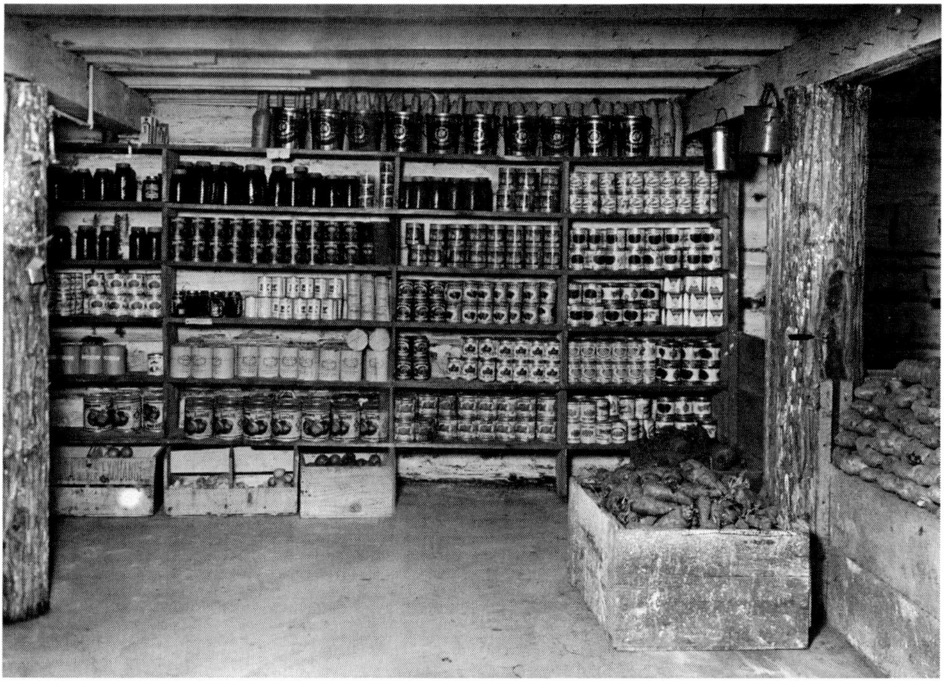

Basement storage of canned food for the hospital.

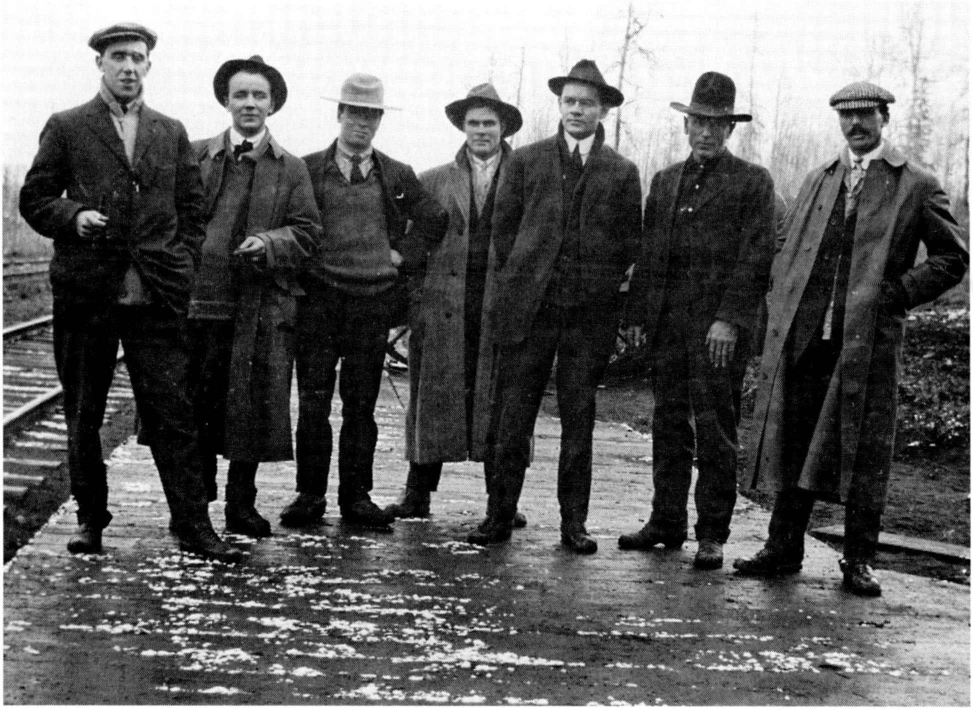

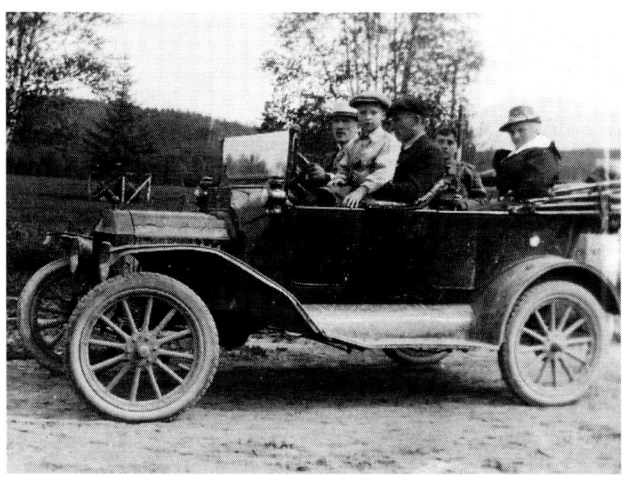

Volunteers leaving for WWI on November 5th, 1914. In no order: G.R. Middleton, John Frost, James Turnbull, Thomas Brewer, John Nesbitt, Andrew Monour and Lorne Fulton. Astonishingly, all came back.

Wrinch family in their automobile.

CHAPTER 9

The War Years
1914–1918

SOMETIME DURING THE First World War, Horace was seen sitting
on a bench in Hazelton, knitting socks for the Red Cross to send to
the boys at the Front. The picture is a charming one. The story sym-
bolizes both his and Hazelton's war effort: a community supporting
its boys at the Front, endearing, but more than a little unknowing
and innocent about the reality of the war. In space, time and understanding, the war in Europe was a long way off. What it was all about
must have been very confusing for Hazelton residents. For most of
the war, the soldiers who joined up were volunteers. The patriotic
enthusiasm the start of the war engendered gradually settled down
into grim acceptance when news of dead and wounded relatives and
friends began to be reported. Canadian casualties were relatively light
until the Battle of the Somme in 1916, but they mounted steeply
thereafter.

Horace was now approaching fifty. Although his children were growing up, they were still far too young to be caught up in the war, which would obviously be over long before they would feel any urge to volunteer. Sons Leonard and Cooper, thirteen and eleven respectively in 1914, would by necessity be going to Vancouver for schooling because at this time Hazelton had no high school.

The *Herald* and the *Miner* faithfully recorded their arrivals home for vacations and their departures back to school, and noted in the Local News section when they won prizes, which they often did. Leonard attended King Edward High School in Vancouver, where he was awarded a Governor General's Medal and, later, a scholarship from the University of British Columbia for the most proficient high school graduate in the province. Cooper passed his examinations for high school. Ralphena and Arthur at home were growing up fast, while Harold was not yet a toddler.

Canada, tied to the Imperial Government in London, was immediately drawn into the conflict. At the start there was much patriotism, jingoism and distortion of what was happening. In August, repeating the slanted news sent to it, the *Herald* announced that the British Navy had inflicted a crushing blow on the German Navy and said that "it is now almost universally looked for that Germany will be smashed in three weeks." In September, a headline announced as a known fact that the "Kaiser is looking for peace."

All over the British Empire, people broke out in a fever of patriotism. As they did from every town and hamlet in Canada, men from Hazelton rushed to volunteer. Stanley Geary and Constable R. Ponder were the first to go. Both were already in the naval reserves and so were called to the colours immediately. After a rousing send-off at the Omineca Hotel at which there were many "patriotic speeches and songs," they left on August 4.

In the first days of the war, the government agent in Hazelton, S.H. Hoskins, received a telegram from John Reid Barker, a telegraph operator at one of the cabins on the telegraph line, that read, "In case of need, please enroll my name among volunteers for active

service. Mounted or foot. Will take about ten days to reach town."
Barker, a man from Brierfield, Lancashire, had fought in the South
African War and apparently did not want to miss this one. Wounded
in the ankle at Ypres, he was later invalided out of the army with
eczema and possibly returned to Canada.

The authorities sprang into action with surprising alacrity. Within
that first week of the war, big guns were brought from Esquimalt to
be mounted on the bluff that overlooked the narrows in Vancouver's
Stanley Park. Canada sent a million bags of flour to England. On the
Skeena River, eight special constables were sworn in to guard the
New Hazelton bridges from fierce assaults from the Kaiser's forces
or, perhaps more likely, some pro-German fanatic. (As fate would
have it, one of the guards, Bert Taylor, was murdered at Sealey Gulch
in October, but this had nothing to do with the Germans, being a
simple case of drunken robbery.)

Premier McBride moved startlingly quickly. Hearing of a conversation in the Union Club in Victoria on July 29 that the Chileans
were behind in their payments for two submarines being built for
them in Seattle (although they had paid ninety percent of the purchase price), he persuaded the Americans to cancel the contract and
sell the submarines to British Columbia instead. Afraid that, once
war was declared, neutrality laws would prohibit the Americans from
delivering them, he arranged for speedy test trials and delivery four
miles outside British Columbia's waters on August 4 — the day war
was declared. For three days, before the Dominion took the submarines over, British Columbia had its own navy.

The community of Hazelton gathered on November 5, 1914, to
wish good luck to a group of volunteers leaving to join the Prince
Rupert Light Infantry. G.R. Middleton was a teller in the Union
Bank, secretary of the athletics association and goaltender for the
soccer team. John Frost was a rancher. James Turnbull and Thomas
Brewer were forest rangers. John Nesbitt, a forest warden, was a veteran from Strathcona's Horse of Boer War fame. Andrew Monour
was a clerk in the Bank of Vancouver, and Lorne Fulton, a druggist

from the Up-To-Date Drugstore, joined up expecting to join the medical corps. Hubert Wrinch, Horace's nephew, who had been managing the Up-To-Date Drug store in New Hazelton, also joined up. And in December, Dr. A.F. MacAuley from the hospital staff left to join a regiment in Prince Rupert.

In June 1917, May Hogan, the lady superintendent and matron at the hospital, left to join the Overseas Nursing Staff of the Canadian Forces. Her friends gave her a good send-off at Hazelton station. After first serving on the staff of the Ontario Military Hospital in Orpington, Kent, she was transferred to "somewhere in France" in January 1918. She served, in fact, at the No. 10 Canadian Stationary Hospital in Calais — still considered in the war zone since Calais was a target for German bombers. That December, she sent back to her mother a German steel shrapnel-helmet as a souvenir. After the war had ended, she remained in England for some months nursing at the No. 3 Canadian General Hospital.

—⁓—

Like every other community, Hazelton endured the war as best it could, trying to keep a sense of normality amidst the ever-grimmer news. Soon, stories of the daily happenings of Hazelton appeared side by side with grotesque news of the war, and this became normal. The *Herald*'s headline in April 1915 that the "Canucks Made Brilliant Charge Saved the Day But Lost Severely," accompanied the report that Dr. Wrinch had secured a lease on a building on Ninth Avenue in New Hazelton and would soon be moving his drugstore to the new location. The *Miner*'s headline in 1916 telling of the "Great Slaughter in the West" — this was the Somme — lay next to the report of the success of the Telkwa barbeque. The following week, the report that Horace, along with Alex Manson, had opened the Hazelton annual fair, deemed a great success for the remarkable display of fruit and vegetables, appeared on the page alongside the headline that "British Troops Again Smash German Lines." A reader could turn from reading about the repulse of the Prussian Guard with heavy losses, again, to the report that the ladies of New Hazelton had tastefully decorated a hall for a patriotic dance.

The people of Hazelton supported their boys at war. They knitted socks. They held a multitude of fundraising events. In the words of the song, they kept the home fires burning and looked for the silver lining as best they could. No fundraising event, concert or canvass was too small for them to organize.

The ladies of New Hazelton met one evening in the home of Mrs. Sawle. Since she was the wife of the publisher of the *Herald*, the meeting, which set up a branch of the Red Cross in New Hazelton, was well reported. The goal of the society was to knit socks and make nightshirts for the men at the Front. Lest one think that the ladies had strange ideas about trench warfare, it should be added that the nightshirts were intended for patients in hospitals.

The Hazeltons throbbed with all manner of societies and organizations to help their men in uniform. What the soldiers craved most of all were newspapers and cigarettes. One soldier in France wrote that he read and re-read the *Miner* four times cover to cover so as not to overlook any news, even though by then the news would have been woefully out of date.

Apart from necessary maintenance, the hospital ticked over during the war with no major improvements. Horace dedicated his fundraising work to the war effort rather than to the hospital. The major changes at the hospital had, in fact, already happened. In the week that war broke out, the electric power plant was turned on. With this, the recently installed X-ray machine became fully operational. Since it was not practical to run the generator during the night, it charged batteries that then had the capacity to light the buildings for a full twenty-four hours.

One evening in July 1915, Horace looked round the Assembly Hall. All was set for the Patriotic Concert. He inspected the decorations the ladies had put up. Flags hung everywhere. They had set out flowers in tasteful and patriotic arrangements of red, white and blue.

The Board of Trade, in common with many small towns across the country, was planning to buy a machine gun for the war effort, and this concert was to raise money for it. Horace was on the committee, together with that other Hazelton pioneer, Richard Sargent. After J.W. Morrison had given a stirring rendition of "The Best Old Flag on Earth" and Mrs. Goddard had sung "Your King and Country Needs You," Richard Sargent spoke about "Canada and the War." Horace then spoke about "Britain and the War" and lauded the generosity of the community in already donating $700 towards the needed $1,100 for the machine gun. The Rev. John Field then moved a resolution, passed unanimously, expressing a determination to continue the war in the interests of right and liberty.

By the first week of August, most of the required amount had been raised. Horace contributed $40 and Leonard, Cooper, Ralphena and Arthur each gave $1. (Voluntary or not, it was Arthur's first contribution to Canada's military effort. After the Second World War, he became a major general in the Canadian army.) The government, with a greater grasp of the realities of the conflict, quashed such well-intentioned initiatives to buy a machine gun and asked for the money instead.

During the war, Horace was chairman of the Hazelton Red Cross. Alice, May Hogan (until she left for the war) and her mother, Mrs. Hogan, living in Hazelton after her husband had died, were on the committee. In recognition of her splendid service to the Red Cross and other laudable causes, Mrs. Hogan was made honorary chairman. She also became the housekeeper at the hospital.

The annual picnic in the hospital grounds in 1916 raised $328 for the Red Cross. This year a midway had been added, boosting the proceeds considerably. In October, a special Red Cross canvass organized a series of social events, at which collections were taken. Another organization was the Soldiers' Aid and Employment Fund, which supplied tobacco and other comforts to soldiers in Europe. It was also to assist them re-establish themselves in civilian life when they returned.

The organizations that raised funds were soon tripping over themselves and duplicating each other's efforts. To improve efficiency, Horace for the Red Cross, S.H. Hoskins for the Canadian Patriotic Fund and A.R. MacDonald for the Soldiers' Aid Committee set up a central body to coordinate their efforts. During 1916, Hazelton's contribution to the Patriotic Fund was over $7,000.

The *Miner* applauded the community:

Hazelton is cheerfully bearing its part in the war for world liberty. No call for men or money has gone unheeded, and our town has fairly earned an enviable reputation for contributions of soldiers and cash. Up to the present time we have sent more than fifty men with various corps, and the list of soldiers from Hazelton and vicinity is being constantly added to. Over ten per cent of our population and approximately half our men of military age are members of Canada's overseas forces.

Proportionately, this ten percent was equivalent to 100,000 volunteers from a city with a population of a million.

The citizens of Hazelton were determined to support the boys at the Front and to "continue to a victorious end," the *Miner* said, "the struggle in maintenance of those ideals of Liberty and Justice which are a common and sacred cause of the Allies." To pass a resolution to that effect, they gathered in the Assembly Hall in August 1917. The proceedings opened with a hymn, followed by a prayer by the Reverend John Field and a biblical reading by Horace, who also "spoke ably to the resolution in his customary convincing manner." S.H. Hoskins then spoke and "disclosed the perfidy of the Huns in relation to the Scriptures." After listening to many more speeches, the citizens enthusiastically passed the proposed resolution. The Kaiser was instructed to take note.

During the war, a law, passed to preserve the meat supply, laid down that meat should not be eaten on Tuesdays and Thursdays. A wartime banquet was therefore held in April 1918, presided over by Horace. The purpose, he said, was not to raise money for the Red

Cross, which it did, but to show how one could eat in a healthy and simple way without eating meat or wheat. The main course was fillet of sole with Spanish rice and beans. "The service was excellent," the *Miner* reported, "and no delay was experienced in the serving of the meat-less and wheat-less food to the diners, no light task, as over eighty people attended."

Horace seemed to be involved in almost everything. He had to be busy. It was a virtue — or vice — that he showed not only then but also in later years when he was a Liberal member in the provincial legislature.

—✺—

Legend holds that Horace never did learn to drive an automobile with any acceptable degree of proficiency and that behind the wheel he became a terror to everyone around him. His son Harold used to relate that when his father had to go to Terrace in the early 1930s, he would be asked to drive him to ensure he arrived home safely. Reportedly, an old-timer in later years recalled with affection and respect that Horace had never owned a car he didn't roll. Here then was one activity at which Horace did not excel!

He acquired a Ford motor car in 1916 and took his newfound ability to drive to heart. New roads — more like improved wagon tracks in some cases — meant that he could move around the district much faster. These roads were still of poor quality and ran only between main centres. Because there was no resident doctor in Smithers during 1918, he went there on a regular basis, usually weekly.

"Dr. Wrinch," the *Miner* recorded on one occasion — though it is not clear if it was said with pride, despair or by way of warning — "has joined the ranks of speed demons. Receiving an urgent call to attend a patient at Smithers who was seriously ill, the doctor made the distance from the hospital to New Hazelton in fifteen minutes in his car. At New Hazelton a gasoline speeder [automobile] was placed at his disposal and, accompanied by two members of the GTP

Engineering staff, he raced to his destination, a fifty-mile journey in two hours."

There were few reports of accidents, but enough to give credence to his reputation for bad driving. On New Year's Eve at the beginning of 1922, for example, his car "had tried to climb a bank, but with poor success. Fortunately, little damage was done and the car was said to be running better than ever now." There is an archness about the *Herald*'s comments about his driving that suggests it was viewed as a shared joke by the community. Later the *Herald* quoted Horace as saying that he did not favour speed limits in British Columbia. "He favours speeding up the slow drivers. The doctor," it said, "will not need speeding up."

———

The Red Cross, home, hospital, nurses training school and the farm all kept Horace busy. Farming was Horace's special interest and gave an outlet for his practicality. Not surprisingly, therefore, he was president of the Hazelton Agricultural and Industrial Association. In October 1914, the *Herald* quoted him as saying that the agricultural experiments undertaken on the hospital farm had turned out to be extremely successful.

Two varieties of oats had grown well and had won first prizes at the Telkwa and Prince Rupert fairs. His millet, he said, had also taken first prize. The oats had grown to over six feet tall. Horace had also harvested forty tons of hay. The wheat he had been experimenting with for several years had taken first prize in both fairs. "What was the most interesting crop to the doctor was the peas," the *Herald* said. "He had been doubtful about them in previous years and had not attempted to grow any. In the experimental plot were the Prussian Blue peas and these did remarkably well." He also grew rhubarb indoors. The *Miner* reported that he had already cut his first crop of the year which was unusually early for rhubarb.

His son Harold recalled that his parents were both lovers of the soil, not only for the practical and necessary production of vegetables and fruits for the hospital, but also for growing flowers. He recalled:

> I can remember my mother gathering armloads of flowers in the morning to put in hospital wards and my father out in the evening, hoeing, tending and admiring the garden. This was his favourite relaxation. . . . As well as providing fresh vegetables and fruit, the garden supplied plenty of food for preserving for the winter months. In small fruits, we had raspberries, strawberries, rhubarb, gooseberries, black and red currants and crab apples. Larger fruits could not stand the cold winters. In vegetables, we preserved peas and beans — originally in glass jars and later in tins. Cabbages were hung up in the root cellar, as well as some potatoes. Other potatoes, several tons, were stored in the hospital basement in bins. The ones to be used in the spring before the new crop was ready were buried in large wood-lined pits in a field. The number fed from this supply was at least sixty persons. . . . In the 1920s there were men looking after the farm and garden and running the power plant. A Chinese man, Chowk, did all the laundry and still had time to puff on a two-foot-long bamboo pipe when he felt the urge. There were two men and one cook in the kitchen.

In delivering the hospital report for 1915, Horace reported that the previous year had been trying. However, the results "surprised and gratified" everyone. He warned that, although the small deficit had been eliminated, necessary repairs in the ensuing year would call for higher expenditures. By the end of 1917, the financial picture had deteriorated. Quite simply, income was much less than the cost of upkeep and necessary maintenance. "It will be impossible," the *Miner* warned, "for this institution to make ends meet without help."

There was, moreover, now an urgent need for a new sterilizer, which would cost $275. In pointing out the need, Horace, allowing himself a note of humour, wrote that necessary sterilizing of instruments and dressings "has been done by the use of small sterilizers having a very small capacity for work and a very large capacity for getting out of order. But for the angelic dispositions of our nurses, they would have gone on strike long ago for a proper sterilizer."

In January 1918, Horace therefore launched an appeal to the community for funds. A series of debates ("Should Women Be Allowed the Vote?" was one of them) and mock trials were held. The first mock trial was so successful, with a hundred people attending in a full hall, that another one was held the following week. In this one, Horace was persuaded to play the part of a "minor witness" and was photographed along with the rest of the cast, looking a little foolish and very self-conscious. In addition, a concert and a comedy (*The Return of Deborah*) were presented and a dance arranged for the Assembly Hall. These raised $200. Horace thereupon announced that the needed amount had been raised and thanked the community for its support.

—∿∿∿—

Horace's Methodist faith was his rock. This was his gold, his silver, his copper; this was the ore he brought to the surface and let enrich his medicine and good works. When he submitted the hospital annual report in "sincere acknowledgment of the overruling power of the Divine Being, in Whose Hand are All the Affairs of men," he meant it.

Whenever he was in Vancouver or Victoria, Horace took time to attend conferences, to give talks and also, when asked, to preach. These cities, though, were too far away for him to be in the centre of Methodist activity in the province. His activities were reported upon intermittently in the *Western Methodist Recorder*. He was active in the church, being on many, if not all, of the Methodist committees in the Skeena district. He was elected chairman of the district at the meeting of Methodists at St. Andrew's Hall in Hazelton in May 1917.

In this capacity, he attended to district business with the Methodist hierarchy. Once again he was selected to be the delegate to the Methodist conference in Vancouver. He took the Sunday services at the hospital, where Alice, May Hogan or someone else with musical talent played hymns on the organ — which was possibly the one that Alice had brought with her from Ontario in 1900. Many patients joined in the singing, a tradition that lasted for many years after Horace and Alice were gone.

His son Harold recalled that, though there was a religious element to the hospital, it was non-denominational. His father did not push religion on anyone. He said:

> He was of course quite religious, though he wasn't narrow about it. We had a good life. He was kind to us and we never seemed to lack for anything. He would bring in crabs and shrimps from the coast and at Christmas we had fresh vegetables like celery and tomatoes. In the early days we had no playing cards because that was gambling, but eventually he accepted that bridge was an intellectual game and we had lots of that. We were not allowed chewing gum, but of course we got that in town anyway.

On the way back from the 1917 Annual Conference in Calgary, Rev. J.H. White, superintendent of Missions at the time, visited the district to discuss co-operation with Presbyterians along the line of the Grand Trunk Pacific (the Skeena and Bulkley River districts). As chairman of the district, Horace represented Methodism at this meeting. White reported that after three very lengthy, deadlocked sessions, "finally, Dr. Wrinch made a proposition which attracted the most favourable attention and, after a full discussion, both in full committee and in denominational sections, a unanimous recommendation was made."

This recommendation led to the redefinition of boundaries and a closer focus on the coming together of churches in the district. Since this was beyond the authority of the delegates, they had to refer it to higher authorities, who approved it. This cooperation was clearly part of the larger discussion that led to the 1925 merger of the Methodist and Presbyterian churches as the United Church of Canada.

In discussing the good work the Methodist Church was doing on the Skeena, Dr. White went on to describe the hospital:

Nothing finer is being done by our Church in B.C. The Hospital is the best equipped in the north, with the possible exception of Prince Rupert. Dr. Wrinch and his staff are held in the highest esteem and are one of the largest factors in the standing which our Church enjoys in the estimation of the general public.

———

Horace may not have been an easy person to work for. He had a reserved and formal manner that some would — and did — see as coldness. More than one person recounted that he could be brusque in his manner of speaking. Fifty years old in 1916, he was, despite his progressive views on many things, in some ways very Victorian. He was a pillar of the Hazelton community and no doubt felt that the hospital was his: he had planned it, built it and run it, so of course he should be in charge. This did not always sit well with the collegial doctors of a younger generation who were coming to work at the hospital. It is noticeable that many of them did not stay for more than a couple of years.

Dr. William Sager and his wife, Hettie, arrived at the hospital in May 1916. Having graduated as a doctor only a few years before, Sager was twenty-nine and waiting to go to China as a medical missionary. He and his wife quickly clashed with Horace. Gregarious and informal themselves, they found Horace overbearing and difficult. Dr. Sager apparently thought that as a professional he should be an equal partner in running the hospital. Just as clearly, Horace thought he should not.

Horace had taken possession of his new Ford automobile the week the Sagers arrived. He met them at the station with this new car, of which Sager said, "he seemed very proud" and drove them over the Hagwilget Canyon, around Old Hazelton and then back to their new home on the hospital grounds. Sager described Horace at this time as a thickset man, with a moustache and a military bearing. "Will could see," Dr. Sager's son later wrote, "that Dr. Wrinch would be a tough taskmaster. He was pleasant enough but he had a cold and formal way of talking and seldom smiled."

Horace took Sager on his rounds visiting the Gitxsan in the district. "Dr. Wrinch seemed to know all of them, and Will noted that his rough manner only partly concealed a genuine interest in their welfare. He was abrupt and his attitude was paternalistic, but he was clearly a popular visitor, and Will had his first insight into the basic humanity of his authoritarian chief." Horace told Sager the names of the villages and places such as Moricetown, the Bulkley River, and Rocher de Boule as well as their original Gitxsan names. Will noted that "Dr. Wrinch expressed regret that so many of these colourful native names had been replaced by flat European ones."

The relationship between Horace and the Sagers did not, however, improve. Hettie, who soon took a strong dislike to Horace, was not at all happy in Hazelton. When she first made a visit into town, she did not like its dirty streets and "the rough-looking men, both white and Indian, around the saloons." Thereafter, she did not leave the hospital grounds except in the company of her husband and had her groceries sent up from Mr. Sargent's store. She was also busy with her young children and the rigours of winter.

At first, mistaking her reserve for coldness, Hettie found Alice to be unfeeling and formal. She soon saw her warmer side, though, and recognized that Alice too cared deeply about the welfare of the community. Her sympathy for Alice, who she said was not in the best of health, led her to believe that Horace dominated his wife as he did those around him. Hettie also blamed the difficulty of her own childbirth on the "ham-handed delivery by Dr. Wrinch," although she reluctantly admitted that the large size of the baby's head might have had something to do with her ordeal.

When Horace went to Vancouver for the annual Methodist conference in May 1917 and asked Dr. MacLean from Smithers to manage the hospital in his absence, Sager was incensed. "Will knew that he could do the job — he was now handling as many surgical cases as his chief and he was sure that Dr. Wrinch knew he could. It was a clear case of enmity, prompted perhaps by jealousy. Will was deeply shocked and disillusioned." Perhaps Sager, twenty-five years younger than Horace and only recently qualified, had unrealistic expectations.

After just over a year, Sager's posting to Hunan Province in China arrived. He preached his farewell sermon in Hazelton on June 17, 1917. He and Hettie were clearly happy to leave Hazelton, and Horace.

Horace's reserved, structured manner, though, could well have offended not only Sager but also other younger doctors coming to work at the hospital. A glimpse of this can perhaps be seen in Horace's relationship with another doctor, although, again, it is difficult to assess the truth of the situation. Horace wrote scathingly of this man, a prospective candidate for a position in church work in Telkwa and Smithers. This was too serious a responsibility, he wrote, to be taken on "by a man not definitely attached to our Church and concerning whose antecedents we know very little." He went on to note that the proposed person, a doctor, although charming and an accomplished violinist, had been undermining him in the hospital, where he had worked for four months, and might not be reliable in church work. Horace wrote that:

> While with us, he, as nearly as could be, wrecked our work by setting the staff all on edge. Thrice I was confronted with the task of reconciling different elements, and so bitter was the feeling that it seemed as if to retain one group meant the resignation of the other. . . . I am on terms of business courtesy with [him] of course and I feel I have been a good friend to him and have been generous with him in many ways. In fact, he professes the highest regard for me. At the same time by insinuation and innuendo, he does not hesitate to belittle and disparage the hospital to serve his own ends. Even while in the hospital, he sought to impress the nurses with the idea that where my ideas and methods did not accord with his own — why so much the worse for mine. But of course he let me down easy by suggesting that for one who had been out of touch with advanced thought and teaching

for so long, every consideration should be given. I am not writing this in bitterness but to give an idea of the character of the man . . . and to suggest that if he would carry on a double character in regard to the hospital and myself, it is not outside the realm of possibility that he might do so with regard to our church work. I would prefer to see one of our staunch and well-tried Methodist pastors at Smithers.

Clearly not the man for the job, if Horace had anything to do with it.

———

The annual celebration of Dominion Day on Monday July 2, 1917, was held on the hospital grounds as usual and was considered to have been the biggest and most successful picnic yet. Leonard had just arrived back from high school in Vancouver and was able to help out. Early in the afternoon and throughout the proceedings, motor cars disgorged large numbers of passengers at the gates of the enclosure, where tagging committees had an increasingly busy time coping with the constant arrivals.

Although the day was a little cool, the refreshment committee served ice cream and cold drinks to a continuous stream of thirsty souls. The shooting range, with a prize of a large box of chocolates for the winner, was well patronized and good score cards were turned in.

There were many sporting events. Young and old, competitors and spectators alike enjoyed the footraces, sack-races and wheelbarrow races. The pillow fight on a wooden horse caused a good deal of amusement to the onlookers as did the highly competitive ladies' nail-driving contest. The afternoon was rounded off by an al fresco supper, served by the ladies of the Red Cross. The dance in the evening was well attended, the music being provided by Mrs. Reid. After expenses of approximately $80, the proceeds for the Red Cross were a satisfying $438.

———

The war dragged on. In Ottawa, despite government promises, Prime Minister Borden introduced into the House of Commons legislation for conscription, provoking an instant crisis in Quebec. In France, General Haig's forces were "again smashing the enemy."

The men from the Hazeltons who had gone to war with such enthusiasm, believing they would miss out on a great adventure if they did not hurry, believing all the wishful thinking about the war being over by Christmas, had by now realized that the reality of war was horribly different.

The intensity of the experience in the front lines gouged a gulf between them and people back home, who had only a vague understanding of what their gallant boys at the Front were enduring. Wipers, Valcartier, seam squirrels, Festubert, Peggy, Vimy, Hill 70, dreams of a blighty, potato mashers, whale oil, Kinmel Park — all these words meant little or nothing to civilians. But for every man from Hazelton who served in the trenches, these words were heavy with meaning and memories of shared experiences and lost friends.

The reticence of returning soldiers to talk about the war is well documented. They seldom spoke about it because they believed that those who had not been there could never comprehend their experience. It was not until the mid-1920s that war memoirs began to be published and only then did most people begin to understand that the war had not been glorious, clean and heroic, that not all men had died quickly, bravely leading their comrades towards a fiendish foe.

Soldiers at the Front wrote home. Many of these letters, sometimes seeming to have been missed by the censors, were published in the *Herald* and *Miner*. James Turnbull, one of the volunteers in that first group of seven who, waving flags, had left in November 1914, wrote that the war was simply scientific murder. The Pats (Princess Patricia's Canadian Light Infantry) had again experienced a gas attack. Only about 150 of the regiment remained on the front line. At the time of writing, he said he had not had his clothes off for sixteen weeks. Then a lance corporal with the Pats in France, he wrote home the following year:

We are living on the lid of hell these days and don't know the minute when she is going to blow up. . . . We have been jumping around from place to place lately and there has been no time for anything. We've had frost and we've had snow, and we have fresh visitation of the white stuff this morning [March 4]. . . . The shells were landing twenty-five yards away last night. Fortunately they were high explosives, which either blow you to bits or miss altogether, so it is all right either way. I saw Lorne Fulton two nights ago and Spot Middleton about three weeks ago. We are quite near each other, but it's hard to get away when things are so nervy as they are now.

The toll on Hazelton men was heavy. Andrew Monour had been wounded in the head but, invalided back home, was recovering in the convalescent hospital in Esquimalt. Private Jack Frost was also invalided home and would have surgery to give him, it was hoped, full use of his injured foot. In September 1916, the *Miner* reported that James Turnbull of the Princess Pats had so far escaped injury, although only seven of the men who were with him when he joined remained in his company. Private James Hevenor arrived home on leave "minus an arm but in good health and spirits." He had gone away with the 102nd and had been wounded the previous September.

In 1917, it seemed that almost every issue of the *Herald* or *Miner* had tragic news. It announced the death of the Stoltze boy in February; Harold Findlay in March; H.P. Blake in April; Charles Helas and Frank Gray, killed at Arras, and H.L. Gibbs in May; and Major Tony McHugh in June. W.F. Brewer had also been killed in action. The death of E.E. Charleson, one of the best-known pioneers of the Hazelton district was announced in December. He was one of those who, years before at the December 1901 meeting, had given support to Horace for the building of a hospital.

Many who went to war from Hazelton did not return, and many of those who did return were injured in body or mind. A feeling grew throughout the war that more would have to be done to help returning soldiers and their families. It would no longer be enough to give each returned soldier the right to a section of land for the $10 allowed under the Homestead Act. War scrip would no longer be enough. Returning soldiers and war widows — indeed why not everyone? — should be provided with some form of health care. It was not as if there were no examples. In England, Lloyd George had shown it could be done. Horace was among those who thought that it was time to adopt similar measures in British Columbia.

In October 1918, while Europe lurched towards the armistice, another killer arrived. This one killed at home. Worldwide, the Spanish influenza pandemic affected up to five hundred million people, killing between fifty and a hundred million. One of the deadliest natural disasters in human history, it was first observed in North America in January (although there are many theories about where it came from), and it spread rapidly around the world.

The first cases appeared in Vancouver on Friday the 4th of October. Within days, the numbers mounted. One morning, Vancouver General Hospital had only a few beds occupied by patients with the flu and twenty-four vacant beds allocated for more. During that day, the hospital admitted forty patients, and the next day had 124 new cases. A call went out for a hundred volunteer nurses to deal with the growing pandemic. Four days later, there had been 1,156 cases, with fifty-five deaths. By early November, doctors were too busy to report numbers. In what must have been a heartrending few days for Horace and Alice, their son Leonard, who was away in Vancouver studying, contracted the flu. He was, though, fit enough — or lucky enough — to survive.

Inevitably the flu slipped along the railway lines, the roads and the rivers to Hazelton, arriving there in the second week of October. By October 25, the *Herald* was reporting that influenza had closed the town. The schools and churches shut their doors, and the railway gangs almost completely stopped working. With the hospital filled to capacity and more sick people being brought in all the time, Horace persuaded the manager of the hotel in New Hazelton to open as an emergency hospital. Harold recalled that his father also arranged for several railcars to be parked on a siding in South Hazelton, where they were used as an additional hospital. "The well are helping the sick," the *Herald* said, "and the doctor and his staff are putting in many extra shifts." Horace reported that he had treated well over a hundred cases and that the flu was now spreading to the Gitxsan.

The emergency hospital was a lifesaver for many. It was not enough, however, for thirty-four-year-old Peter Dale. A worker at the Silver Standard Mine, he had volunteered to accompany a sick couple to the hospital. Admitted to the hospital himself on November 8, he died five days later. His fellow workers at the mine redirected their Red Cross contributions for October and November to his widow. The flu then infected Dale's widow and four children. These all survived, though, and were discharged a week later, alive but without their breadwinner.

By November 15, the *Herald* reported that the Spanish flu, which had caused so much sorrow and suffering during the previous three or four weeks, was on the wane. It added, with an almost audible sigh of relief, that fortunately most of the cases in town had been mild. It stated:

> The checking of the disease locally is credited largely to the introduction by Dr. Wrinch of an anti-influenza serum. He had tried the provincial health department for assistance or advice, but was informed that there was no preventative and that the disease was asymptomatic. Finally the doctor got in touch with Dr. Ferrier, who was on his way here, and a supply of serum was secured in Winnipeg. Since then more has been secured. At the time of writing, not a case has developed among those treated.

How effective this vaccine (from the Provincial Bacteriology Laboratory in Winnipeg) really was is debatable. It has been said that there was not an effective flu vaccine until the 1930s and 1940s. However,

Horace and his patients believed that the vaccine he was administering did give protection against the disease.

The *Herald* said that Dr. Wrinch had reported 150 cases, excluding First Nations, in Hazelton and New Hazelton, sixty cases in Smithers and six in Telkwa and Moricetown. In all, only seven of these patients had died. By way of comparison, eleven percent — about 900 — of the flu victims in Vancouver had died.

As for the First Nations, Richard Loring reported to his superiors in Ottawa that at the end of October the Gitxsan communities had so far been immune to the malady. This, he said, was largely on account of their "being mindful of contagion and having resorted to a lesser extent about the town here and more at home on their locations." At the end of November, he reported that seven out of fourteen villages had remained "perfectly immune from the contagion."

Nonetheless, by the end of December there had been forty-three deaths among the Gitxsan in the whole district. In Gitanmaax, on the first bench above Hazelton, there had been eight deaths, including those of Martha Oakes and Sam Patsey. In Kispiox, there had been eight deaths, including Kum-kul-la-klak and Elfie Wilson. No children of school age, Loring wrote, had contracted the disease.

Jessie Gould, who had come to Hazelton in 1909 and knew Horace well, related that he was working all the time and "was often found asleep on the side of the road in his cutter [automobile], wrapped in his fur robes. After being out on all-night calls, he would be back in the hospital at 6 a.m." He did not spare himself and would pay a price.

Horace wrote about these times for the *Missionary Outlook*:

Uppermost in the thoughts of many will, no doubt, be the question as to how the work of the hospital was affected by the epidemic of Spanish influenza. It was naturally impossible, with our normal accommodation being fairly taken up with general work, for us to find accommodation for a big rush of epidemic cases. At the first onset we set apart accommodation for fourteen influenza patients, but this was taken up within a day or two. We realized then that other arrangements must be made, for influenza patients were being brought in on almost every train and they must be taken somewhere. Fortunately the managers of the Northern Hotel of New Hazelton were found to be willing that a portion of their rooms should be used as an Emergency Hospital. . . . It is a cause of profound gratitude that, while several members of the hospital staff were subject to attacks of influenza, they were all mild cases and no one has suffered either from the disease or its after-effects. . . . Surely in the face of all the difficulties and adverse conditions under which everyone has labored during the past year, we have the greatest reason for gratitude that, by the hand of Divine Providence, this hospital has been able to carry on its work in the manner it has.

Here we have classic Horace — the bare facts, the benefit done, consideration for others, thanks to God and no mention of himself.

Dr. H.C. Wrinch, the *Herald* said, summarizing the crisis, proved himself one of those supermen whose ambition in life was to administer to the sufferings of humanity. He was the only medical man in the district several hundred miles in extent. The *Herald* went on to comment that many people had been inclined to laugh at the disease rather than respect it. Horace, it said, faced great odds, but had set to work night and day. He had to make use of far too few resources to deal with the large number of cases, being called to a dozen places at once.

For a time, it looked hopeless, bright young lives were being blotted out and the number of sick was increasing. He kept going, covering many miles by car and by train. For three weeks he laboured, getting sleep on the road and meals where he found them. "Dr. Wrinch has always been worthy of the esteem of the local people," it said, "but he is now held in reverence by all. To him is given that which money cannot buy — the love of his fellow citizens."

In November 1918 came the end of the war. Amidst the rejoicings and flag waving, the *Herald* struck a quieter, albeit vindictive, note:

When the news came over the wire that the armistice had been signed — that the yellow had shown up in the cur and he had come to the Allies with his tail between his legs whining for peace — there was no shouting or cheering or flapping of flags, but there was a joy and a relief greater than would permit of noisy celebrations. While the hostilities have ceased, the war is not over, nor will it be until the articles of peace have been signed and the German Empire, with its newly established separate states, are deprived of every means of again waging war and until they have begun to pay for some of the damage they have done.

Here is the energy and the feeling, held widely across the victorious nations, that pushed the statesmen of the day into the Treaty of Versailles, thereby laying the foundations for the war that followed twenty years later.

By the following summer, those of Hazelton's soldiers who were coming home were back. Although May Hogan is the only woman named, over a hundred volunteers (mainly) from the Hazeltons had donned a uniform. Forty-three-thousand British Columbians, from a population of 450,000, had served overseas. Of these, approximately 6,000 had been killed and over 13,000 wounded.

Hazelton honoured its soldiers with a gala banquet in July 1919. Originally it was planned just for people from the Hazeltons, but there was so much interest that people came to honour them from Kispiox and Smithers and from as far away as Prince Rupert.

Once again the ladies had decorated the Assembly Hall with flags and flowers. Horace, as chairman of the organizing committee, surveyed the twenty or so chairs placed for the soldiers they were honouring. As Gray's Orchestra from Smithers played in the background, Horace and the committee formally greeted the guests at the doors. Practically everyone from Old Hazelton and New Hazelton was there. The agenda for the evening unfolded. There were songs and speeches, with Harry Broadfoot delighting the crowd with his renditions of Harry Lauder songs.

Horace gave the main speech and presented the soldiers with certificates of honour and appreciation. Captain Thomas Brewer expressed the thanks of the returning soldiers to the people of the district, not only for the night's entertainment but also for the manner in which they had worked and supported them during the whole war. After the formalities, there was dancing until three in the morning. Present also, perhaps, were the ghosts of those who had not returned in person.

Remarkably, all seven men who had joined the Prince Rupert regiment in November 1914, in the first enlistment from Hazelton, had survived. Four of them were present that evening: Captain Thomas Brewer, Captain J.F. Frost, Corporal James Turnbull and Sergeant L.D. Fulton. Spot Middleton was still in England with the Soldiers' Settlement Board and Andy Monour was with Molson's Bank in Victoria. Monour, though, like many others, never really recovered from the wounds he suffered in 1916. He died in October 1920, aged only twenty-nine.

Lieutenant May Hogan returned home in September 1919, arriving in Hazelton at the same time as the Rev. Willan, the new Methodist minister. The community welcomed them both at a reception in St. Andrew's Hall, "beautifully decorated with greens and flowers." There were speeches and songs, and everyone was glad the war was finally over.

A silence fell upon the land as it staggered out of the horrors of a war that should never have happened. And what of the world the soldiers had returned to, wounded or not? Many politicians made splendid speeches with fine words. Soldiers' Aid Societies were changing their plans to deal with peacetime activities. The government was again giving first options on farmland to soldiers. But not all returning soldiers wanted to farm. The government was giving each one a war gratuity, but that was not going to be enough. "Make the Returning Soldier Welcome," the Ottawa Repatriation Committee said in its advertisements. "Don't let the welcome die away with the cheers." For many people the time had come to go beyond statements of welcome and pious sentiments and to provide better health services for them and, indeed, for the population at large.

New ideas about community health were topics for discussion at the well-attended annual meeting of Hazelton Hospital's patrons in February 1919. Snow was lying thickly upon the ground. Many from Hazelton and New Hazelton had come to the hospital by sleigh, "where Dr. and Mrs. Wrinch and the nurses made everyone welcome and feel glad to be alive," as well they might be after a war in which twenty million had died and after a flu pandemic that had killed between fifty and a hundred million.

The patrons met in the main floor ward of the hospital, which was "prettily decorated and . . . filled to capacity." Before the meeting, Miss Uren, the lady superintendent of the nurses' training school, gave a demonstration of the new sterilizer and "made her accompanying talk most interesting." There was, as usual, a musical program followed by "dainty refreshments in an abundance that over-taxed the comfortable consuming capacity of the gathering and made everyone feel glad the war was over." The Valentine pie that the nurses had baked proved particularly popular.

Mr. Cairns from Vancouver, the representative of the Indian Department on the hospital board, praised the work of the hospital. He also spoke about the growing movement to make all medical and hospital treatment free and predicted this was coming in the not-too-distant future.

An editorial in the *Herald* the following week reported on the movement that was gaining ground — state control of hospitals with free treatment, medical services and advice to all. In Alberta, it said that there were already community hospitals that were proving beneficial. The *Herald*'s editorial writer would have been present at the meeting and he reported what he had heard. "The object today is to treat the largest number of cases at a given point where accommodation, equipment, and medical, surgical and nursing skill can be provided."

At a convention of the new British Columbia Hospital Association in Vancouver the previous summer, one of the themes had been that the hospital should be a community service. This, clearly, was what Horace had been thinking for a long time.

The strain of dealing with the Spanish flu pandemic had taken its toll on the fifty-two-year-old Horace's health. He fell ill, having what the *Herald* called the only serious illness of his life. Whatever it was, it forced him to take time off, but not for long. By the end of January 1919, he was, the *Herald* reported, back in town for the first time in a couple of weeks, "although he is still far from being his old self." No doubt exhausted, Horace likely would have looked forward to some peaceful years with Alice in a world made safer and happier by the struggles of the previous four years. But it was not to be.

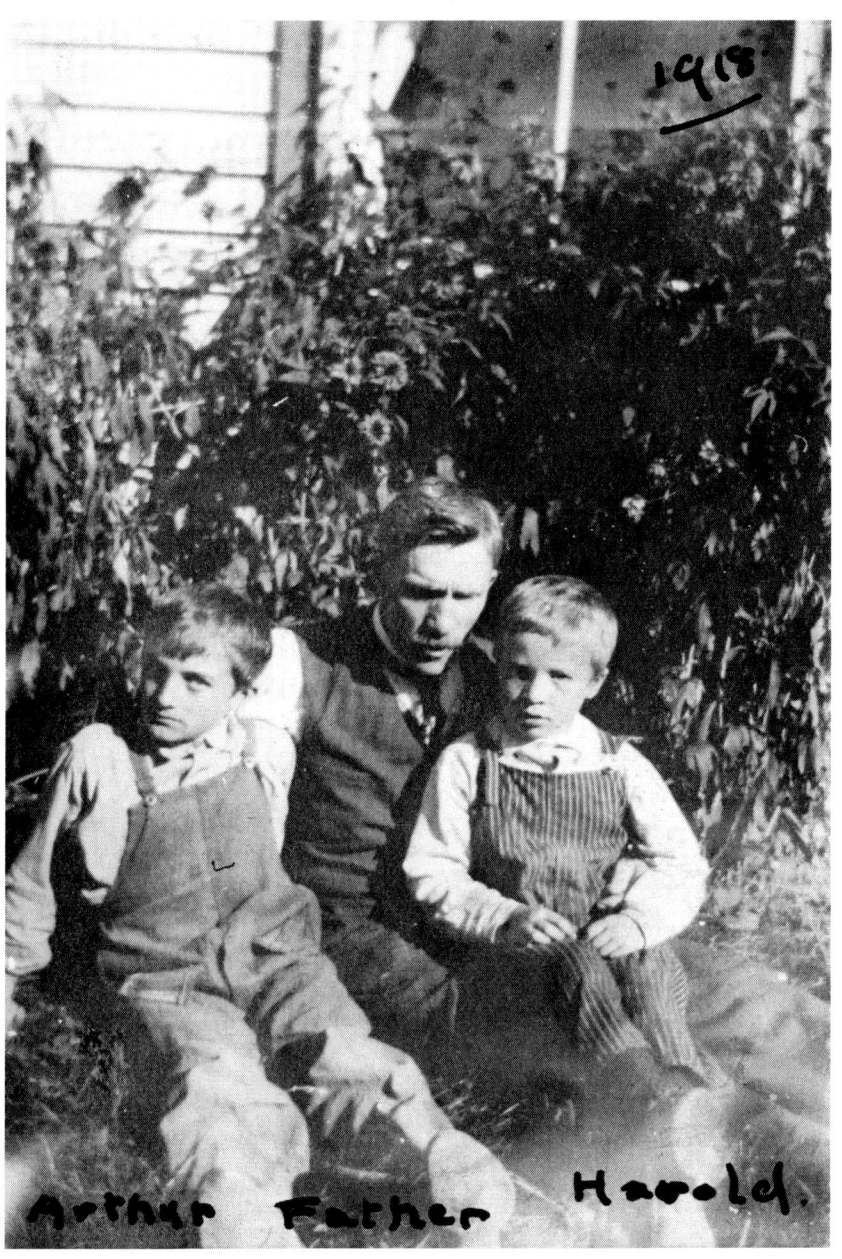

Horace with sons Arthur, left, and Harold in 1918.

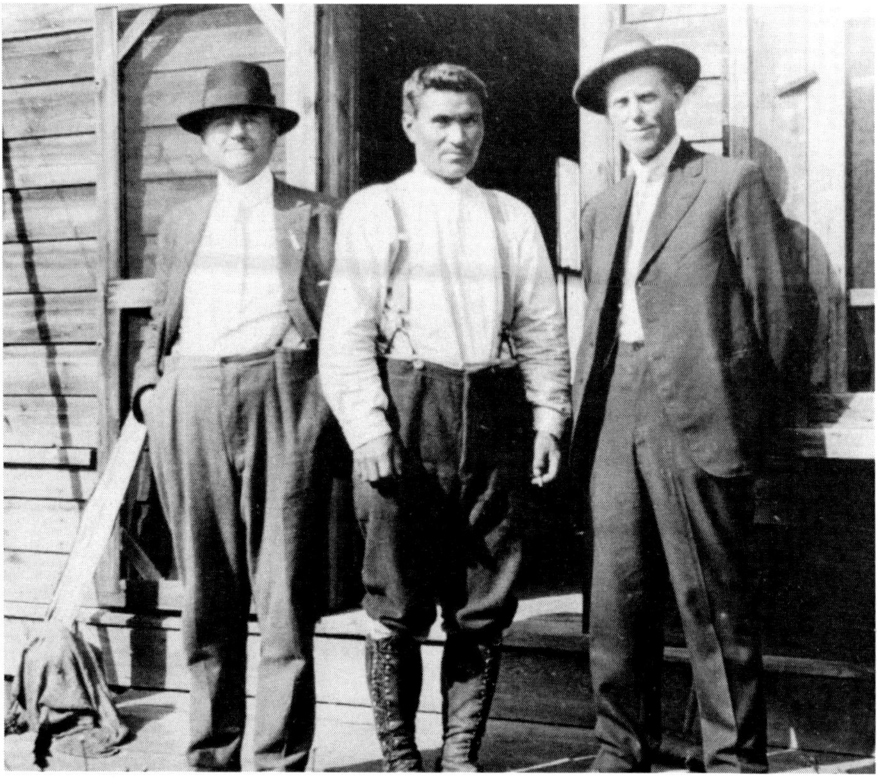

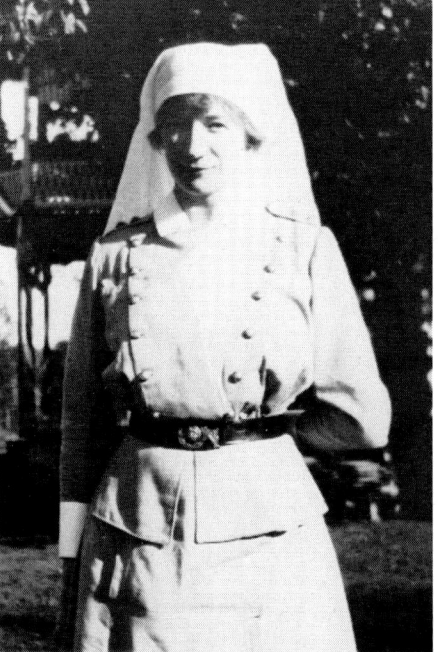

▲ Simon Gunanoot, centre, after his surrender in 1919. Stuart Henderson, his lawyer, at left and George Beirnes at right.

◀ May Hogan, later Horace's second wife, when she joined up in WWI in 1917.

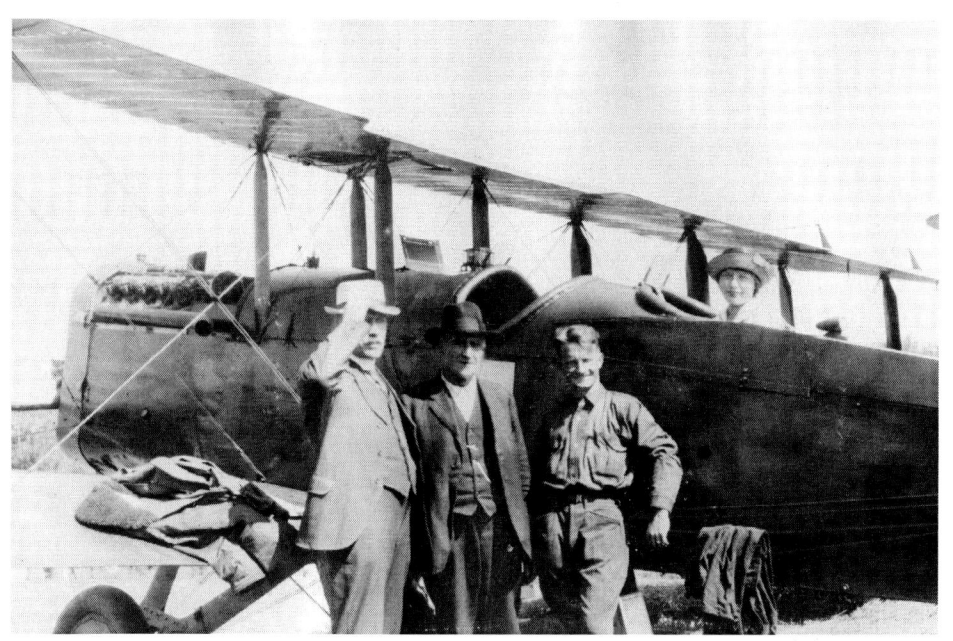

Horace with Captain St. Clair Streett and the first aeroplane to
visit Hazelton, in 1920, on its way to Nome, Alaska.

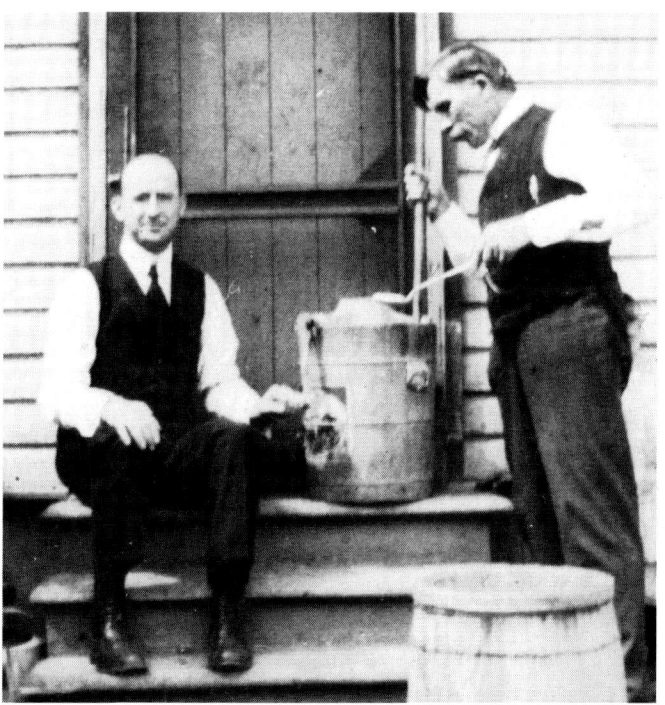

Making ice cream for a Hazelton Hospital picnic.

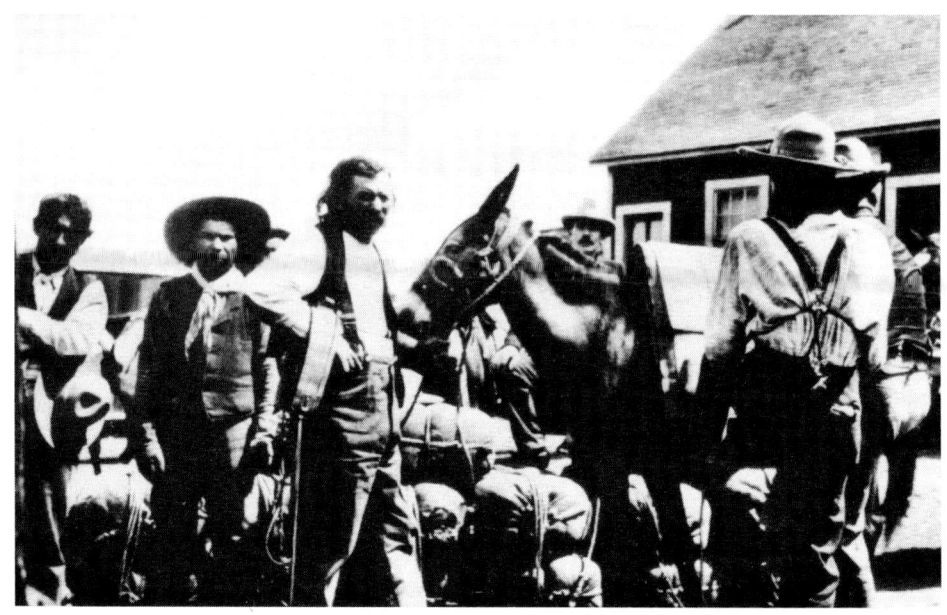

Cataline (Jean Caux), third from left, the famous packer.
He died in the Hazelton Hospital in 1922.

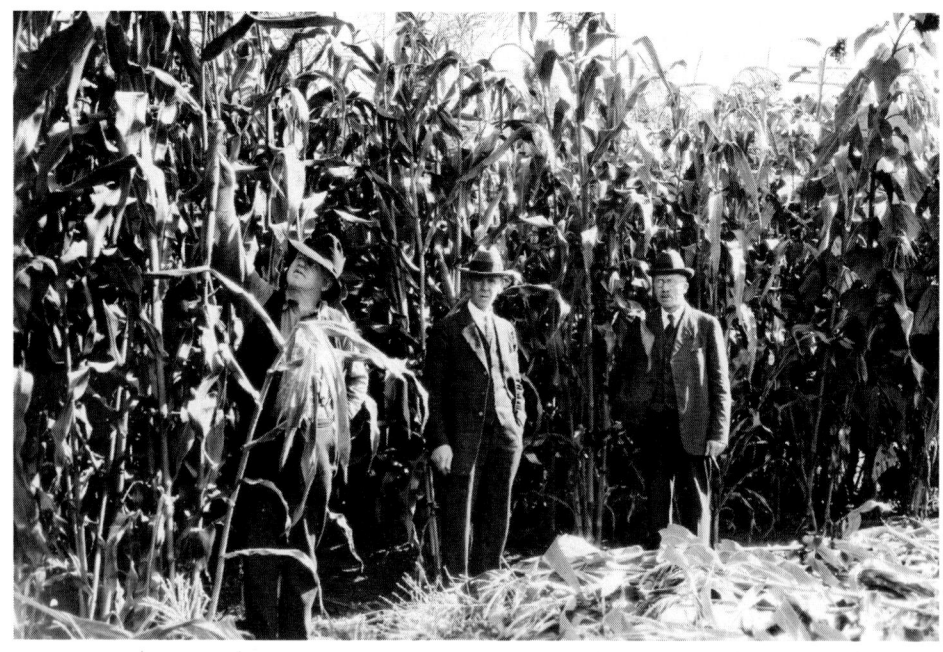

Sperry Cline, Richard Sargent and Horace in front of the crop of corn and
sunflowers Horace grew on the triangle lot in Hazelton in 1925. The corn was
12½ feet high, the sunflowers 13 feet high.

CHAPTER 10

Brave New World
1918–1923

HORACE AND ALICE, aged fifty-four and fifty respectively, celebrated twenty years of marriage in June 1920. She was his pillar and his staff, his assistant and his companion. She had given their children the nurture that Horace, always busy and a little distant at times, perhaps had not. The two eldest boys, now adults, were well able to stand on their own feet. In January 1919, Leonard, who was finishing his first year at the University of British Columbia, took his brother Cooper back to Vancouver so that he could attend King Edward High School. Leonard did well, earning the highest marks during his first year of university and winning the Royal Institute Scholarship. Deciding to study medicine, he went first to complete his undergraduate degree at the University of Alberta, where he obtained his Bachelor of Arts degree with honours. Meanwhile, the *Herald* faithfully reported that Harold, Horace's youngest son, had won the race for the under-tens at the 1921 Empire Day celebrations in New Hazelton.

Harold remembered his father as a tall man, broadly set but not portly. "I never saw him, I think, without a collar and tie," he said. "He was always formally dressed. A strong person." Settled well into familiar clothes — old friends such as his homburg hat and favourite neckties — Horace would also have been settled in his ways and convictions. There was much in this brave new world that would strike him as not being right, not being the order of things as they should be. Times indeed had changed.

His children were bringing to him all the noise and bustle of new ideas, new ways of thought and new moralities. His flashing missionary zeal of the 1890s had mellowed into mature service to the community and to his Methodist Church. Horace had reached the point in his life where he would have understood that there were more years behind him than ahead. He would have thought that the hospital, the farm and the church and a quiet and settled middle age with Alice at his side would be what the future held for him.

In February 1919, soon after the annual meeting of the hospital patrons, Horace and Alice went to Rochester, Minnesota, so that he could study the latest methods in surgery at the Mayo Clinic. He welcomed this chance to rest, away from the demands at Hazelton and also to recover from his exertions of treating the Spanish flu. "I am very glad I came to Rochester," he wrote in late March. "The surgery that is being done here is of the highest character, and there is such a great amount of it that the visiting surgeon can be profitably engaged every hour of the day." They returned to Hazelton in April after a successful, restful and instructive time away.

Horace's work as chairman of the Red Cross continued. Although it still had a large and enthusiastic membership, now that the war had ended it no longer had a defined purpose. At the annual meeting in November, Horace, as well as Alice, were thanked, "it being conceded that no other occupant could have been found to give such whole-hearted and able attention to the duties thereof." Helpful as always, Richard Sargent proposed that the branch should direct its efforts towards the Hazelton Hospital, financially and otherwise, while holding itself open to assisting with relief after disasters. This, the *Herald* said, was a "very worthy move." It helped, of course, that, as everyone knew, Sargent was chairman of the hospital board. Full disclosure cures many a conflict of interest.

Horace continued his work in Hazelton, balancing his medical practice with the business of managing the hospital. As always, he seemed unable to refuse an invitation to be on any committee for the public good. In 1919, he was elected to the Soldiers' Aid Committee, which, like the Red Cross, was adjusting to what it should do in peacetime.

Horace was still very much a farmer, not only on the hospital farm but also in the Bulkley Valley. While visiting his brother Leonard, now settled on a farm at Chilliwack, approximately sixty miles east of Vancouver, Horace took a closer look at the farming in the Fraser Valley. He went to see the Timms tomato greenhouses, which had several acres under glass. He also went to the Vancouver nursery farms to investigate seeds and to the milk corporations in the Valley to learn how the farmers had banded together to cut out the middlemen and supply the Vancouver market directly.

As secretary of the Hazelton District Stock Breeders Association, he had written to C.W. Peck, V.C., now a local member in the federal parliament, asking for money for fences to keep cows in the Hagwilget area from straying onto First Nations reserves, thereby causing mayhem and increasing the likelihood of conflict. At home at the hospital, Alice imported ten white Leghorn chickens, trying as always to keep them safe from marauding dogs.

In 1919, the Advisory Board of Farmers Institutes had been gathering information about agriculture in the North. Mr. Burrow, the minister of agriculture, was chair of a committee that came to inspect the prospects for farming and to listen to farmers' concerns. Horace was one of those who made presentations to the committee in Smithers, and he used the opportunity to inform it that there were not enough doctors in the North. Times had changed, he said. If they wanted farmers to settle in the Bulkley Valley, they would need to make better medical care available. His written submission on this need was attached to the committee's report.

In 1920, perhaps inspired by his friendship with the Large family, Horace became a Mason. He was initiated in the Tyee Lodge No. 66 in Prince Rupert and raised to membership in October 1923. Richard Geddes Large, the son of Horace's friend from Trinity Medical College, and soon to come to the hospital as a young doctor, in later life would become a Grand Master.

———

Whenever anyone important came to Hazelton, it fell to Horace to plan the event and act as host. In September 1919, the Governor General, the Duke and Duchess of Devonshire, together with a vice-regal party, came to visit. With others on the committee, Horace welcomed them at the New Hazelton train station. Under clear blue skies, the vice-regal party climbed into eight cars for a drive around the district, stopping at the Hagwilget bridge to admire the canyon and meet local First Nations.

They visited the school where Miss Wallace had arranged for the children to build an arch of flags and maple leaves. The children presented the duchess with a bouquet of sweet peas and locally grown roses. The Governor General then declared a holiday for all. The guests came back to the hospital for a tour and lunch, after which they chatted with patients.

Later they inspected the collection of Gitxsan art, tools and cultural objects that Horace had acquired over the years. After another stop in Hazelton — more gifts, more speeches, more bouquets — the party returned to the station to continue their journey. "To Dr. Wrinch," the *Herald* said, "is due the credit for the successful planning and carrying out of the program." All had gone well except for the fact that the car in which the duchess was riding had stalled at the top of a hill. She cheerfully jumped out, the *Herald* said, and put her shoulder to the wheel to help the car over the top.

The *Herald* was a cheerleader for Horace, partly because Sawle, the publisher, was an old acquaintance from before the war. If there was any criticism of him at this time, it was not reported, at least, not yet. In February 1920, the paper gave this assessment of him:

> Dr. Wrinch is remarkably well balanced. He has worked up a big job for himself, and he developed himself along with the job. Today he is a successful farmer, a successful financier, a successful manager, a good student, a successful doctor and an exceptionally clever and successful surgeon. In the first and last mentioned labours he might be classed as a specialist. Dr. Wrinch is modern in his ideas and surrounds himself with the very latest equipment and perfects himself in its use. At the same time, his enthusiasm and thoroughness permeate the entire staff, which results in the unqualified success of the Hazelton Hospital. The *Herald* holds no brief for Dr. Wrinch and our only object is to point out to the public some of the essentials to a successful hospital.

In this recital of Horace's virtues, rather obviously designed to help the hospital's fundraising efforts at the time, the *Herald* made no mention of his activities as a Methodist minister. The one thing that motivated him more than anything else, the one thing that gave him the soul and spirit for all his activities, it missed completely.

——⁓——

In 1920, Horace almost became the medical superintendent of a second hospital. He was drawn into the rivalry between Smithers and Telkwa regarding the best location for a new hospital in the Bulkley Valley. If Dr. Wallace had established a hospital there, it did not survive, perhaps being destroyed by the disastrous fire of April 1914. Nevertheless, with the population in the district growing and with the railway opening it up for commerce and farming, there was a clear need for a new hospital. Horace himself had made the point the previous year to Mr. Burrow, the minister of agriculture, when he was touring the district. Settlers in the Bulkley Valley wanted more medical services. Horace had more work than he could manage at the Hazelton Hospital, and he therefore favoured a new hospital. Smithers and Telkwa, however, each wanted its own hospital.

Citizens in both communities set up committees, knowing well that even with government grants only one hospital could survive. A fierce competition developed between the two, each boosting its own claims and disparaging those of the other.

Both sides even acquired properties for their proposed hospitals. The Telkwa committee, supported by the Rattenbury Land Company, which was developing its huge land holdings in the district, said that the building Smithers had acquired was an old boarding house on a swamp without drainage. Telkwa itself had acquired the old Aldermere Hotel, situated on five acres on a five-year lease at $6.50 a month, with an option to purchase.

Horace, who had been asked to look at the proposed building and assess its suitability as a hospital, reported to a public meeting in Telkwa on April 6 and recommended proceeding. Dr. Wrinch, the Telkwa hospital committee said, had advised that the old hotel was admirably suited to be a ten-bed hospital. Horace confirmed to the government that the proposed building would suit very well:

> This site could hardly be improved upon for hospital purposes. . . . At the urgent request of the people who feel themselves entirely at sea in the development of the Hospital project, I consented to act as Medical Superintendent and assist them in laying out the interior of the building in a suitable manner, and generally getting the Hospital into operation. The time is certainly ripe for the establishment of another hospital east of Hazelton for the service of the people in the Bulkley Valley. . . .

The *Herald*, from Hazelton sixty miles away, told its readers that the Telkwa hospital was definitely going ahead and that government assistance was now assured. This, though, was premature. Smithers, with apparently more persistence than Telkwa, pressed on and announced that its hospital would in fact open in May. The *Interior News* in Smithers made a personal attack on Horace on April 21. Warner, the editor, accused him of being behind a recently published article, almost certainly in the *Herald*, which denied the need for any hospital in the Bulkley Valley and that suggested starting two small hospitals in the Bulkley Valley was absolutely wrong. The *Interior News* claimed that the author of the article in the *Herald* was afraid that two hospitals in the Bulkley Valley would only result "in lessening the efficiency of a hospital that provides medical treatment at a price and makes a nice fat living for Dr. Horace Conscience Wrinch [this was a reference to Hazelton Hospital]."

Warner continued his attack and speculated:

Our various enterprises were nauseous to that great apostle of all that is pure and true as well as to his humble satellite, the scion of righteousness and wisdom. Had the 'super-man' signed his name to the article the apparency of its source would have been none the more pronounced. Two weeks ago a movement broke out in our neighbouring town of Telkwa for the establishment of a hospital, a movement in which all attempts to get information met with 'Dr. Wrinch suggests this' and 'Dr. Wrinch advises that' and 'Dr. Wrinch intends' etc., and it is only reasonable to assume that Dr. Wrinch is no inconsequential spirit in the latest enterprise.

Horace's thoughts about this odd personal attack are not known, but they did not stop him from assisting the Telkwa hospital committee.

Soon after the article appeared, both committees wrote to the government, arguing their respective cases. Somewhat inconsistently, Warner accused Horace of supporting "lots of hospitals, so many indeed that they would all go broke and the business would still go to him." Horace wrote letters and when in Victoria met (or tried to meet) with the appropriate government representatives. He sent his draft floor plans for the proposed Telkwa hospital to the government in late June.

The inspector of hospitals, E.G. Arthur, wrote to the government on July 2 and assessed the merits of both hospital proposals. Everything Dr. Wrinch said about the Telkwa hospital was true, he said. It was a much better building and was on a better site, and Telkwa was more centrally located. However, in his view, Smithers would probably grow in proportion to the railway. Telkwa, being more rural, was a community "less likely to give effective maintenance to a hospital, than is one in which the majority of the population is industrial and commercial." Although Arthur seemed to be favouring the Smithers proposal, which he was reported to have provisionally approved some time before, he advised the government to wait and see. Perhaps, though, his advice on population growth was persuasive.

Smithers, in any event, pressed on. Its hospital committee perhaps realized that the first hospital to be finished and taking in patients would be the survivor. Accordingly, its Bulkley Valley District Hospital hired a matron, a Miss G.E. Eveleigh, and proceeded to complete the hospital, taking in its first patient in the third week of August 1920.

Premier John Oliver, in Smithers at the beginning of September on an electioneering tour, was invited to visit this hospital and officially open it. The premier said that the hospital was worthy of every support, and he promised the government would do its fair share in supporting it. That would have effectively ended the debate. Who was going to close a hospital the premier had opened? The Telkwa and District General Hospital Committee did not, though, give up and was still trying to get the necessary grant as late as October. However, it must have known it had lost the contest.

The Telkwa hospital disappeared from the record and may have settled down as a community nursing home. In December 1922, a nursing home was certainly in operation in Telkwa but appears to have been short-lived. In November 1924, a new nursing home was built in Telkwa, and Elizabeth Nock, a recent graduate from Hazelton Hospital Nurses Training School, was engaged as nurse-in-charge. When Horace visited the nursing home for the first time a little later, he found it "a most complete and comfortable institution."

—⁓—

A nearly forgotten figure from Hazelton's past re-appeared in 1919. So many settlers, railway workers and miners had come into the Skeena and Bulkley river valleys that some did not even know who he was or they thought of him merely as a legendary figure of myth and mystery.

Constable Kerry, on duty in Hazelton police station one morning, looked up at the man who had just walked in. Identifying himself as Simon Peter Johnson, he said he had come in to fight his case. Not knowing either who he was or how carefully this surrender to justice had been orchestrated, Kerry told him to return the following week when Sperry Cline, for some time a provincial policeman, would be back. When Kerry's confusion about the man's identity was sorted out, Simon Gunanoot surrendered to justice.

For thirteen years, Gunanoot had lived as an outlaw in the forests, lakes and mountains of northern British Columbia. He had become a legend, first as a savage murderer and then as a heroic outlaw. All the police, all the Pinkerton's men, and all the bounty hunters had failed to catch him. By 1919, though, Gunanoot was tired. He wanted a freer life. There had always been people, both Gitxsan and non-Indigenous, in touch with him, and they had kept him supplied with his ammunition and other necessities.

Some of them had contacted Cline, and together they helped negotiate Gunanoot's surrender. Cline had arranged to be in Prince Rupert when the surrender happened because, had it all gone wrong, he would have had to testify and his role in the affair might have caused him problems.

Gunanoot's surrender caused great excitement in Hazelton among those who remembered the story. Much of the townspeople's sympathy was in Gunanoot's favour. Would a Vancouver jury, though, agree? The authorities took him there to be tried for the two murders.

Gunanoot was defended at his trial by Stuart Henderson, a well-known defence lawyer who often appeared for the underdog. Horace was required to give evidence but added nothing new to his earlier medical testimony. Obviously, he could give no evidence about whether Gunanoot had committed the crimes or not. By now, Gunanoot was being described by the press as a valiant folk hero — a veritable Robin Hood. Few, it seems, wanted to see him hanged.

The jury, after retiring for only ten minutes, returned a verdict of not guilty, and Gunanoot walked free, to return to Hazelton. Richard Loring, still the Indian Agent in Hazelton after thirty years, reported to his superiors in Ottawa in September that Simon Naghun (Gunanoot) was back in Hazelton "much relieved and concerned that his children (4) attend school and come under better influence and conditions of life."

When Gunanoot died in 1934, a well-known but anonymous citizen who had known him well was quoted in the *Herald* as saying, "So Simon Gunanoot is dead, eh? He was a good fellow, just as fine a fellow as anyone would wish to be on the trail with. I knew him and made several trips with him before his trouble occurred. There was nothing bad about him."

After the first couple of years, Simon was often in Hazelton, it was said. Both First Nations and non-Indigenous people, including the Hudson's Bay Company bought his furs. He had even been down by train to Prince Rupert and then down to Vancouver by steamer. "The years that were spent by many posses and by individuals hunting the 'bad man,' Simon was watching them all the time and was kept posted by his friends, so that he knew every move of the enemy, which at no time seemed to be of a very serious frame of mind. They [the hired searchers] were having a good time and the government was paying liberally for it. Simon was a great favourite of the Indians and at no time was in danger of betrayal."

—⁓—

As ever, Horace had his official duties outside the hospital to attend to. Not only was he still a medical officer for the province, but he was also one of the three magistrates handling cases in the police court in

Old Hazelton. The *Herald* reported in June 1919, perhaps with some amusement, that the Victoria police office had asked for a report on the morals of Hazelton residents. Someone had complained. "Practically every person in town," the report on the complaint said, "is accused by the unknown informer of either frequenting immoral houses, gambling or some other crime." The time had come, it was said, for a thorough investigation by the magistrates, but nothing seemed to come of this.

Horace and Richard Sargent, a fellow magistrate, had a busy time in February 1920. "Almost nightly," the *Herald* said, "the Justices of the Peace, Dr. Wrinch and R.S. Sargent have been on the bench. The cases vary in seriousness, but are mostly of the ordinary police court variety. . . . The offenders have got the notion that a lawyer is a pretty good defence against the enforcement of law and order, regardless of costs. However, the local judges seem to have pretty good ideas of the multitude of laws and how to assist in the observance of them."

One of Horace's cases reached the appeal courts. James Kramer appeared before Horace in 1920 charged with having seventy beaver pelts in his possession out of season. In spite of a skillful defence by Stuart Henderson, Kramer was convicted. Horace fined him $20, with the pelts to be confiscated. On his client's behalf, Henderson appealed on a technicality to the British Columbia Supreme Court, which overturned Horace's decision. After a further appeal, the Court of Appeal vindicated him and restored the original verdict.

———

Because the hospital had admitted more serious cases than usual and was at capacity, the 1920 annual meeting was held in St. Andrew's Hall in Old Hazelton. In his report on the previous year, Horace gave a description of the hospital, which had by now become a compound in itself. In addition to the hospital and his own home, there were two cottages for use by employees, an engine house, storerooms and an ice house, a garage, a stable, a drive house and a poultry house.

The farm had fifteen Jersey cows and 150 fowl. A bungalow had been erected a little distance from the hospital for infectious cases. All buildings were lit by electricity — this was still four or five years before Hazelton itself had electricity. The old acetylene gas plant, though, was still in use when needed.

The hospital farm and gardens supplied fresh milk, eggs, vegetables, fruits and flowers year round. The staff consisted of two attending physicians and surgeons, two trained nurses, six nurses in training, a housekeeper and assistant, an engineer, a caretaker and gardener, a laundryman, a ward assistant and a part-time secretary. Later that year, May Hogan became the secretary at the hospital.

However admirable and sound the hospital was, its finances were once again coming under pressure. Throughout its history, the hospital's finances see-sawed between loss and profit. Horace ran a tight ship and so the swings were never great nor were they out of control.

With costs rising and fees and other income staying the same, there was, nevertheless a constant strain on the budget. When built, the annual maintenance had been $3,500. By 1919, it had reached $20,000 a year. Although the average cost for each patient had risen to $2.88 a day, fees had not been increased during the previous six years. Nor had provincial government grants. Although the population of Old Hazelton itself had fallen to approximately 250, the population of the surrounding district had increased, as had the cost of living (including, inevitably, the cost of all supplies), and this suggested that a financial crisis might be coming.

Horace made another appeal for public donations. Supporting this was a two-page article in the *Herald* on the history of the hospital and its importance to the district. The hospital needed at least $2,000 by the end of 1919, Horace said, otherwise he would have to consider increasing fees. The Red Cross, of which he was chairman, donated the proceeds it had raised at the summer picnic. The church bazaar in December, at which Alice was in charge of the ladies' work stall, raised $300. The hospital also organized a sleigh-ride in the snow to the Silver Standard Mine that raised $80. Six sleigh-loads of people from Hazelton and New Hazelton, paying $1 each, went in beautiful weather out to the mine, where sandwiches, cake and coffee were served in the cookhouse. Some brave souls even ventured into the tunnels. Despite the generosity of the community, with rising costs, no increase in fees and an increasing numbers of patients, in 1919 the hospital had a deficit of — $23.81.

The nurses training school was still operating successfully. Miss Eva Martin graduated in 1920 with the highest marks ever awarded. Times though were changing. The provincial Nurses Registration Act that came into effect in April 1919 had implications for the school. It required every hospital with a nurses training school to employ two registered nurses on its school staff. As a consequence, Horace reported, the school had hired another staff nurse, Miss Andrews. To meet a new requirement for more extensive written exams for nurses, Horace admitted two more student nurses and shortened the nurses' working day to eight hours to allow them more time to study.

The following year, he reported that the school had affiliated with Vancouver General Hospital to allow nurses to take their final year of training there. Miss S.K. Phillips and Miss M. Collier, the first two nurses to go to Vancouver, acquitted themselves creditably. Later, Horace proudly reported that all three nurses in training at his hospital had successfully passed the licensing board exams and were now entitled to style themselves as Mrs. McCutcheon, R.N., Miss King, R.N. and Miss Bates, R.N. All this, however, resulted in a considerable additional expense.

Horace was always looking for ways to boost the presence of the hospital in the community. Social events such as Dominion Day and picnics in the hospital park had always been part of his style. He could be expected to embrace National Hospital Day. This took place on Florence Nightingale's birthday of May 12 every year, and was held all over North America as a way to celebrate the contribution of a hospital to its community. Eight thousand hospitals in Canada and the United States participated. In an article in the July 1922 edition of *Hospital Management*, a continent-wide journal published in Chicago, Horace wrote, ". . . the idea of a 'National Hospital Day' caught the hospitals' and also the public's [imagination] and it ran like wildfire. Some institutions and communities were not satisfied with a day, but spread their event over a week, and in some cases even more than that."

The purpose was to educate the public about hospitals and their usefulness in maintaining public health. Horace adopted this movement with enthusiasm, and he became chairman of the provincial committee for National Hospital Day. Commencing in 1921, he arranged a celebration at the hospital every year until the financial constrictions of the Depression forced him to end it. In that first year, he organized an open house, with nurses and staff acting as hosts. Residents of the district toured the hospital and the hospital grounds. Tea was served on the veranda, where visitors remarked on how the hundreds of daffodils displayed everywhere gave a pleasing effect.

Hospital Day in 1922 was celebrated with an extended program of four days. On Thursday, a moving-picture show, loaned by Wiggs O'Neill, was presented at the hospital, entertaining a large number. On Friday, there were addresses about the hospital in all the schools and also a concert in the Hazelton Assembly Hall with a six-piece orchestra that later provided the music for a dance. On Saturday, there was the usual open house with light refreshments, a baby show, ice cream, and a draw, the prize being a donated hundred-pound pig. On Sunday, all the churches in Hazelton made the need to support the hospital a theme at their services.

With some forgivable hyperbole, the *Herald* reported on these celebrations: "The Hazelton Hospital is regarded as a part of the district and it is one of the chief social centres as well as the great human dry dock where barnacles are scraped off, leaks and breaks are located and repaired and where the body and mind are given a general overhauling before the ship is allowed to continue life's voyage. . . . For whatever purpose one goes to the Hazelton Hospital, one comes away with a brighter outlook." More to Horace's immediate purpose, the celebrations raised $450, of which $129 had been raised in the draw for the pig.

At the meeting of the hospital patrons in February 1923, Horace was able to report a much improved financial position. The balance on hand at the end of 1922 was $165. Revenues had increased because the provincial government had increased its grant. Furthermore, the Rev. Ferrier had made an independent assessment of the hospital's finances and had persuaded the Methodist Board of Missions to increase its grant. This enabled the hospital to do some of the important maintenance work that had been postponed during the war.

In fewer than ten years, Hazelton moved from steamers clawing their way up hills of water on the Skeena River and from horseback and dog-sled travel to airplanes landing on Mission Point. In 1920, it was announced that Hazelton was to be put on the air route between New York and Alaska as the last stop before the final dash to Nome. Two representatives came from Vancouver to investigate possible landing sites and declared that the lower field of the hospital would be an excellent choice. The town became very excited. Fences on the proposed landing field were taken down. The crops were cut early.

The day chosen for the landing, July 20, was then declared to be Aviation Day, and a town picnic was arranged. People planned to come from Prince Rupert, Smithers and Burns Lake to watch the airplanes arrive. Four American Air Force De Havilland 4-B type airplanes were to come, stopping on their way at Saskatoon, Edmonton, Jasper and Prince George.

They were delayed, however, by strong winds and the need to make repairs. The picnic had to be postponed, causing great disappointment. Then Captain St. Clair Streett, the pilot in command, came by train from Prince George and declared the hospital landing ground was too narrow, too wet, and should never have been chosen in the first place. He thought the flat ground on Mission Point would be preferable. After considerable frustration at the delays, the planes finally arrived almost unannounced in the second week of August.

Taken by surprise, Hazelton residents scrambled to find ways of getting over the river to Mission Point to see the planes land. One party driving furiously up from Smithers was too late but had seen the planes chugging through the air towards Hazelton. "The 'planes left Prince George at five minutes past nine," the *Herald* reported "and the first machine landed at eleven minutes past twelve, thus the speed averaged about seventy miles an hour. . . . No. 4 was the first of the 'planes to land and it took to the ground like a swan and was parked like an auto."

That evening there was a banquet for the aviators in St. Andrew's Hall, followed by a dance in the Assembly Hall. Nothing much of a regular service seemed to come out of these exploratory flights, although by late 1922, the monoplane *Hazelton* was using Mission Point as an airfield to take parties to hunt big game in the mountains.

Fire was a huge risk to all towns in those days. As has been seen, Horace was always worried about fire at the hospital, not only for the safety of the patients but also for the safety of the nurses living on the top floor. He had every reason to be concerned as there had already been one minor fire at the hospital.

One September night at the beginning of the war, Horace had woken just after midnight to the sounds and smells of what he feared most — fire. The oranges and reds of the blazing building flickered on his bedroom walls. He heard the crackling and roaring and smelled the acrid, tangy smoke. His barns were ablaze! No one knew how it had started. In the darkness, the silhouettes of those trying to put it out were mere black shapes against the flames. The Harris brothers came across the road from their farm and helped to prevent the flames from spreading. Horace would have wept as the big horse and his favourite little bay, the one he used for trotting around town, perished. The hay crop and all the tools stored in the barn were gone. All in all, the loss was about $1,000, which would have been a grievous blow to the hospital. Later, however, young men from Hazelton stepped up and volunteered to rebuild the barns, saving the hospital much of the otherwise unavoidable cost.

In December 1919, a block of old buildings in the centre of Old Hazelton burned down. This fire started in a Chinese restaurant at about nine in the morning, and it destroyed a part of the town that had seen many of the prospectors, grubstakers, speculators, greenhorns and gamblers meet and strike deals. At Christmas in 1920, another blaze started at midnight at a Chinese barber's shop, burning down two blocks and nearly destroying Horace's Up-To-Date Drugstore.

In February 1921, a fire destroyed the building in which the Royal Bank was situated and burned Sam Lee, a Chinese resident, to death. Horace had the gruesome task of examining the victim's remains, which appeared to have been cut apart before the fire.

With this suspicion of foul play, the police became interested, but nothing seemed to come from their investigation. Horace's drugstore across the street was only "warmed" this time, having some paint peeled off by the heat. Another fire in 1922 started at one in the morning and destroyed the Hazelton Hotel, two cottages, a residence, a two-storey building across the road and the B.C. Café.

—◦◦◦—

Horace participated in church activities whenever possible. In 1919, he was one of three ministers to ordain a new minister in Hazelton. This was Brother James Evans, who worked mainly in Smithers and Telkwa, and had obviously proven himself worthy. One of the ministers gave a fine sermon and Miss C. Goddard and Miss Gladys Davis sang solos at the service, after which the ordination was conducted by the brethren. "Here in the great North, a good soldier was being commissioned," the *Western Methodist Recorder* said, "for the better accomplishment of his task."

When the Methodists celebrated the opening of the new Union Church in Old Hazelton in January 1922, it was, surprisingly, the first Methodist Church in town. As has been seen, Old Hazelton was largely an Anglican town, the Anglican St. Peter's Church having opened in 1900. Horace had held Methodist services in the hospital until 1912, when a Methodist minister came down from Kispiox to hold services in rooms above the Up-To-Date Drugstore rented from Horace. This, though, burned down, and so local Methodists raised the necessary money and built the new Union Church.

It didn't have lighting or heat and the outsides needed painting, but it was at least open. Horace was on the platform as the first missionary, together with Rev. J.R. Hewitt, the minister. "This is the first church we have had in Hazelton," Rev. Dr. White, Superintendent of Missions, said, continuing, "of course it could not have been done without Dr. Wrinch. Our dear Dr. and his family have put their very heart's love into it."

Horace's friends back east had not forgotten him. Victoria University in Toronto, which was affiliated with Albert College, his old college in Ontario, awarded Horace the honorary degree of Doctor of Divinity in 1921. In reporting the award, the *Western Methodist Recorder* described him as "an unobtrusive man, of few words and of quiet genial demeanour, Dr. Wrinch is of stalwart physique and of equally stalwart character.... He continues to be an ardent missionary and minister of the Gospel, rendering constant and loving service to both the bodies and souls of his fellow-man and without distinction of voice and colour."

The *Missionary Outlook* also acknowledged the role of his wife, Alice, in Horace's accomplishments: "Any account of Dr. Wrinch's life-work would be incomplete and ungracious if it failed to refer to the splendid inspiration and support which he has received throughout from Mrs. Wrinch.... In the midst of manifold duties, this remarkable couple have maintained a Christian home and home life of simplicity and charm. A family of splendid children is not the least of their contributions to the church and community."

The Methodists in Hazelton held their last district meeting as Methodists in May 1925. When next they met, they would be part of a larger church. On June 10, the three churches, the Methodist, the Congregational Church and a large portion of the Presbyterians, merged to form the United Church of Canada. This new church would be the spiritual home of twenty percent of the country's population and would have 8,000 churches. There were appropriate — and probably teetotal — celebrations in Hazelton.

Although Horace had been interested in hospital administration and ways to finance health care for as long as he could remember, he probably had been thinking about it with more focus once it was seen that the Lloyd George reforms in the United Kingdom were functioning well. This had shown that progressive change was possible, and would have led him to think of how to reform the province's health care. His thoughts found expression, first, in his work for the British Columbia Hospital Association and, second, in his drive for publicly funded health insurance.

Always active in medical circles, he was a member of the British Columbia Medical Association and was its representative in the Grand Trunk Pacific District, that is, the area along the Skeena and Bulkley rivers. He would also have been in regular correspondence with the other Methodist Mission hospitals in the North, such as the ones at Bella Bella, Port Simpson and Port Essington. He would have seen the benefits of cooperation and sharing of information among the hospitals in the province.

Approximately five hundred institutions provided medical care in British Columbia. They were of every size and every type. Some were mission hospitals, some were private hospitals, and some were big city hospitals such as Vancouver General and the Provincial Royal

Jubilee Hospital in Victoria (the name at this time). There was a great need for standardization and coordination of resources, educational standards and efficiencies. Most of their administrators would also have seen the need for reform in the way they were financed.

Horace had been a member of the American Hospital Association since 1909, being at that time one of the two members from British Columbia. By 1917, there were five members from British Columbia, including Dr. George Darby, Horace's Methodist colleague at Bella Bella, Miss Jessie MacKenzie, who was ladies superintendent of the Provincial Royal Jubilee Hospital, and Dr. Malcolm MacEachern, who since 1913 had been the general superintendent of Vancouver General Hospital. MacEachern and MacKenzie had joined the Association in 1915 and 1914, respectively. Both Horace and MacEachern were also the British Columbia representatives on the Editorial Board of *Hospital World*, which was the official journal of the Canadian Hospital Association.

Here was a core group of hospital administrators who could see the benefits of an organization for hospitals in British Columbia. In the American Hospital Association, they had a working model that would have been useful for them when they formally established the British Columbia Hospital Association at the 1918 convention. MacEachern, at the centre of things in Vancouver, was probably the prime mover for its establishment, but he would have drawn on the experience of like-minded reformers around the province. Horace would have shared his knowledge and experience about community hospitals. That he was elected to the executive in the first year suggests that he had been involved in its planning and establishment. Later, he was to serve two terms as its president.

It was June 1918. Horace placed a hand on the railings of the suspension bridge to steady himself and looked down into the depths of the Capilano Canyon in North Vancouver, which would have reminded him of the Hagwilget Canyon. Other delegates to this first convention of the British Columbia Hospital Association were on the bridge and strolling on the paths alongside it, some chatting, some merely putting in time before dinner. The deep canyon was awe-inspiring, with the river a few hundred feet below and huge trees soaring up, almost blocking the sky above. He noticed MacEachern, MacKenzie and MacLean (later a premier of the province) — a formidable group of medical Scots — discussing some point of the day's proceedings with great animation. MacEachern was, it had been agreed, to be the first president of the new Association.

The three days had gone well. The proceedings, in what the *Daily Colonist* called the spacious auditorium at the University of British Columbia, then situated near Vancouver General Hospital on Fairview Slopes, had been informative and useful. In addition to laying down a path for the standardization of hospital procedures throughout the province, they had formed the basis for a coalition of hospital administrators that could influence government thinking on such matters as hospital finance. They had shared information and had benefitted from the displays of new medical devices and procedures. The *Daily Colonist* rightly said that it marked a new era for hospitals in the province.

The goals of the new British Columbia Hospital Association were to promote hospital efficiency in the province and to unite all hospitals in co-operative efforts in development — all goals close to Horace's heart. The convention had discussed such matters as the hospital as a community service, hospital architecture, cost-saving measures, standardization of hospital equipment and supplies, the X-ray department, financing and the modern-trained nurse. Jessie MacKenzie gave a talk on "Small Economies in Hospitals."

Horace's own address on the problems small hospitals faced had been well received. And he had enjoyed Dr. Young's talk on the hospital as a community service. In saying that the days of state control of medical services were coming, Young may have gone too far for many delegates, but it was surely, he said, only a matter of time. The present ad hoc system of private payments and per capita grants could not continue.

After the business sessions, a convoy of cars had brought the remainder of the delegates, some of whom had been on a tour of inspection of the Royal Columbian Hospital in New Westminster, to the Canyon View Hotel at Capilano Canyon for a formal dinner. MacEachern spoke, and Dr. Riggs proposed a toast to the graduating class of nurses, who were among the guests. After dinner there was lively dancing.

Strongly of the opinion that the state should be doing more for the health of its citizens, Horace wrote a front-page report for the *Herald* in August 1919 under the headline "Financing the Hospitals and All Free Treatment." He reported on two papers given to the convention that year, one by J.J. Bamfield, chairman of the board of directors of Vancouver General Hospital, and the other by Robert S. Davy, chairman of the board of Victoria's Provincial Royal Jubilee Hospital. The government, they said, had accepted responsibility not only for the health and welfare of the insane and for the prevention of disease, but also for the health and safety of workers through the Workmens' Compensation Act.

Therefore, Horace wrote, it was logical that it "becomes the function of our government to place within reach of every one of its people adequate facilities for restoration to health no matter what may have been the cause of their disability. . . . The funds necessary should be contributed in an equitable manner *pro rata* by every man and woman during their earning period of life, e.g. 18 to 60."

Here then is the basis upon which Horace later argued for public health insurance when he was in the Legislature. "If free hospitals, then why not also free medical and surgical treatment," he wrote, "just as has been and is being done for our soldiers." The executive of the Hospital Association, he reported, was preparing a recommendation to the provincial government to that effect.

Horace made sure that the voice of Hazelton Hospital was heard in the Association. He wrote in the hospital's annual report for 1921:

> . . . our most valuable national asset, the health of the people is, to a
> large extent, entrusted to the hospitals. Viewed from this standpoint,
> surely there could be no policy more short-sighted than one that

would parsimoniously limit the service and efficiency of these institutions. . . . Our own Hospital has held membership in the Provincial Association every year since its inception four years ago. This year we have no less than fourteen individual members also in this association.

Hospitals in the province were running out of money. The old ways of raising funds were not good enough in the post-war world. On February 11, 1921, Horace, now president, called an emergency meeting of the Hospital Association, to be held in the Empress Hotel in Victoria. The purpose was to discuss the "distressing financial conditions most of the public hospitals in British Columbia were facing." He said that every public hospital in the province was in a financial crisis and could not carry on much longer.

Mr. McGregor, from the Provincial Royal Jubilee Hospital, agreed and cited a recent instance in his hospital where board members had to give personal bonds to maintain the supply of milk for patients. All cost-cutting measures had been taken. It was only a matter of time before banks stopped giving them credit. Horace announced that he had therefore arranged a meeting with the government for the following day. MacEachern and McGregor helped Horace draft a letter to be delivered to the government explaining that hospitals in the province urgently needed help.

The next day, Horace led a delegation across the street to present the letter. During the meeting with Premier Oliver, he requested that the government provide emergency funding for hospitals while a more permanent basis for public support could be worked out. The time had come, he argued, for the government to do something. The United Municipalities and the United Boards of Trade gave their support to his proposals. The delegation asked the government for action to disburse forthwith the deficits of public hospitals in the province, to double the scale of per capita grants and to bring in a measure at the earliest opportunity to provide a universal basis of taxation for the adequate financing of all hospitals receiving aid under the Hospital Act.

Horace complained to the premier that the Hospital Act imposed duties on the hospitals but did not recognize that the cost of compliance had increased. The premier promised to put their proposals before the executive council (the cabinet) and said they would consider the matter carefully and sympathetically. "Your statements with regard to the condition of the hospitals," the premier said, "are about as strong as language can make them. You must remember, however, that the government is paying a larger share of the expenditure on hospitals than ever before. . . . The trouble is that the people demand services which they are not willing to pay for."

The Hospital Association met in convention annually. At the 1922 convention held at the Royal Columbian Hospital, Horace, even though president, was not able to attend because Alice was ill. Richard Sargent read Horace's speech. The members present passed a resolution expressing their sympathy. They noted his thorough knowledge of hospital affairs and his sound judgment in dealing with the technicalities of the hospital situation. Despite his absence, he was re-elected as president for a second term.

The second topic that concerned Horace in these years was more aspirational — the need to introduce publicly funded health insurance in the province. His actions on this ran concurrently with his activities for the Hospital Association.

His was not a lone voice. Many in Canada had been carefully watching the Lloyd George reforms in the United Kingdom. Discussions for and against the introduction of public health insurance in Canada had started even before the First World War. The debate had been rigorous and at times rancorous. Ernest Hall wrote to the *Victoria Daily Times* in December 1916, arguing that health insurance was one of the next great social reforms and one that the medical profession should advance. "Universal health insurance would," he wrote, "without greater expense to the worker, provide burial insurance and also medical, nursing and hospital care and two-third of wages during sickness up to a maximum of twenty-six weeks a year."

Dr. J.W. McIntosh delivered a paper on the topic to the Vancouver Medical Association in 1916, following which a committee had been set up to explore the subject and report back. McIntosh had left the Liberal party to form what was loosely called the Soldiers' Party, made up of ex-soldiers and supporters who wanted more assistance for soldiers returning from the war.

The following year, the *Daily Colonist* reported that "the nationalization of the medical and nursing profession of Canada is not far off, according to the belief of Dr. J.W. McIntosh, MPP, [Member of the Provincial Parliament, a term used in British Columbia at the time] of Vancouver, as expressed to some fifty British Columbia nurses at the Victoria Club last night." The *Daily Colonist* reported him as saying, "Many doctors here are now ripe and ready for state control of medicine." A growing body of opinion in British Columbia was calling for the adoption of some form of state health insurance.

After the war had ended, the demand for health benefits had grown, not only for returning soldiers and their families but also for the population at large. Trade unions, farmers' organizations, women's organizations and friendly (fraternal) societies became more insistent in their demands for some form of state health insurance. The militancy of the trade union movement in British Columbia meant that the province would be in the forefront of the push for change.

One of the many organizations pushing for reform was the Hospital Association. Its members were vocal supporters of publicly funded health insurance. Horace informed the executive committee in August 1923 that he would be recommending that a special committee be set up to investigate the state financing of hospitals and health care in other provinces.

Nor was this just a British Columbia movement. Across the country, many shared the view that state health insurance was necessary, beneficial and long overdue. In 1917, Dr. Blackader, president of the Canadian Medical Association, argued that some form of health insurance was coming and that the medical profession should make sure its voice was heard to ensure it was appropriate. A symposium on health insurance was held in Ottawa during the 1917 annual meeting of the Canadian Public Health Association, and in 1919

Canada's first commission on health insurance was established.

In 1919, the federal Liberal Party adopted a program of adequate health insurance "so far as may be practicable, having regard for Canada's financial position" as part of its election platform. When Mackenzie King came to power as prime minister in 1921, he did not, though, act on it decisively. Federal initiatives became trapped in parliamentary committees for the whole decade. Several other provinces took their own steps along the same path. In Saskatchewan and Alberta, municipal doctors' schemes were set up. In Alberta a municipal hospital plan was started at the Lethbridge Hospital in 1919.

But the voices in British Columbia seemed to be the loudest and have the most support. In a speech at the 1918 Hospital Association convention, Dr. A.S. Monro, a director of Vancouver General Hospital, referred to the Lloyd George reforms in England and the need for something similar in Canada. "A beneficent socialism that would provide, at the expense of the State, for the care of the sick and injured is as yet too Utopian for realization," he said, "but the trend of events is along these lines."

J.J. Bamfield, another director of Vancouver General Hospital, addressed the topic in his talk entitled "The Duty of the State to the Individual." In this talk he maintained "that all should have the inalienable right to a free diagnosis and should then have the option of receiving treatment in a state ward free of charge or accept other hospital accommodation for which they would be required to pay."

This was the warm-up. The Hospital Association met again in July 1919, this time at the Empress Hotel in Victoria, with an opening address by Lieutenant Governor Sir Frank Barnard, who later acted as host at a garden party at Government House. Not to be outdone in hospitality, the Rotary Club of Victoria organized motor tours of Victoria beauty spots for the delegates and their friends. At this convention, D.G. Stewart from Prince Rupert proposed a specific resolution that the government provide a free dispensary in connection with each public hospital, free medical examination and all free nursing and medical services. This led to strong disagreement from the representatives of the Vancouver and Victoria Medical Associations. Horace, jumping into the discussion, said:

> I am almost filled too full for utterance. It has raised the whole question that has been simmering away in our conscience ever since we have had to do with hospitals. There has always been that limitation. Someone says: Why haven't you this and why haven't you the other convenience and facility for giving proper and adequate treatment? And the answer has always been: "We would be delighted to have it but we cannot afford it." . . . We must have the government step in and do more for us than we are getting at present.

Dr. McIntosh then joined in the discussion, saying that he was strongly in favour of a state health insurance scheme coming in as quickly as possible and "we have an assurance also that the government of British Columbia has realized that the people of British Columbia are demanding some form of state health insurance, so much so that they have promised to bring in a measure of insurance at the next session."

Horace then added his full support to the scheme, saying, "Health insurance is an ideal condition. It is a big thing. . . . I am very much in favour of putting through a resolution along those lines. Let it go before the government and be thrashed out and let the medical men unite; then let careful and wise committees sit on those measures and discuss them and get all the consideration necessary. I would like to see us get a resolution through." McIntosh then added a cautionary and prophetic note. "I wish to put myself on record," he said, "that without the support of the medical profession I do not think the scheme will carry at all."

Despite this concern, on February 16, 1919, when he was in the Legislature as head of the Soldiers' Party, McIntosh had, together with his colleague Frank Giolma, raised the matter in the House with "a strong plea" for universal, compulsory and contributory state health insurance. He referred to both the Bismarck legislation and the Lloyd George legislation. The medical profession in England, he said, which initially had been strongly opposed, had swung round to support it. It was time that British Columbia followed suit. On Thursday, March 6, 1919, Dr. MacLean, later to succeed John Oliver as premier, moved an amendment motion in the House to the effect that early consideration should be given to state health insurance.

As a result, and after some procedural wrangles, a Committee of the House, later changed to a Royal Commission, was established in November to investigate state health insurance and pensions and to make recommendations to the government. It got down to work with its first meeting the same month. E.H. Winn, the chairman, said the main points to be investigated were members' pensions, maternity benefits, state health insurance and public health nursing.

This commission, entitled the Royal Commission on State Health Insurance and Maternity Benefits, but often called the Winn Commission, heard from representatives of the public, including those from fraternal (friendly) societies, miners' and teachers' associations and the medical profession. The proposals for health insurance had broad social support in many sectors of the province. The Winn Commission delivered two separate reports, one on maternity benefits and one on health insurance. Its report on health insurance, tabled on March 18, 1921 stated:

> Health begets happiness, happiness prosperity, and with happiness and prosperity, our Country cannot help but reach the height of success in the commercial world. Finally, we may expect Health Insurance to help forward industrial peace, for it will provide machinery for continual conference between employer and employee. It is believed that Health Insurance is needed in British Columbia in order to tide the workman over the grave emergency incidental to illness, as well as in order to reduce illness itself, lengthen life, abate poverty, improve working and earning power, and diminish the cause of industrial discontent. There is no other measure now before the public which equals the power of Health Insurance toward social betterment.

The Winn Commission went on to recommend that there should be province-wide compulsory health insurance. This should apply to all wage earners under the age of sixty-five who had been bona fide residents of the province for at least eighteen months and whose income was not in excess of $3,000 per year, with insurance benefits to extend to families and other dependents. Insurance would be voluntary for those with greater incomes.

Implementation of the recommendations, though, was unlikely. The government majority was slim, and British Columbia was already $50 million in debt. Moreover, opposition from many in the medical profession was certain. The Winn Commission's report was not even printed. Notwithstanding this, on November 30, 1922, the Legislature did resolve to consider state health insurance with a view to discussing the advisability of appointing a committee to bring in a bill in that session. Somewhere among this series of hurdles, however, the proposal died.

In the early 1920s, the appetite for adoption of health insurance reforms in Canada seemed to diminish. Earlier tentative approval of state medical insurance in the United States had turned sharply to firm disapproval, and the economic recovery of the early 1920s placed it on almost everyone's back burner. Trade union influence and also industrial and social unrest declined. In his study "Canadian Medical Insurance — Private Practice, Public Payment," C. David Naylor wrote that "The tenor of the times had clearly changed. . . . Only in British Columbia, it seems, did a sizeable segment of the profession take concrete action in the matter of health insurance."

In British Columbia, then, the discussion did continue. Horace, for one, was not going to let the matter drop. Throughout the 1920s, he continued to advocate for health insurance "which would provide medical and hospital insurance for everyone." As president of the Hospital Association in 1921 and 1922, he was, of course, firmly in the debate and had a platform. After his election to the Legislature in 1924 on the government benches, and again in 1928, when he sat on the opposition benches, he had a bigger platform and there he became its standard-bearer.

With the passing of the years came the death of old friends and acquaintances. In December 1919, Helen Bone died in Guelph, Ontario. She was a link to those days of medical studies in Toronto, when she had been Alice's roommate at Grace Hospital. She was also a link to the early days of the Hazelton Hospital. The old packer Cataline died in 1922. He had always said that he did not like hospitals and that people only went there to die. Despite such talk, though, he had in fact contributed to the hospital's appeals for donations over the years. He had resisted going there for as long as he could. His friend Sperry Cline took him eventually, grumbling and groaning, and there he did die.

They buried him in the cemetery on top of the bluff. Horace and Cataline were hardly friends, but Cataline was a link to the distant past, to the days when Hazelton was cut off from the outside world for four or five months of the year. He was, moreover, a link to the gold rush days of the middle of the previous century.

In the middle of June 1922, the *Herald* reported that Horace and Alice were going to the Mayo clinic in Rochester, Minnesota, again "on account of the continued illness of Mrs. Wrinch. They will be away some weeks, and it is hoped by all that when they return Mrs. Wrinch will be in much improved health." As the family knew only too well, however, Alice had cancer. That was why Horace had not attended the convention of the Hospital Association, even though he was president. They returned from Rochester after the treatment in mid-July with an optimistic report on her health. She was, it was said, showing a material improvement, but in fact the cancer within Alice had continued to grow.

In the second week of March 1923, after an illness that had lasted four years, Alice died. Her cancer had hung over Horace like a black cloud, darkening everything with anxiety and foreboding. The care and treatments would have absorbed much of his emotional and physical energy. Her death, when it came, was intensely distressing. Here was the person he had shared his life with, the person he had married at the "pretty ceremony" at her brother's house in far-away Merton, the person he had relied on for counsel and support, now gone. She had helped Horace over the years, had supported him in everything he did, and had been for him a source of strength. A tribute in the *Christian Guardian* said:

> A long journey, a serious operation, a considerable recovery, were followed by a glad return to the happy circle of her family and her share in the tasks of her husband. Even when her right hand had lost much of its strength, she still fulfilled the duty of superintendent of the hospital, guided the affairs of the family, exercised benevolence towards those in need, aided and encouraged the growth of the congregation, rejoiced with the happy and sorrowed with the distressed without distinction of race or creed or colour, and went forward courageously into the unknown future, whose possibilities she well understood.... So upon the cold, chilling aspects of frontier existence, the life of Alice Breckon Wrinch shone with the warmth of noble and inspiring womanhood; and the cold and cheerless, the dry and parched avenues of human souls became transformed with the flower of Christian integrity in lives made nobler by her presence.

The family came together at this sad time. It had lost one of its pillars. Not least among Alice's accomplishments was that of being a mother. While Horace was perhaps a little reserved, Alice was nurturing and nourishing. She provided warmth and, in the way of strong women, held the family together in Horace's many absences. Ralphena and Harold were still living at home, as was Cooper, who at that time was working as a clerk in the Union Bank. Arthur was attending high school in Vancouver and was unable to return home. Leonard, studying at university in Edmonton, was able to get back in time for the funeral.

The whole district mourned. A writer in the *Western Methodist Record* said, "The different tribes (six) sent representatives to call on the doctor in order to convey their sympathy with the family and for the doctor in the hour of their sorrow. Before leaving the house they left wreaths of flowers, and such a profusion of flowers I have rarely ever seen before." The *Herald* described the funeral procession, with mourners trailing after the coffin like frail fingers as if reaching to keep her with them. "The remains," the *Herald* reported, "were conveyed from the residence to the church where the population of the district turned out almost *en masse* to pay their last respects to the departed."

The Rev. J. Hewitt, one of the half-dozen clergy at the funeral, preached the sermon on "Everlasting Life," after which he delivered the eulogy. Following the service, Robert Tomlinson spoke about Alice to the First Nations in their own languages. Then the Salvation Army and other choirs sang. In addition to those from Hazelton and New Hazelton, there were representatives from Kispiox, Terrace, Smithers and Telkwa. Six tribes of First Nations from the different parts of the district were present. She was buried on the bluff of the hill overlooking Hazelton, among the Gitxsan grave houses and graves of many friends and acquaintances.

The *Herald* paid tribute to her, saying that with her death "early on Sunday morning, one of the happiest and brightest lives that ever lived on the frontier came to an end." It continued:

> . . . she had been a great, but a very patient sufferer, and even during the past several months when needing constant care, she was bright, cheerful and optimistic, although her family and friends knew that the end was not far off. . . . During the past twenty odd years she saw many changes in population and in conditions, but she never deviated from her ideal of Christian service. She was an ideal wife, a grand mother, a true friend, a great worker and generous and kind to a degree. . . . Her work was a success and this district owes much to her efforts. . . . Until four years ago Mrs. Wrinch enjoyed excellent health, but since then had been unable to take the active part to which she had so long been accustomed. But at no time did she lose interest in the people of the district and their doings. Even in her last hours she discussed plans for the future development of the school children.

The following week the paper printed, in addition to the long list of names of those who had given floral tributes, a letter from Horace and his family:

Dr. Wrinch and his family take this opportunity of conveying their most sincere and heartfelt gratitude to the very many friends, who, in so many ways, gave expression to their sympathy with them in their bereavement. The sadness of this experience has been softened, and if it were possible entirely effaced, by the memory of this wonderfully kind and spontaneous expression of appreciation and esteem of the one who has just passed out of our present associations into the higher life.

Words could not express the depth of Horace's grief. But life had to continue. There was the hospital to run, surgeries to perform and community affairs to attend to. The hospital held its third National Hospital Day in May. This was said to be very successful "but perhaps a trifle cool for ice-cream." The baby competition was as successful as ever, with the judges taking half an hour to decide which of the seven entrants would be awarded the prize. The Hazelton First Nations football team defeated the settlers 5 to 1. The dance that the Ladies Auxiliary arranged in the evening was a great success, with piano solos and songs as usual. But — and it was a big "but" — for the first time, Alice was not there by Horace's side.

Not long after, Horace announced that he would be leaving Hazelton to attend a conference in New Westminster, and then would be going to California to visit his brother Frank. He needed time away.

CHAPTER 11

Stepping into Politics
1924–1928

CHRISTMAS 1923, the first after Alice's death, was a sad one for Horace and his family, but it was not necessarily quiet. Arthur and Ralphena returned from Vancouver, and Leonard from his studies in Edmonton. Horace hosted the traditional turkey dinner at his home for all the staff, thirty-two of whom sat down to enjoy it this year. Traditionally, the nurses decorated the reception hall and sitting room, and placed a Christmas tree in the corner. As was his custom, Horace gave a gift to every member of staff and to every patient in the hospital. On Christmas Eve, the Gitxsan band and choir paraded through Hazelton, singing and playing carols.

Horace was now a widower entering middle age. His children were growing up, leaving home and making their own way in the world. He would have foreseen that the coming decade would bring many changes for the whole family. Without Alice, though, what else was there for him to do but soldier on? He was still very much a community leader. While labouring for the public good with the Hospital Association in Vancouver, he worked also for the public good at home in Hazelton. As well as running both hospital and farm, he still had a busy practice as town doctor and government medical officer.

The war had changed the world in which he lived. The post-war world needed, it seemed, to forget those four terrible years, to close that book and start another one, one that was fresher, brighter and more optimistic. The nineteenth century had really ended in 1914, and then, after the savage interlude of the war and the flu, the modern age had started. Where change was possible — in communication, transportation, labour-saving devices, clothing, music, literature, dance and social mores — change happened.

With all its varying fashions and new social customs, the coming years would provide more leisure time than ever before. The effervescence of the times, more muted in rural areas perhaps and scarcely touching some, gave many people, in particular the young, a sense of optimism and a joyous relief to be alive. New standards of morality, albeit a response to the grimness of the previous war years, might have offended Horace's sense of what was appropriate. As an eminently practical person, however, he would have accepted what he could not change.

The end of the war, the treaties and the establishment of the League of Nations promised everlasting peace. Even though the United States had not joined the League and had shrunk into isolation and money making (with the chief business of the American people being, as President Coolidge said, business), there was an optimism, some would say naivety, in many people's understanding of international affairs that held good for almost the rest of Horace's life. Over the horizon, though, unseen by the residents of Hazelton, as elsewhere, the darkening clouds of the Depression and the next war were already beginning to form.

In May, not long after Alice's death, Horace went on a six-week driving holiday. Taking Arthur and Harold with him, he visited his brother Frank at Visalia, in the San Joaquin Valley of California.

There he examined the grape and prune farming enterprise his brother had recently taken up. Harold remembered that on the long journeys, his father had put him in the back seat of the car "punching a counter to see how many cars we had met that day."

Naturally, because this is what he always did on vacation, Horace visited medical centres to keep his skills up to date. He visited his old friend Robert Peers at Colfax, California, where Peers ran the School for the Tuberculous. A Canadian and a classmate from Trinity Medical College, Peers at that time was one of the leading tuberculosis specialists in the United States.

On his return, Horace declared that the North was good enough for him and he was glad to be back. Having seen modern X-ray equipment in California, he recognized the need to upgrade his equipment at the hospital. Consequently, he bought a quartz lamp, which was an improvement, he said, on the ultraviolet ray they presently had. It was also time for major renovations to the hospital buildings, the first since the war had broken out. He set about installing a new roof, building an office where he could examine patients and painting the interior and exterior of the building. It all cost money, of course, this time being about $5,000.

He also came back from his travels with new ideas about farming. In August, he started construction of a silo, the first to be built in the western end of the district. He filled it with a heavy crop of corn, averaging, the *Herald* reported, ten feet in height. This promised to be a good source of stock feed. He believed, he said, that no other ensilage corn gave the yield he had achieved on an acre and a half at the hospital farm. "In addition to potatoes," Harold recalled some years later, "there were vegetables for the cattle and horses because we had horses for transportation and a dozen cattle for milk." He also remembered that in 1924, the first year they had the silo, his brother had chopped up the silage vegetables by hand, a task that was not difficult for him because "he was such a strong person with a broad axe."

On the hospital farm, Horace sowed a new species of Red Bob seed that had been recently developed by the University of Alberta.

He distributed some of the seeds to half a dozen farmers in the Bulkley Valley. He also planted the small triangle lot that he owned in the middle of Old Hazelton. From this small lot he harvested seven tons of sunflowers and corn. The corn, the *Herald* reported, was twelve-and-a-half-feet high, and the sunflowers planted around the edge were six inches higher. He was proud enough of it to be photographed in front of the crop, standing with Sperry Cline and Richard Sargent, the sunflowers and corn towering over them.

One of Horace's hobbies — and perhaps his chief relaxation — was gardening, and he often won prizes for his blooms. In 1924, he established the Hazelton Horticultural Society, and was duly elected its first president. As a public service, the Society placed fresh flowers in the dining cars of trains that stopped in New Hazelton. His son Harold remembered having to get up early when the Wrinch turn came to pick flowers and deliver them to the steward waiting on the station platform.

To open the Horticultural Society's first annual show, a parade of flower-bedecked cars processed through Hazelton. The 200 flower entries filled the Assembly Hall with a "riot of bloom and colour." Gray's Orchestra was brought in from Smithers to play for the dance in the evening. Horace and his family exhibited at the flower show for many years, usually walking off with prizes. In 1930, the family took more than half a dozen of the prizes, with Horace coming first, second and third in the dahlia category.

Robert Tomlinson, the first patient in the hospital, had given up his mission at Kispiox. In 1924, he joined the staff of the hospital with the title of Steward to manage the farming, gardening and maintenance. Harold recalled that Tomlinson was a fine man who had worked in many places in and around the North, and "at one point he was looking for a job, and my father asked him if he would help at the hospital." He was a solid, dependable deputy for everything non-medical. Dr. Geddes Large, the son of Horace's old friend from Trinity Medical, also came to work at the hospital in 1924 and stayed for two years.

Horace was proud of the nurses training school and always made a fuss of nurses when they graduated. There was usually a dinner for the graduating nurse — Miss Ruth Bolivar, for example, in 1924 — which staff and patients attended. The graduate was presented with a bouquet of roses on behalf of the board. Horace usually gave a speech, as did the Chairman of the Hospital Board — Richard Sargent in Miss Bolivar's case. "R.S. Sargent presented the diploma and Mrs. Mathieson presented the pin, heard the obligation, and presented the graduate with a bouquet of magnificent 'mums on behalf of the nursing staff. A round of cheers was given and the exercises [graduation exercises] were bought to a close with the Maple Leaf and the National Anthem."

Hazelton was becoming widely known as a beauty spot. Increasing numbers of tourists were coming by train or by automobile to admire the Hagwilget Canyon, look at totem poles or fish in the Kispiox River. In 1924, the Hazelton Horticultural Society invited Sir Henry Thornton, president of the Canadian National Railway, to visit. Horace met his special train and party of thirty at the station with a fleet of fifteen cars. Richard Sargent drove Sir Henry in his car, with Horace acting as what the *Herald* called the "entertainer," or guide, and they went to the lookout point at the Silver Cup Mine.

They were given the usual tour: the view of Hazelton from the cemetery bluff, the totem poles at Kitwanga, a tour of the hospital, inspection of Gitxsan art, tools and cultural objects laid out on Horace's veranda, and then tea. This time, Horace's daughter, nineteen-year-old Ralphena, was the hostess, a duty she performed in what the *Herald* called "a charming and hospitable manner." Horace naturally made sure that Sir Henry's railway car was filled with flowers for the rest of his journey to Prince Rupert.

Sir Henry, though, was not merely there to view the scenery. One of the reasons he had come was to explore the possibility of bringing more tourists to Hazelton in association with the railway. To that end, while he was at the hospital, he had a lengthy meeting with Horace. Probably not coincidentally, F.H. Williamson, deputy commissioner of national parks, was in town as Horace's guest at the same time. A plan was afoot to establish a national park in the Hazelton district. Although there were, it turned out, too many obstacles, it shows that the community leaders of Hazelton were actively looking at ways to develop local tourist attractions. In another attempt to bring in more tourists, Horace called together local businessmen to discuss other opportunities, and they struck a committee, with Horace and Richard Sargent as members, to investigate this further.

In July 1925, the Governor General again came to town. This time, though, it was Lord Byng of Vimy. Horace asked residents to welcome the vice-regal party by hanging out flags, and he invited everyone to attend the reception on the hospital grounds. Horace, along with Sargent and Sawle, met Lord and Lady Byng and their special train at the South Hazelton station and, after stopping at the Hagwilget Canyon to watch the First Nations spearing fish 250 feet below, brought them to the reception on the hospital grounds.

"I particularly want to meet the boys who served overseas," the Governor General said at the reception. "I want to learn how they are getting on. I owe it to them." Horace officially welcomed the Governor General and his wife and presented them with a book of photographs of the region. Mrs. Mathieson, the lady superintendent, presented Lady Byng with a bouquet of flowers from the garden.

Horace watched as the veterans lined up to speak with the Governor General. For many of them, Lord Byng had been their commanding general at the battle for Vimy Ridge. Later the Governor General and Lady Byng mingled with the large crowd that had come to meet them. When chatting with the veterans, Lord Byng recognized in the crowd Mrs. Houghton, his music teacher from his schooldays in England, and they happily reminisced for a while. Lord Byng and Horace found that they had Essex in common: Lord Byng owned a mansion, Thorpe Hall, in Thorpe-le-Soken, the next village to Kirby-le-Soken, where Horace had spent his childhood. So convivial was the conversation that Lord Byng invited Horace to come and see him when he was next in England.

After the reception, the plan was for them to drive to the bluff in the First Nations cemetery to admire the view of Hazelton and the confluence of the two rivers. Then it would be on down into Hazelton where the First Nations Chiefs would welcome them and where Gitxsan dancers would perform a welcome dance and blow eagle-down feathers over them.

—⁓—

At times, it seemed that the *Herald* followed Horace's every move. In the May 15, 1925 issue, for example, he or the hospital featured in nine of the stories on the front page: one of them, admittedly, being no more profound than the beautiful baby contest at the Hospital Day celebrations. Earlier in the year, it reported on his participation in a debate at the Union Church. The Rev. Pound and Mr. Archibald argued that the League of Nations could prevent international war. Horace, together with Geddes Large, argued that it could not.

Obviously the doctors' arguments were more persuasive because when the ballots were counted, it was evident that Horace and Large had won. The evening ended with community singing, which everyone enjoyed thoroughly despite the now pressing necessity for the great nations on Earth to heed Horace and Large's advice and re-organize their affairs to make the League of Nations work.

The hospital had enjoyed electricity since mid-1914. This was necessary to power not only the X-ray machine, lighting and other utilities, but also the receiving radio that Horace had bought in 1924 that brought the outside world closer. Hazelton itself still did not yet have electricity, but in September 1925, it was just weeks away. "Hazelton People to Bask in Glow of Electric Light Soon," the *Herald* headline announced. The accompanying article noted that, "Poles were distributed around town the end of last week and they are now being erected. This old town is passing from the pioneer and frontier stage to modernism. The pack-dog, the canoe, the pack-horse (except for isolated trips), the freighting outfits, the steamboats, have all gone and now the wax candle . . . and the coal lamp are to go into the discard." Into the discard perhaps went the candles and coal lamps, but after years of official neglect the town of Old Hazelton was not going with them. It was not going to wither and fade away like Aldermere. For a while, there had been a concern that it would.

—◦◦◦—

The second week of May 1924 was a busy one for Horace. On the Sunday, he preached in the New Hazelton Church on man's dependence on others. And then on the Monday he hosted the annual celebrations for Hospital Day, followed by a nurses' graduation celebration for Miss McCall and Miss Nock. Down in Old Hazelton, the Liberal party for the newly formed Skeena riding was holding a convention to choose its candidate for the provincial election in June. Horace was not attending. Although a progressive with liberal inclinations, he may have thought he had better things to do.

Premier John Oliver — Honest John as he was called — was a colourful, folksy, farmer with rural roots and an anti-establishment attitude. Premier since March 1918, he governed a province undergoing profound social change. The first years after the war were turbulent. Soldiers returning from the war as heroes could not find jobs. Markets for minerals had declined substantially, and companies were laying off workers, not hiring them. Fish stocks were down. "The Fraser is fished out," an assistant commissioner of fisheries said. "Its present condition is a monumental record of man's folly and greed." The lumber and shipbuilding industries were doing well but were mainly closed shops to non-union members. Many returning soldiers were suffering in body and mind, and with them their families. Socialism and even Communism seemed attractive and were gaining adherents.

By mid-1924, though, the economy was recovering. The markets were buoyant, and provincial revenues were up. Returned soldiers had settled down and found work, with road building providing much employment. Nevertheless, the problems Premier Oliver was facing were daunting: what to do with the Pacific Great Eastern Railway (from Vancouver to Prince George), which had become a nightmare of debt and delays; how to get better terms from the federal government; how to get freight rates reduced; what to do about prohibition; and how to deal with the business and professional elites in Vancouver.

Honest John Oliver was not a member of those Vancouver elites. Sneering at his folksy ways, they were causing him trouble. He was losing touch with this urban world, where new money, new sophistication and political machines on the right and left were eating into his votes.

On his left were the Socialists and Communists, not perhaps as strong as in 1920, but still with appeal. On his right were the Conservatives under William Bowser, who had taken over as party leader when Premier McBride had died. Turmoil in the party had led some younger Conservatives to defect and join with the Farmers' Party, the Soldiers' Party and other smaller parties to form the Provincial Party. This was led by General McRae from Hycroft, his mansion in Vancouver. During the war, McRae had been director of supply and transport in Canada and then, in the United Kingdom, director of administration in the Ministry of Information.

The Provincial Party attacked both Bowser and Oliver for corruption in connection with the building of the Pacific Great Eastern Railway. Believing, perhaps, that the rising tide of prosperity favoured him, but that the increasing clamour about integrity in politics did not, and with his political foes apparently divided, Oliver called an election for June 20, 1924. All was set for a lively time.

Delegates came to the Liberal convention in Old Hazelton from all over the district — fourteen from Smithers, ten from Terrace and a few others from elsewhere. One group wanted E.T. Kenney from Terrace to represent them; another group wanted Olof Hanson from

Smithers. The convention, going on all afternoon, became dead-locked. Neither side was prepared to accept the candidate of the other. Nor could they persuade anyone else present at the convention to run.

What about Dr. Wrinch? He was one of the most respected people in the community. Could he be persuaded to run in this election? A committee was struck to try to persuade Horace to accept the nomination, and the meeting was adjourned while the delegation went up the hill to the hospital to find him.

Horace, watching the automobile come into the hospital grounds, would have seen that the men who stepped out of it had a purpose in their steps that wasn't medical. Alex Manson, the Attorney General, was accompanied by Mason Adams, president of the local Liberal association, as well as by Olof Hanson and E.T. Kenney. Horace would perhaps have realized that their presence at the hospital meant the convention was deadlocked.

If Horace suspected that they were going to try to persuade him to stand as the Liberal candidate in the next provincial election, he would have been right. Alex Manson, running in the Omineca riding, was an experienced Attorney General. In an election in which every seat counted, he would have known that with Horace they had a good chance of winning the Skeena riding. Was it not Horace's duty to run?

After a few hours, the delegation reported back. Horace had agreed. He would fight the election as the Liberal candidate. Saying he had never belonged to a political party but if elected he would represent it as a Liberal, Horace made his consent conditional on his not being a machine voter. He reserved the right, he said, to use his own judgment when occasion arose. The convention accepted his nomination unanimously. Both Hanson and Kenney heartily endorsed him as the Liberal candidate.

In many ways, Horace was a political innocent. On the Sunday after the convention, for example, where a more determined and aware candidate would have been speaking to delegates, rounding up support, castigating opponents and promising the impossible, he

264 / Service on the Skeena

preached in the Union Church in Hazelton on flowers and their influence on life.

The *Herald*, supporting him in an editorial, said: "The Liberals of Skeena have been particularly fortunate in securing Dr. H.C. Wrinch as standard-bearer. He was first mentioned as a candidate in 1920, but he could not be induced at that time to enter the contest. . . . He has always possessed a high sense of public duty and during his twenty-five years of residence in this immediate district has never failed to carry a large share of work and responsibility."

Horace's opponents were old acquaintances: Richard Sargent for the Conservatives and Frank Dockrill for the Provincial Party. Sargent was one of the few who had been in Hazelton longer than Horace, and Dockrill was a successful mining man who had lived at Telkwa for a number of years. Dockrill said that he had great respect for Dr. Wrinch, whom he knew from his work on the Telkwa hospital project a few years before, but he thought that "if he went to Victoria under a Liberal Government he would have to change his moral views to those of the political machine or he would soon be cast aside."

Horace began campaigning. At the start, Manson accompanied him, presumably to coach him and give advice. In a letter to the electors of the Skeena constituency published in the *Herald*, Horace declared that his interests were practically entirely within the district so that its success was his success, and that he had no axe to grind other than to promote its furthest and fullest development. He then went down the Bulkley Valley to Smithers and Telkwa where he received a good reception. He met the boys at the Duthie Mine on Friday morning, went to Kitwanga in the afternoon and met with another group in the schoolhouse at Woodcock in the evening. On Monday, together again with Manson, he went to Usk and then on to Terrace.

"At every place Dr. Wrinch appears," the *Herald* reported, "he is met with enthusiasm and large gatherings." He spoke in Terrace at the Progress Hall, which was filled to capacity, and his remarks "were characteristic of the candidate, being of that straightforward, honest and positive nature, slow but sure. . . ." He was, it reported, promising to continue the same policy of uprightness and fairness to all in his political position just as he had followed in his profession. The *Herald* said he had a successful meeting at Moricetown and gave a fine address there.

The Liberal party had more advertisements in the *Herald* than the other parties, but then it was a Liberal-leaning paper. Its full-page advertisements proclaimed Oliver's record of helping the population ("Oliver Government gave Women Minimum Wage and 15,000 Women and Girls have Benefitted") and the dastardliness of the Conservatives ("Conservative Speakers have Threatened to Interfere with the Minimum Wage Act!"). The advertisements of the other candidates were, in comparison, sober and unimaginative. Richard Sargent, the Conservative candidate, published a short statement merely promising sanity in the Legislature, honesty in administration and lower taxes.

To no one's surprise, Horace won his own seat handily, although the Liberals barely managed to hold onto power. "Late Hour Returns Show Liberals Return with Small Majority. Dr. Wrinch is elected in Skeena," the headline of the *Herald* proclaimed. Total votes cast were 1,567, of which Horace won 791, Dockrill 530 and Sargent 246.

Horace at once sent a telegram to Premier Oliver, who had lost his own seat, offering to resign if he wanted to run in Skeena in a by-election, but Oliver declined this offer and later ran successfully in the Nelson riding. There was no escaping it. Horace was now the member representing the Skeena riding. The campaign in the riding was declared by the *Herald* to be a clean one, and "the candidates are as good friends today as they were before nomination. . . . We do not particularly congratulate Dr. Wrinch on his election but we do most heartily congratulate the voters," the *Herald* said, "on the wisdom of their choice."

For the times, though, the election across the province had been nasty, with allegations of dishonesty and corruption flying as quickly as the newspapers could carry them. As a result, when the votes were counted, it was found that not only Oliver but all three party leaders had lost their seats. Bowser soon resigned as Conservative leader, and McRae left provincial politics to enter federal politics. Oliver, though, was still premier and was able to form the government, albeit with a reduced majority. His government had a solid bench of five Liberal representatives from the North, one of whom was Horace.

At the election party held to thank the voters, Horace moved through the crowd of about two hundred who were milling around on the lawn in front of the hospital. He chatted with one then the other, thanking them for their support. The evening was a little chilly, but at least the rain was holding off. It all looked very festive with Chinese lanterns strung from the trees. This evening, anyway, was a time to celebrate. Everyone seemed to be enjoying the flower gardens and the homegrown strawberries and cream, cakes and sandwiches. Leonard, Cooper and their friends had been playing tennis earlier.

In his speech, Horace thanked the voters and said he was honoured by their choice. He hoped he would serve their interests as best he could. He invited anyone who wanted to have a social of their own to use the hospital lawns. The more people he drew into the hospital community the better.

After the speeches there was to be a musical program. Leonard had threatened to play or sing something, and Mr. Connon would be giving one of his monologues that everyone enjoyed so much. Afterwards, Horace knew, the young people would be singing well into the night. It was a satisfying evening.

Before going to Victoria to take his seat, Horace had a meeting with Prime Minister Mackenzie King. On a tour of the West, the prime minister came by train along the Skeena River to Prince Rupert. After the journey, he wrote in his diary:

> This has been a wonderful day. I have seen nothing anywhere comparable to the scenery along the Skeena River as we have enjoyed it all day long. I fairly shouted for joy when I awoke at eight and looked out at the mountains and valleys and streams. It would be impossible to describe the grandeur of the whole scene, the rugged vastness,

exceeding the Rockies in charm and strength. . . . I sat on the back of the car most of the way, both morning and afternoon just feasting my eyes and soul. For the appeal is to one's soul. I sang hymns, the old Presbyterian psalms and paraphrases. It was a day of worship of God through the glory of his handiwork.

The *Herald* reported that Horace went with Olof Hanson onto the prime minister's train car for lunch and spent some time talking about the Skeena district and its requirements. It is possible that they may have boarded the train when it stopped at New Hazelton and travelled with the prime minister to Prince Rupert. "Dr. Wrinch told the Premier," the *Herald* said (at that time, the title was used interchangeably with prime minister),

that he would not be swamped with requests from the interior for little local concessions, but that the big interest of the interior was tied up with the railway and the Pacific port. He urged the premier to do everything possible to help the development of the railway and the port, for these were the two great markets for most of the produce of the interior. With all the facilities provided for handling freight, the interior could get along nicely by developing the resources. . . . Dr. Wrinch impressed very strongly on the Premier that it was not the desire of the people of the north that the wheat and other products of the Peace River country be taken to Vancouver, with a haul of several hundred miles greater than that required to allow the traffic to take its natural course to Prince Rupert. Vancouver and the south may have more votes and thus might easily influence a government to adopt a policy disastrous to the country, and the North was now making its representations to avoid any such mistake.

The prime minister, wily, subtle and smoothly noncommittal, admitted that the doctor had indeed voiced his own personal opinions as to future developments in the North. The *Herald* was a little more skeptical of the prime minister's sincerity. It did not think taxpayers would be satisfied until "the Premier's sincerity takes form in an elevator, wheat trains, trans-Pacific boat service, at least one new boat to be built at Rupert, an outlet at Rupert for the Peace River wheat, and a railway that is more than a branch with one blind end."

—◦∿◦—

Premier Oliver's Liberal party had won only twenty-three seats in a forty-eight-seat house. The revolt of the electorate that had nearly brought down his government reflected the changes that were happening in society after the war. Old-style politics would no longer work. New policies had to appeal to reformers, soldiers and farmers. He saw clearly that his government's survival was now dependent on the Labour party in the Legislature, and that much of his program would have to be progressive in order to maintain its support.

Oliver stood up to his critics inside the party and pushed on with a radical program. This included constructing university buildings at Point Grey in Vancouver, extending workmen's compensation benefits, spending money on bridges and roads, introducing new old-age pension measures and, of great interest to Horace, taking up the matter of public health insurance.

When the legislative session opened in October 1924, Horace did not wait long to make his maiden speech. He would not have been shy. Although reserved, he had over thirty years' experience of public speaking. In early November, therefore, he rose to his feet and seconded the motion on the budget. After talking of the accomplishments of the government in health care, he described in detail the Skeena region and its potential.

He spoke about the importance of transportation for the North. Transportation is British Columbia's greatest need, he said, and it is time that the Province realized this and stopped chasing outside capital to develop its resources. When completed, the new Trans-Provincial Highway would open up the North for tourists and link Victoria to the Grand Trunk Railway country. He predicted a marvellous future for the ports of Vancouver, Victoria and especially Prince Rupert, behind which, he said, lay a vast undeveloped territory.

The *Victoria Daily Times* congratulated Horace on his maiden speech. He was new to the experience, it said, and he had acquitted himself as if he were thoroughly at home in the legislative atmosphere. Dr. Wrinch, in his comments about the North and the need for better transportation, it noted, had "left much material for reflection in the minds of his fellow members of the House." The *Herald* liked the speech so much that it published it almost in its entirety over two editions.

When in Victoria for the weeks of the parliamentary session, Horace often stayed at the James Bay Hotel and walked to and from the Legislature. As a backbencher, though, he spent only such time in Victoria as was necessary for legislative business. Even apart from his inexperience of the House and its procedures, there would have been no question of his being in the cabinet. He had a medical practice to maintain, as well as a hospital and farm to run.

Horace's venture into politics did not, of course, go unnoticed by his Methodist friends. Some questioned whether it was appropriate for a minister of the church to enter politics at all. A clerical colleague, defending him, wrote that Horace's answers to his critics were unanswerable, saying, "When opportunity came for him to enter politics, some of his friends criticized his decision to do so, on the ground that the activities of the Church are on a higher plane than those of the state. His reply was to the effect that in a representative form of government, Christian interests ought to be represented, and that therefore an avowedly Christian worker had a rightful place in the Legislative Assembly."

At the end of his first session, Horace recorded his impressions of the House. He wrote to his constituents, the *Herald* reported, to dispel the notion that members did not work when bills were not being discussed in the House. He outlined how much work on legislation was done in various committees at times when people were perhaps wondering when the Legislature would get down to business. Wanting to dispel the impression that all members did was to hand out contracts to friends, he said that, in his experience, members actually worked very hard to balance the needs of their constituents with the interests of the province as a whole.

Horace took his duties as an elected politician seriously and involved himself fully in the business of the House. He spoke on many measures in the next few years. His long journeys by train and steamer to and from Victoria gave him ample time to brief himself thoroughly on the issues. In addition to advocating for health insurance legislation, he spoke on topics that evidenced the thoroughness of his research and the wide range of his interests.

The *Province's* legislative reporter described Horace in an article in December, 1925:

> The discursive debate was continued this afternoon by Dr. Wrinch of Skeena. . . . He brings with him a suggestion of the North country, where he is physician in ordinary [in regular service or attendance] to a far-scattered community. Tales are current in this House which do honor to the service rendered by Dr. Wrinch to the ailing humanity of that northern country. He is a serious-minded man, but there is a touch of quiet humour in him, too, and there is no member who commands a greater respect among his fellow members of this House. These qualities of his were conspicuous in his quiet, grave speech today. . . . He left the impression, as he always does after his infrequent interventions in debate, that if the riding of Skeena can ill afford to lose his medical services during the term of the session, the House and the country benefits by his presence in the legislature.

In 1925, his farming knowledge too valuable to be wasted, Horace was appointed secretary to the agriculture committee but, sniffed the *Herald*, "unless the minister of agriculture changes his plans the committee will not have much to do." Horace's contribution, however, was such that he became chairman of that committee. He was not above political theatre at times. In February 1928, he brought samples of Bulkley Valley cheese into the Legislature for the members to try. Reportedly they declared it delicious. As a farmer and belonging to farming organizations in the Skeena district, he was much concerned about the dairy industry. He took up the problem of milk distribution when he met with the Board of Trade in Prince Rupert in March 1925.

His proposal was that the government should establish a depot there for the handling and marketing of milk and cream. The government would control this for five years to give farmers the opportunity to build up their herds and build the necessary plant. In due course, farmers would receive part of their money in the form of stock in the distributing depot, eventually to own the entire business. The government would receive full return for its investment. The farmers would manage the business themselves, and the public would get a sufficient supply of milk, cream and butter.

He went to Victoria to discuss the proposal with the government. Returning to Hazelton in mid-April, he reported on progress. Although the Ministry of Agriculture had agreed to continue the Vanderhoof creamery for that season, it was not persuaded by his ideas about a depot at Prince Rupert. It was perhaps a little too progressive.

The Produce Marketing Act of 1927 was one of the more controversial pieces of legislation of the Oliver government. Fruit farmers in the Okanagan Valley were losing confidence that the free market system could give them a reasonable profit on their produce. Many believed that they needed to have a more co-operative system and that the government had to enforce it. The directors of the Associated Growers in November 1926 and the members of the British Columbia Fruit Growers Association in January 1927 therefore asked the government to set up a committee of direction. This would regulate the grading, packing, shipping and marketing of the entire crop and require all shippers to be members of a new Growers and Shippers Association.

Oliver did not like this proposal, partly because he was a classic free-market Liberal, partly because he thought it could be unconstitutional and partly because he thought it could cost him votes in Vancouver. However, he did accept that it would be popular in agricultural districts and in particular in the Okanagan, where he needed votes. Politically, he was not in a strong enough position to prevent many in his caucus from supporting it. He therefore compromised by allowing it to be introduced as a private member's bill.

As chairman of the agriculture committee, Horace introduced the Produce Marketing Act in the House. Although he did not like excessive state intervention in the economy, he was pragmatic enough to realize that, without it, the produce industry was in danger of collapse. It was, in any event, in tune with what he had already proposed in the North for the Bulkley Valley dairy farmers. The minister of agriculture then complicated matters by proposing that the bill be expanded to cover milk and other dairy products. Including milk in its bill made it even more unpopular in Vancouver, where there were numerous Liberal members.

Since the minister owned, or had recently owned, a dairy farm in Chilliwack and may have had a conflict of interest, he probably should not have intervened. The legislation ignited fierce opposition from some small producers, who felt they had been left out of the decision-making process; from large independents, who did not need it; and from those who, like the premier, on principle did not agree with the state's intervention in the economy.

At this time, it was not thought to be the role of the state to intervene so directly, a role it took on in great measure only during the 1930s and thereafter. Milk was taken out of the Act, reportedly at the demand of the Liberal members in Vancouver as their price for voting in favour. After fierce debate, the bill became law on March 3, 1927. The premier and numerous Liberals voted against it, but the left-wing members and the Conservatives, delighted at an opportunity to split the Liberals, supported it. Opponents criticized the Act as being communistic.

"I have never seen in this House," Captain MacKenzie, a Liberal, said, "a piece of legislation so repugnant, so repulsive, so subversive of the principles of economics. It is the most reactionary piece of legislation brought into this House in the past seven years, and I do not see how anyone with regard to the principles of liberty can conscientiously support it." MacKenzie said it would be setting up a "soviet dictatorship under the control of the minister of agriculture" in the Okanagan and Fraser valleys. The legislation, which did bring some stability to the industry, did not survive a legal challenge, being struck down by the Supreme Court in 1931 as being unconstitutional. Nevertheless, the Act opened the way for increasing government intervention in the economy.

Horace did not confine himself to farming and health matters in the Legislature. He supported, for example, students at the University of British Columbia. Legislation that had established a provincial university in 1890 had been repealed the following year after disagreement about where the university should be located. It was re-established by legislation in 1908. In 1910, land on Point Grey in Vancouver was chosen for the campus. Construction started but slowed down during the war.

In 1915, though, a temporary site was opened at the McGill college facilities adjacent to Vancouver General Hospital on Fairview slopes. These quickly became over-crowded when students returned from the war, which led to students marching in 1922 — the famous Great Trek — to put pressure on the authorities to hurry up. Eventually the Point Grey campus opened in 1925.

Horace stood up for students and the university in a debate in the House in December 1925. "University training," he declared emphatically, in answering attacks on higher education, "makes a man more fitted for any job than he would be without it." He recommended that employers should be sympathetic towards employing them, saying that a qualified student was of far more value to them and his country than he was before. "He should be invited into industry, there to take his place in the economic life of the Province."

Horace was an advocate for teachers' pensions. Some provision for pensions had been established earlier, but it had not been effective. He introduced a motion, supported by the finance minister, John MacLean, to encourage the request of teachers for pensions. The motion, which was passed unanimously, recommended that all necessary assistance be given to teachers by the finance department to prepare carefully worked-out legislation on an actuarial basis. This was to be completed in time for its presentation to the House sufficiently early in its next session to be given full consideration.

Back home in March 1927, Horace was "in high spirits," the *Herald* said, "over the way in which the government met all the attacks of the opposition and the way in which the government got through all of its important legislation." It also reported that he had been able to get $120,000 from the new road fund for the road between Skeena Crossing (Kitseguecla) and Terrace.

Horace's work as a backbencher should be seen within the context of Premier Oliver's progressive social program. Horace believed in these policies — health insurance in particular — but he did not initiate them against the grain of his party. He had been arguing for public health insurance for many years. Now that he was a member of the governing party, he had the opportunity to persuade his colleagues in the House and in Committee to move the project forward. As a result, he became known province-wide as the standard-bearer and champion for public health insurance.

In an address to the governors of Vancouver General Hospital in 1924, Dr. E.H. Young, the provincial health secretary, said, "For a number of years 'care of the sick' by the state has ... been a petty [that is, small] hobby of Dr. Wrinch of the Hazelton Hospital and as President of the British Columbia Hospital Association for two years, he advanced that scheme before the Association and had it presented to the government," which, however, after a promising start, had not acted on it.

Horace persevered. He stood in the House on the afternoon of February 7, 1927, and described in detail how the health insurance scheme he was proposing could and should work. "Dr. Wrinch," the *Daily Colonist* reported, "declared that the necessity of health insurance legislation was a matter of vital importance to the Province." He was convinced that the majority of people in the province wanted it, and that it would be quite feasible to devise a satisfactory plan. Saying that it would have to be compulsory, he went on to explain that a tax would be levied on men between sixteen and sixty earning certain levels of income. Legislation should provide for medical attention in the home, medical attention as needed in a hospital, and support for dependents of those incapacitated by sickness.

In his view, he went on, the British legislation was too limited in scope, as it did not provide for special surgical services, hospital care of dependents, X-ray treatments or visiting nurses. He proposed a plan for British Columbia whereby payment for services performed by both hospitals and doctors should be based on a fair scale agreed by joint interests through a commission. With perhaps a touch of na-ivety, he noted that in discussing these ideas with "sensible people" he had failed to hear one cogent argument advanced against the project.

In February 1928, Horace once again raised his proposal in the House and tabled a motion to appoint a special committee to con-sider it. He stated that the need for health insurance had been gener-ally accepted by labour organizations, advisory boards of farmers' institutes and by the Hospital Association, as well as by many others.

Moved by Mr. Colley and seconded by Horace, this resolution was passed unanimously by the House immediately before prorogation on March 14, 1928, and the matter was sent to a committee for consideration. Mr. Colley said that the committee should consider the evidence of the Winn Commission's report and the collected ex-perience of many others. After so many years of public advocacy, Horace seemed to have the wind in his sails.

Then, however, Premier Oliver fell ill. During a visit to the Mayo Clinic, he learned he had terminal cancer. He offered to resign, but his caucus persuaded him to stay on as premier in name while John MacLean took over his duties. When Oliver died at the end of August 1927, MacLean became premier.

When Premier MacLean called an election for July 1928, Horace would have wondered what the Conservatives would do with this health insurance initiative if they gained power. Might they abandon it? Given that possibility, Horace decided to stand for re-election. There was still so much to do.

Horace had always been a temperance advocate. In his Ontario years, he and his brother had organized meetings of the Sons of Temperance. He approved therefore of prohibition and wanted stricter controls. Over the years, he had given many talks on the evils of liquor, having seen its effects on the health of the First Nations. He would have been pleased when prohibition was introduced in British Columbia in 1917 (after a disputed referendum) but saddened when it was repealed in 1921. He probably saw, however, that it wasn't working. That did not stop him, though, from arguing for restrictions on the sale of liquor.

When in the Legislature, he often spoke against the relaxation of liquor laws. In August 1925, he spoke at the presbytery of the United Church in Prince Rupert about the problems with the system of liquor control that had replaced prohibition. Noting that in some cases, prohibition had been successful, he declared "emphatically that all recent experiments with the handling of the liquor traffic, including Government control and the beer parlours, had been a failure." Archbishop de Vernet of the Anglican Church, also present at the meeting, agreed with him.

In February 1927, the *Western Recorder* praised Horace's work at the hospital and his work in the legislature, especially in working to destroy the liquor traffic. "The only right thing to do is to stamp the traffic out of our national life," it said. They all tried, but it was a battle doomed to failure. The laws against selling liquor to First Nations, nevertheless, remained in place. Although, as a correspondent had pointed out as early as 1904, the First Nations were quite capable of filling out a mail-order blank at the Hudson's Bay Company for what they required, not forgetting the all-important whisky. It must at times have seemed a hopeless task.

"Everyone," the *Western Recorder* said, "knows of Dr. Wrinch's earnest and sincere desire to destroy the liquor traffic." In 1927, Horace made what was described as a thoughtful contribution to the discussion. Far too much legitimate and illicit liquor, he had said, was available. He advocated, amongst other things, closing down the export warehouse, because liquor was being exported and then imported back into the province illegally at marked-up prices. He also argued that educational programs should be put in place in schools to discourage the young from drinking alcohol.

His zeal even in this, however, appears to have been tempered by his ever-present practicality. Hazelton was a town of hard drinkers, and Horace knew, within the limits of the law, he had to accept this. When Jimmy May, an old prospector, was sick and in great pain, he had refused to go to the hospital for necessary surgery. Knowing that Jimmy was in the habit of going to the Hudson's Bay Company every morning for a tot of rum, Horace promised him that in hospital he would also be given a good drink of rum every morning. "That young feller Wrinch is a smart doctor," Jimmy said. "He's the only one [who] could find out what was wrong with me."

As Horace had often explained, he did not run the hospital as a profit-making business. One year, there would be a small surplus, the next year a small loss. A useful line of credit with the bank kept him going. The nature of the hospital's finances made these swings unavoidable. When economic times were bad, there was always the potential for revenues to decline in two ways: first, through the decline in revenue because sick people stayed away and, second, through the decline in per capita grants from the governments. These conditions reduced revenues at a time when costs were rising. Although Horace was always trying to persuade the provincial government and the Indian Department to increase the per capita grant, the problem remained. The hospital's finances were to come under most severe pressure when the Depression arrived at the start of the next decade. Meanwhile, Horace had to manage the swings.

By the beginning of 1925, the finances were in "about as low a condition as ever in its history." Largely as a result of circumstances beyond the control of management, the situation had become serious.

Enterprises such as the pole business were closing, and the prospect of a decline in the number of patients was ever-present. Furthermore, people fell behind in paying their bills.

Notwithstanding this, Horace reported that 1924 had been the largest in the hospital's history in many respects — largest attendance, largest revenues but also largest expenses. The number of patient days had, in fact, increased fifteen percent from the previous year, which amounted to an extra 1,000 days of treatment. All who applied for treatment, he said, were admitted even though their cases might be hopeless.

Horace was concerned that a number of people who could well afford their hospital fees were slow in their payments. In his report for 1925, he noted that the amount unpaid by such people was $7,500 — a huge sum that, if it had been paid, would have put the hospital in "a wonderful financial position." One of his unreported and least pleasant jobs was visiting wayward debtors to persuade them to honour their obligations. There was no point, though, in bringing legal action against those who had no money. Happily, with all his measures of economy, there turned out to be a small surplus for 1925. Then, providentially, a new system of workmen's compensation payments was put in place, and the Missions Board and the Department of Indian Affairs increased their grants. This significantly improved the hospital's financial position and continued to improve it for the rest of the decade.

The desirability — indeed necessity — of a new residence for the nurses had been talked of for many years. The present quarters had become inadequate in every respect. Nurses still lived on the top floor of the hospital and, apart from the crowding, this was increasingly being seen as a fire trap. Now it was time to take action. At the annual meeting in February 1924, therefore, the patrons of the hospital authorized Horace to investigate the cost and feasibility of building a new residence.

In April, the patrons agreed to furnish the interior of the new residence if the Methodist Missions Board agreed to pay for construction of the building. The Missions Board agreed to pay $5,000 towards the cost of construction. The Hospital Board thereupon made the formal decisions to build a nurses residence and also to build a new house on the grounds for the house surgeon.

Nothing much could be done over the winter except to raise the additional funds required. The provincial government agreed to pay $2,000, and this was used to lever the Department of Indian Affairs also to make a contribution. During the winter a canvass was made in the community to pay for the furnishings and decoration. The Ladies Auxiliary stepped up to the challenge of raising some of the needed money. By mid-November, the amount in the fund had already reached $2,023, Horace himself giving $85 and his son Cooper $10.

Once the decision had been made and funding secured, everything happened quickly. Planning started, the site was chosen and design settled. Full architectural drawings were prepared. Tenders were issued for the construction in early August 1925. Bids, the tender documents said, were required by August 12. The building, using only northern lumber, was to be thirty-by-thirty-eight feet, with two storeys. Hot and cold water were to be provided on both floors, with thirteen rooms and accommodation for fourteen nurses if necessary. This would open up twelve much-needed beds in the hospital. A Terrace firm, H.M. Wilson, won the construction contract for an agreed cost of $9,000. Work was to commence immediately.

By January 1926, the building was erected and was ready for painting and furnishing. "The new residence," the *Herald* reported, when it opened in March, "is a handsome structure, not so much from the outside appearance as from the interior finish and the furnishings. There is nothing lacking that would add to the comfort and happiness of the nurses, and this in turn will reflect on the nurses' services to the patients in hospital." So, with a modern residence for the nurses and a hospital enlarged by a dozen beds without having to make major renovations, Horace was ready to face the rest of the decade.

———ᐧᐧᐧ———

Apart from his commitments in Victoria during the legislative sessions and his travel on constituency business, Horace was always thinking about new ventures for Hazelton. This included what to do with the land at Mission Point, which he still had the responsibility of managing. Since it was now easy to reach this land across the low-level bridge built towards the end of the war, Horace toyed with the idea of leasing part of it for a summer resort and auto camp. He approached local businessmen, but nothing seemed to come from that. Other ideas were considered, including using it as an airfield and a golf course.

In 1925, Horace bought a new car. The *Herald* continued to find entertainment in his driving, implying that it was a cause of some amusement, and perhaps some apprehension, for citizens of the district. This can be seen in a report of an incident in June. No one was harmed and it wasn't really Horace's fault. The *Herald* reported:

The Doctor was sailing along serenely at a rate quite to the public danger (were there any public) and at peace with himself and the world. Suddenly a culvert gang and an open culvert hove in sight. The boys filled in enough to let his car by and all he suffered was a puncture. His first aid kit hanging to the back of the car provided a new tire and the heavens looked bright once more. Such bliss was not for long. Another culvert hove in sight, wider and deeper than the first. The car refused to make the jump so he tried a detour and got tangled up in roots, stumps, brush and the bottom of the ditch. The brake linings were just new, and the low gear refused to grip. It was embarrassing, but the culvert gang volunteered assistance and hauled the car out of the ditch, but bang went that — spare tire. There was nothing to it but to put on a patch. So . . . he sat upon the roadside and whistled a barmy [silly] air while operating on the spare tire. By the time the tire was fixed and the brake bands were tightened, the culvert had been completed and the gang gone home to supper. The member for Skeena was still many miles from his steak and onions.

As mentioned earlier, the *Herald*'s publisher, Sawle, was an old acquaintance, and probably enjoyed teasing him.

In June 1926, Horace received the welcome news that Leonard,
his eldest son, had passed his medical exams at the University of
Toronto with honours and had been accepted for the staff of St.
Michael's Hospital. This must have brought back memories of his
own internship there, when he and Alice had been planning their
missionary life together and wondering what Kispiox would be like.

Not long after, it was arranged that Leonard would return to
Hazelton to work at the hospital. He joined the staff the following
September, having completed post-graduate studies in California.
Immediately, he started to take some of the workload off Horace's
shoulders. Soon it would be Leonard who was being reported in the
Herald as making public health announcements for Hazelton, tend-
ing to the sick and, in one sad case, diagnosing a child with infantile
paralysis.

That same month, Ralphena went to the Provincial Royal Jubilee
Hospital in Victoria to commence her training as a nurse. In 1924,
Cooper had left the Union Bank and had taken over management of
the Up-To-Date Drugstore. He also took over the postmaster's job
from Richard Sargent. The following year, he married Briseis Rock
in Hazelton United Church, with Horace himself officiating. Soon
their daughter, Leonora, arrived, and Horace became a grandfather.

Horace went on a vacation to visit his brother Frank in California
again. On the way down, as always unable to resist the opportunity to
add to his knowledge, he stopped in Victoria to hear Dr. Banting, the
discoverer of insulin, speak at a convention. When he was visiting his
friend Robert Peers in Colfax, California, he accompanied him as a
guest to the July meeting of the Placer County Medical Society in
Hobart Mills. The assembled physicians heard papers on such matters as "Skin Disturbances Due to Food and Drugs" and "Medical
Aspects of Fifteen Cases of Murder." (He could, no doubt, have
contributed his stories about Simon Gunanoot.)

From California, Horace travelled to Ontario, where he visited family and friends. While there, he went fishing in Bass Lake near Orillia and, the *Herald* noted, caught a big black bass. He visited the Toronto Exhibition and declared it one of the "wonders of the world." Noting that the only British Columbian products exhibited there were timber resources and seeing this as a missed opportunity, he promised to recommend to the government that it expand the province's participation in such exhibitions to include other mining and fishery products to help them find markets in Ontario.

Hospital Day celebrations came and went. The May 1927 event was as successful as in previous years. There were tours of the hospital and the new nurses residence, there were songs, and there were speeches. In the baseball game, "as per usual the Indians" beat the settlers this time by a score of 13 to 6. "At no period did the whites even have a look in." At the end of the day, after the national anthem, there was a dance. One of Horace's duties on Victoria Day of 1927 was to crown the Queen of the May at the New Hazelton celebrations. Placing the crown on the head of young Jessie Smith, he said he hoped her reign would be long and happy. Following this there was a Maypole dance and a baseball game and a tug-of-war — both of which Old Hazelton won.

In mid-September, the *Herald* routinely noted that Horace had left town a few days before and gone to Vancouver. This time, though, his journey was not routine. On Thursday, September 15, 1927, Horace quietly married May Hogan in Chown United Church, far away from the fuss and attention that a wedding in Hazelton would have attracted. The groom was now sixty-one years of age, while the bride had turned forty-six a few weeks previously. His brother Charles, then living in Vancouver, was his best man. Horace had known May for many years. It is possible that he first met her when he came up the coast on the *Queen City* and visited Port Simpson with Rev. Whittington all those years before.

The newlyweds spent a few days in Victoria before returning to Hazelton. The news of their marriage, the *Herald* said, would be received with general pleasure by their friends. Back home in Hazelton a week later, the new Mrs. Wrinch announced that she would hold a reception at her house the following week. Horace, meanwhile, was back at work. He was assisting Dr. Hall in his federally and provincially sponsored study of First Nations health, which was examining in particular how better to deal with the scourge of tuberculosis. There was so much work to be done.

Horace had much to look forward to. His children were now adults, marrying and starting to give him grandchildren. The hospital was on a firm financial footing for perhaps the first time in its existence. It was even possible to think of replacing it with something more modern. He would stand for the Skeena riding in the provincial election to be held later in the year. If re-elected, he could continue to pursue his ideas of health insurance in the Legislature. And, of course, he could settle down with his new wife to enjoy their future together.

CHAPTER 12

Health Insurance Advocate
1928–1933

AT THE LIBERAL PARTY convention held in Terrace in June 1928, the forty-one delegates present again unanimously chose Horace as the candidate for the Skeena riding. In his speech supporting Horace, Duff Pattullo said that "Dr. Wrinch would grace any cabinet as one of the first ministers of the Crown."

Premier MacLean, who had also been at the convention, then accompanied Horace and Pattullo back to Hazelton for an election rally. As leaders do in constituencies when campaigning, MacLean praised the local candidate. Describing Horace as one of the outstanding men of the province, he repeated what Dr. Sutherland had said of him when Horace was speaking in the Legislature on his favourite topic of health insurance. "Dr. Wrinch is a wonder. That old fellow never stands up but what he says something." Whatever his thoughts on being called an "old fellow," Horace in turn praised the premier, in the way candidates do of their leader when he is in town. The following week Dr. Simon Fraser Tolmie, the Conservative leader, was in the Hazeltons campaigning with Frank Dockrill, now back in the Tory fold. The *Herald*, in a fence-sitting editorial, said that both Dr. Wrinch and Mr. Dockrill were good, respected people, but that the election would be won on the policies of the parties rather than on the personalities of the representatives.

Horace may have been hurt, or even irritated, by a letter in the *Herald* at the end of the previous year signed by many of his friends and acquaintances — William Larkworthy, John Willan, Fred Goddard, Sawle among them — threatening not to vote for him if he continued to support his government's decision to replace the aging high-level Craddock bridge at Hagwilget by building a new one somewhere less convenient. They said this would destroy New Hazelton. Did Horace want to do that? In an election year?

Horace was caught between camps. In the one was the government he represented and its plans for the new bridge and in the other were leading citizens of Old and New Hazelton with vocal complaints about the location and the planned lower elevation. By February, however, Horace had prevailed on the government to build the replacement bridge in almost the same place as the existing 1913 bridge. He had also suggested that it be built at the same height above the river as the old bridge, thus eliminating the steep approach roads that had bedevilled the 1906 pack-train bridge. This was a significant victory and one that no doubt helped his re-election chances.

Horace campaigned hard. He held rallies — including a large one in New Hazelton with Duff Pattullo. He travelled the riding. He listened. He delivered more speeches. "The Doctor put up a good campaign and left very little undone," the *Herald* said. "He not only did a lot of work himself, but he had a whirlwind finish. . . ." He was at the election night dance in New Hazelton when he heard the results. Although Horace won his own seat by a large majority, the Liberal government of Premier MacLean was defeated. MacLean even lost his own riding and soon resigned as leader. Dr. Tolmie consequently became the premier in the new Conservative government. The electorate, economically prosperous, benefitting from new social welfare legislation and government spending on roads, bridges, a university, art galleries and theatres, had wanted change.

Back in Victoria, Horace moved from the government backbenches to the opposition backbenches. He would, the *Herald* said, be a good opposition member and would not allow party prejudices to blind him to the welfare of his district or the province. He was one of twelve Liberals elected, only seven of whom had been in the previous House. Horace would thus have been an experienced member of the caucus that chose Duff Pattullo as the next Liberal leader, a choice ratified by party members at the following convention. The new leader, a northerner, had been mayor of Prince Rupert and was an old acquaintance of Horace's.

Showing, as always, the Wrinch passion for "doing things" that his sister Mary had written about, Horace continued with his many causes when he was in opposition. Although his main interest in these years was still the promotion of state health insurance, he was active on many files. Since there were fewer Liberal members in the House than in the previous session, he had more to do. He was appointed to the agriculture, fisheries, forestry and mining committees. "That will, or ought to, keep the local member out of mischief while at the capital," the *Herald* opined.

And busy he undoubtedly was. Taking up the cause of protecting the sockeye salmon fishery on the Skeena, Horace advocated for new barriers at the entrance of rivers. These would allow sockeye through but prevent species such as dog salmon (chum) and pink salmon (humpbacks) from travelling up with them and destroying their spawn and young. He for one, he announced, did not consider the sockeye salmon industry to be dying. The government, he said, had asked the opposition to be constructive in its criticisms, and, well, here he was, being constructive.

On the other hand, he had no hesitation in holding up bills to ensure they would be effective. He was accused of delaying — being obstructive, it was said — a number of bills so as to insist on changes he felt strongly about. He held up, for example, the passage of the Contagious Diseases Act in committee. The government proposal, he said, would repeal some useful sections of the current legislation that gave power to the authorities to regulate the cleanliness of cows and milk. He had also concerns about the proposed Apiarists' Act. Both bills needed improvement. If more careful thought was obstruction, so be it.

In 1929, he tried to save the kingfisher. This bird, having a reputation for killing salmon hatchlings, was on the list of birds open for hunting. Pattullo called it a beautiful bird, and he too wanted to save it. Horace moved an amendment to the list that would have resulted in its remaining protected. "He argued," the *Daily Colonist* said, "that there was a disposition to be somewhat careless in the protection and in the destruction of wildlife." His amendment, however, failed, and the indiscriminate hunting of the beautiful kingfisher continued.

In a sketch of those making laws in the new Legislature, the *Victoria Colonist* said of him:

Dr. Wrinch is very highly esteemed among the members of the House. While he is an ardent Liberal in his convictions, the member for Skeena is able to throw aside his party feeling when he deems it wise in the interests of the country to do so. He prefers to view questions from the standpoint of their effect upon the general welfare of the province and the Dominion than from the narrow point of view of party advantage. He has, since he entered the House, manifested a deep interest in the subject of state health insurance, and served on the special committee that investigated the matter in the last House.

Horace was not going to let sitting on the opposition benches stop him from promoting state health insurance. Much like Cato the Elder in the Roman Republic, who added "Carthage Must Be Destroyed" at the end of most of his speeches, relevant or not, Horace seemed to add the need for health insurance into many of his speeches. And if Cato's audiences grew tired of the old man's speeches and the repetition of a well-worn theme, then perhaps, at times, so did Horace's.

When the Legislature assembled in January 1929, Horace proposed a motion that the House re-affirm its 1928 resolution and appoint a committee of the House to look into state health insurance. A headline in the *Vancouver Sun* proclaimed, "Wrinch to Insist on Health Action" and went on to say that "Dr. Wrinch of Skeena does not intend to let the new government escape responsibility for dealing with the problem of state health insurance. . . ."

In this he was successful. The House gave unanimous approval to the resolution, as amended, to establish a Royal Commission, which was to investigate and report back. "Dr. Wrinch," the *Vancouver Sun* reported, "said that he was glad to see the government so favourably disposed to his resolution. . . . He hoped it meant state health insurance was within measurable distance."

The Royal Commission met, travelled, received briefs and heard over 290 witnesses. It came through the North in August of 1930, stopping at Prince Rupert on August 16, Smithers on August 19 (where Horace made his own submission) and Prince George on August 20. In his submission, Horace said:

> I am speaking now as a resident of one of the more remote portions of the Province, and having lived over thirty years in this district, as a medical man and hospital administrator, I am expected to have a working knowledge of conditions and of the needs of the people. . . . I have only too often had to deal with people who, had there been a system of state health insurance in effect in this part of the province, would have been spared much suffering at the time they required help. . . . Dreading the expense of such attention, many do not seek help from doctor or hospital when they imperatively need it. I have long since reached the conclusion that a state health insurance system would be the solution of the problem of the people's health.

In its report, the Royal Commission recommended the adoption in British Columbia of publicly funded health insurance. Horace commended it in the House and pressed for swift implementation of its recommendations. The report, he said, was a classic, the best report on the subject yet. He said he hoped to see it implemented in the province in the following year. It all seemed to be about to happen.

The initiative, however, now lay with the Conservative government, and it did not — or was unable to — act on it. Premier Tolmie took no further action on health insurance. Beset by problems caused by the Depression, he had run out of ideas, energy and, when the election came, votes. It was left for the succeeding Pattullo government to accept and implement the Royal Commission's recommendations.

Horace himself seldom let pass an opportunity around the province to advocate for state health insurance. In June 1932, for example, while talking to farmers at Telkwa, he said he wanted to extend insurance benefits to farmers and their families. In August, he was talking about it in a reply to a toast at a banquet at a Board of Trade meeting in Fort Fraser. And at the Liberal party convention in 1932, he spoke in favour of it again, where it appeared that there could be strong opposition.

"Dr. H.C. Wrinch," the *Herald* reported, "was there with his advocacy of state health insurance. It met with divided support. At times the debate got quite heated. But the doctor has been at it for some years and he will stay with it for some more years until it becomes an accomplished fact." He was sufficiently well-known for his advocacy on this topic to be featured in a front page cartoon in the *Vancouver Daily Province*. The caricature of him ran with the caption "Dr. Wrinch, Skeena, sure started something when he introduced health insurance."

After one of Horace's speeches in the House, Bruce Hutchinson, staff correspondent for the *Province* and later long-time editor of the *Vancouver Sun*, wrote an affectionate but penetrating article about him as a politician:

Dr. Wrinch is one of the most useful and honoured members of this assembly, and his quiet enthusiasm for public business is only matched

by his almost child-like innocence of party politics. He takes no interest in partisan manoeuvres and accepts every proposal which comes
before the House at its face value, seeing in it none of those ulterior
motives that his colleagues invariably suspect. Dr. Wrinch spoke on
health insurance, and, as usual, his speech was admirable in its con-
tents, but not the kind of stuff to stir the passions or even make the
House listen very attentively. One could understand Conservative
members not paying much attention to a Liberal address on what
must be a dull subject, but it did seem rather disloyal when most of
the Liberals drifted out of the House. If they had listened they would
have learned a great deal more about health insurance than they are
likely to find out otherwise. In brief, Dr. Wrinch wants insurance
now and not a year from now.

—∿∿—

The time arrived when it became necessary to replace the 1904
hospital. It was no longer appropriate, the hospital inspector had
reported, for so many patients, many of them helpless, to be housed
in a wooden-frame structure. Maintenance of an old building was
expensive, and the costs of fuel and gasoline for heating and energy
were increasing. The threat of fire was ever-present. Horace would
have remembered the fire that had totally destroyed the Methodist
hospital at Rivers Inlet in August 1904. It might even have brought
back memories of the fire at St. Francis Agricultural School in Richmond all those years before. The need for a new building had long
ago been identified. Now action was required.

The annual meeting of the hospital patrons in April 1929 authorized the construction of a new hospital. (This was before the stock
market crash in October.) Horace had been planning this for a while,
it appears, and had presented a well thought-out and costed proposal
to the hospital board. Thanks to workmen's compensation payments
and increased grants, the hospital finances were, for once, healthy.
With forthcoming grants from governments, they could afford
$75,000 for a new hospital.

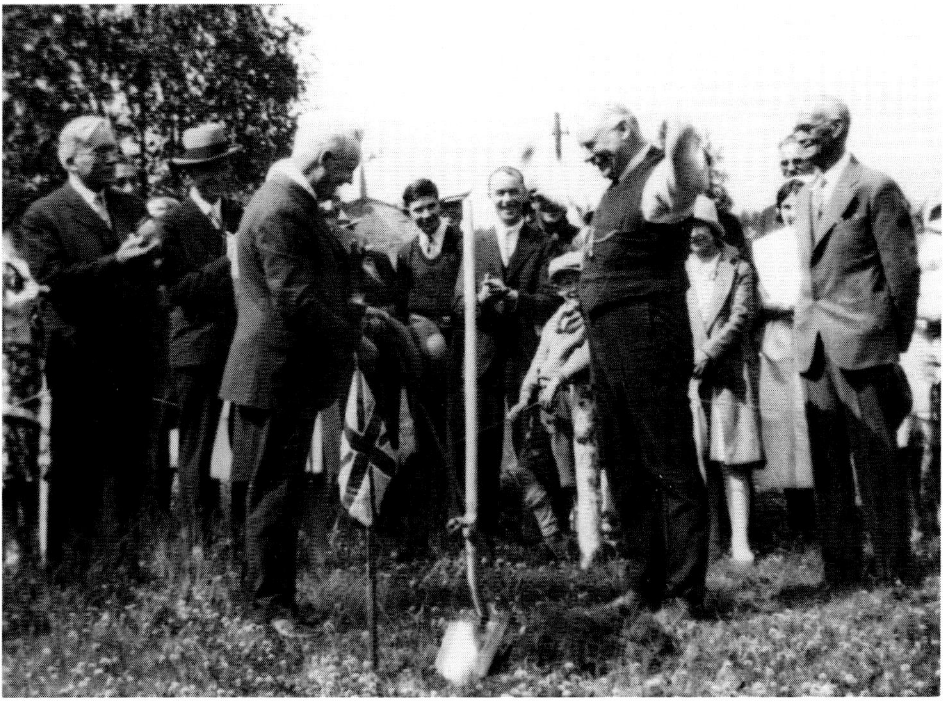

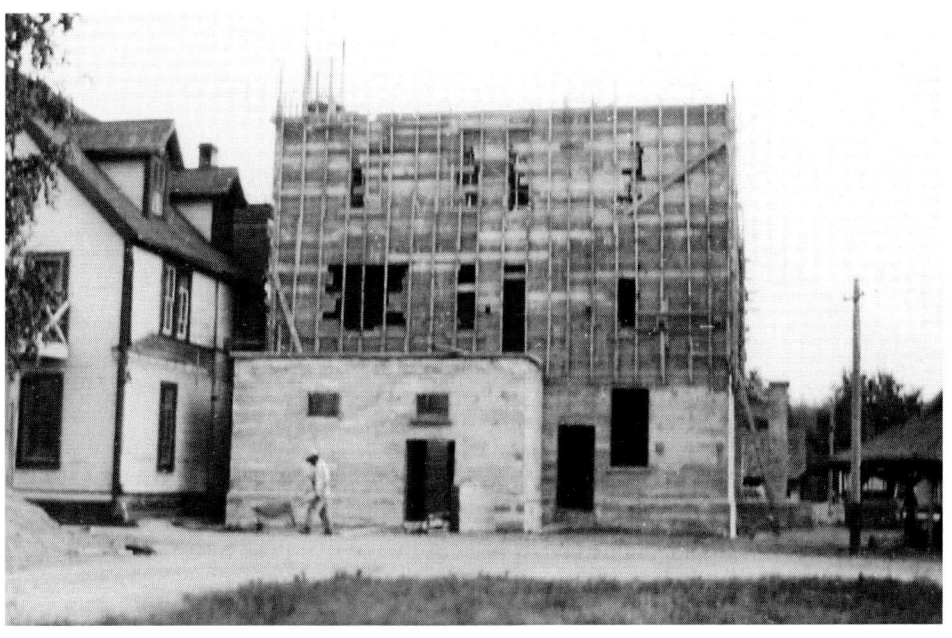

Lieutenant Governor Bruce, centre right, having successfully turned the sod
for the new hospital on June 22, 1930. Horace is on the left.

Construction of the new hospital in 1930.

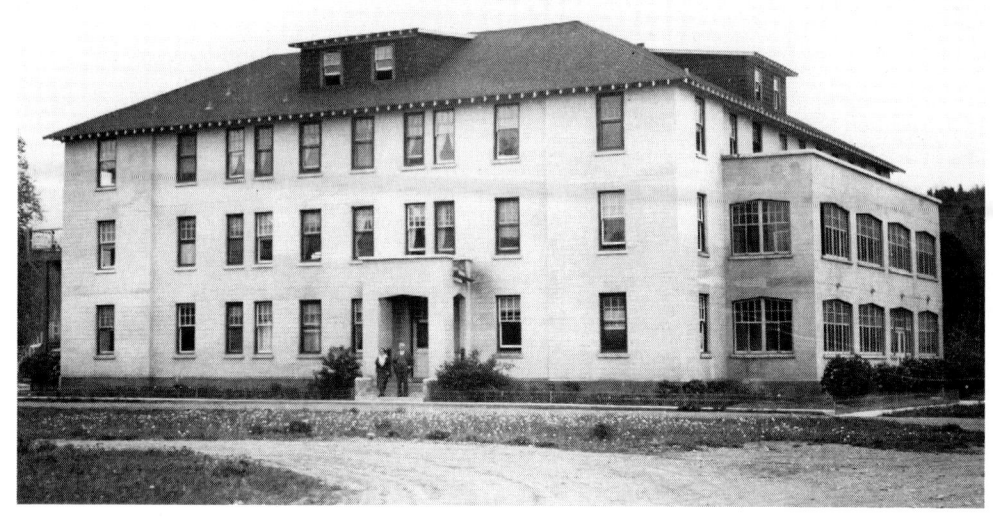

The new Hazelton Hospital, 1931.

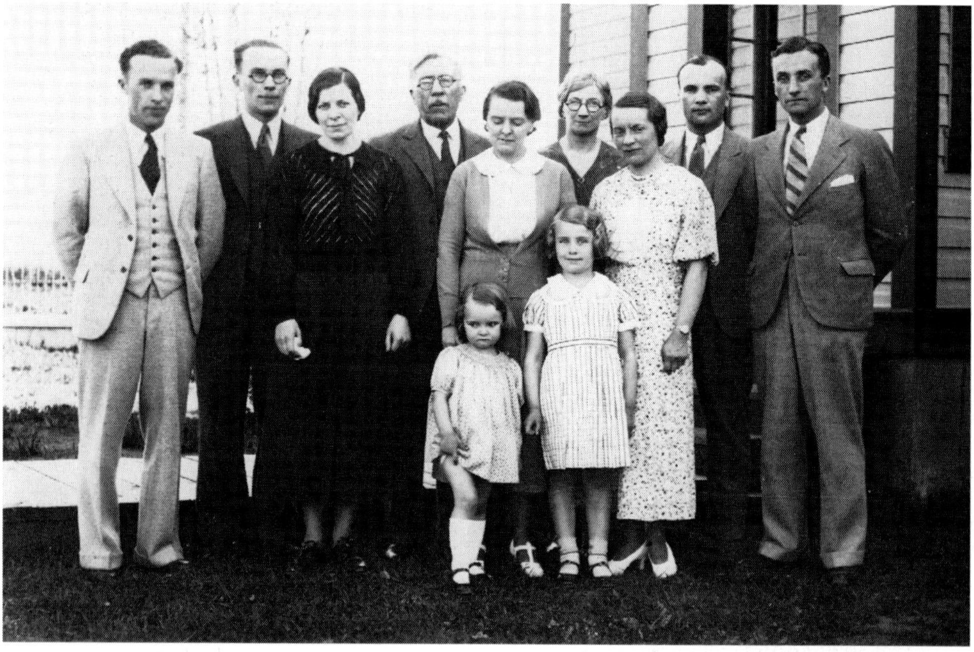

Horace's family in the mid 1930s. From left to right: Harold, Cooper with his wife Briseis, Horace, Frances (Leonard's wife), Horace's wife May, Ralphena, Leonard and Arthur. Leonard's daughter Mary and Cooper's daughter Leonora are in the front.

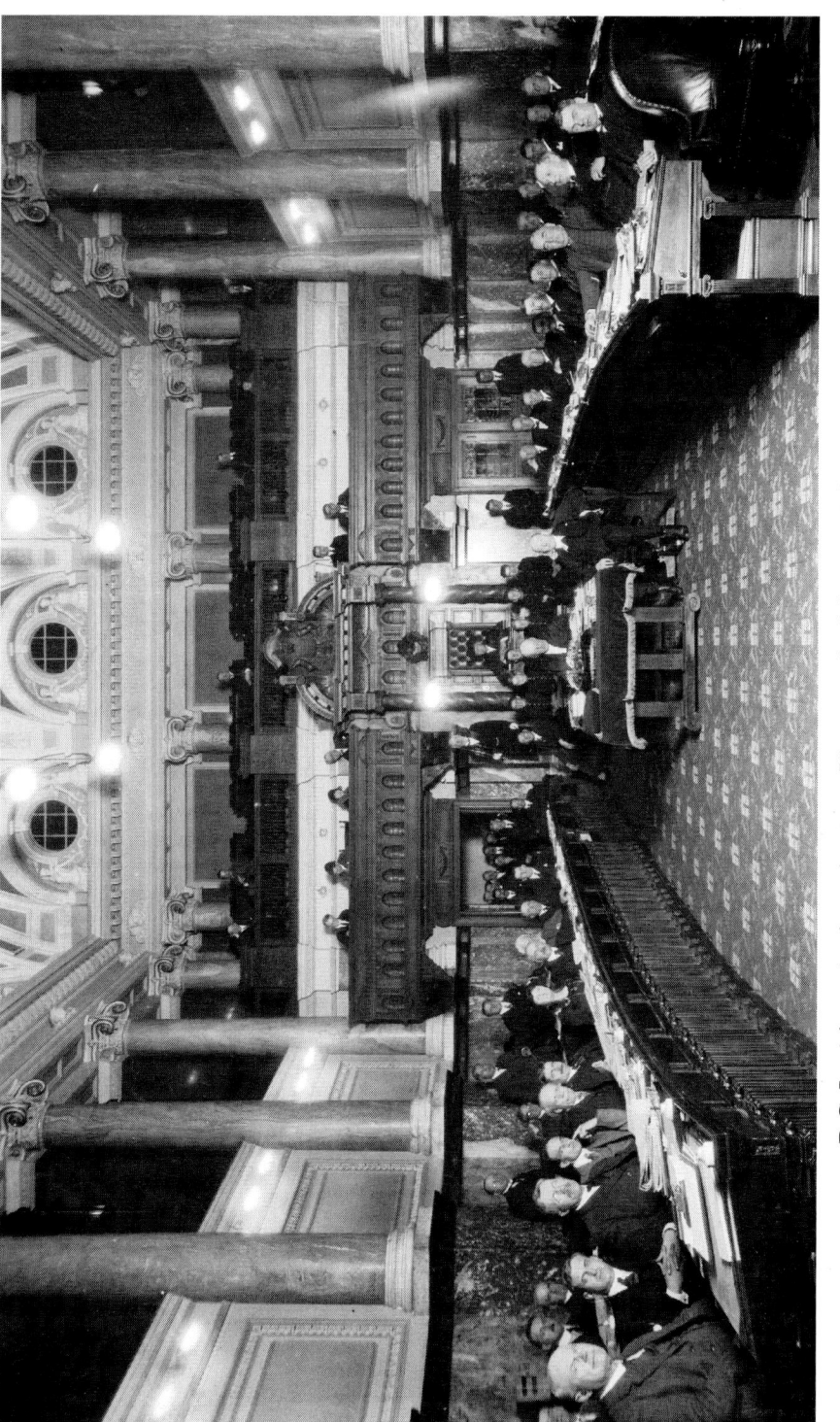

B.C. Legislature in the early 1930s. Horace is third from the left in the front row.

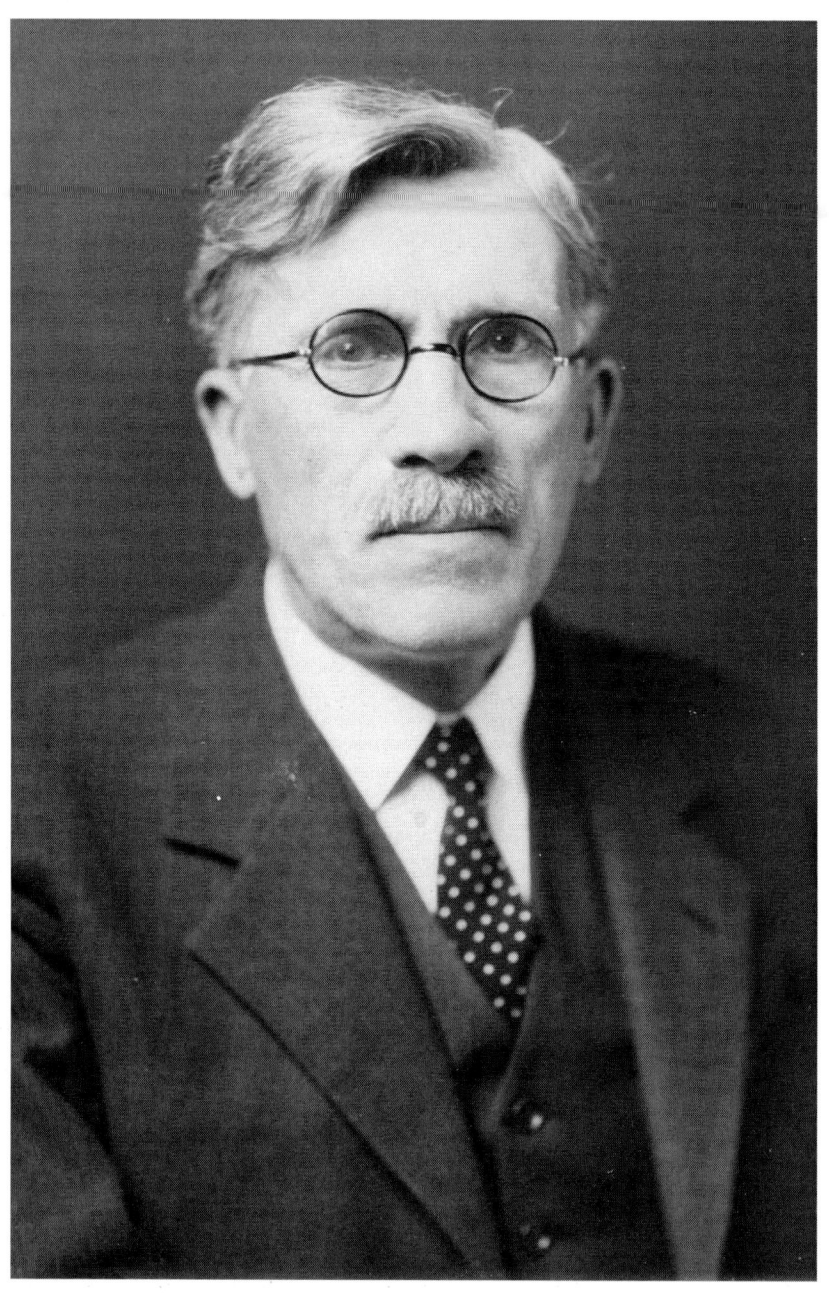

Horace Wrinch at the time of his retirement
from the hospital in 1936.

In December 1929, Horace and R.B. Cochrane, the secretary to the Missions Board at the time, met with Duncan Campbell Scott, deputy superintendent in the Department of Indian Affairs in Ottawa. Presenting him with the proposal, complete with Horace's draft plans, they persuaded the Dominion government to contribute $15,000. This was added to the $15,000 the Church had agreed to pay. The provincial government would pay $25,000 and the remainder was to be borrowed from the Royal Bank. Horace and his wife May themselves contributed more than $500.

The plans for the hospital, changed and approved by the two levels of government, were ready by the end of January 1930. The new hospital was to be built immediately in front of the existing one and would be two storeys high with a full basement. The Department of Public Works in Victoria then changed this plan to a three-storey L-shaped building, with a long side to the south. They issued the tenders at the beginning of April, with occupation required by October. Three tenders were submitted, and the contract was awarded to F.H. Shockley of Prince Rupert.

——

Horace seized a unique opportunity in June 1930 to bring attention to the new hospital. The occasion was the arrival in Hazelton of the most illustrious gathering of dignitaries ever to visit the town.

The parade entered New Hazelton under an evergreen arch. First Nations and non-Indigenous residents alike stared at the procession with intense interest, giving it a rousing welcome. No one in the Hazeltons had ever seen anything like it before. Leading the procession was piper Bob Richardson from Chilliwack, brother of Jimmy Richardson, the bagpiper Victoria Cross winner. After two red-coated mounted police on horses and three khaki-clad members of the provincial police on motorcycles, came P.E. Sands, driving the same Flanders 20 that he had driven into Hazelton on that epic journey in 1911.

Behind them, in a parade of cars that had started its journey in Vancouver almost 800 miles away, came Premier Tolmie and his wife, thirty to forty representatives of boards of trades and motoring organizations, and approximately fifty-five members of the press. Amongst these was Bruce Hutchison, who recorded the events for the *Province*.

Premier Tolmie's Caravan, as it was called, arrived on June 21, 1930. But this wasn't all. In Hazelton, they met a party arriving by train from Prince Rupert that included Lieutenant Governor Randolph Bruce of British Columbia, Governor Parks of Alaska and Ernest Sawyer, executive assistant to the United States secretary to the interior in Washington, D.C., all with their staff, and also many businessmen.

This important group had come to inaugurate the construction of a much-needed highway from the United States to the territory of Alaska. Premier Tolmie wanted this road built to open the northern part of the province for settlement and economic development. The road was to start in Hazelton, and, at that time, was planned to go up the Kispiox Valley. One of the subsidiary objectives was to create one of the greatest tourist highways anywhere in the world. Even though he had a reservation about the cost, Horace supported the project. The *Province* called him "one of the most influential Liberal members of the Legislature" and suggested that his support of the Alaska highway was "particularly significant."

During the official welcome, everyone was invited to a dance in New Hazelton that evening, an invitation accepted by all with great enthusiasm. The party then dispersed. Since there were not nearly enough hotel rooms in the Hazeltons to accommodate them all, many stayed with local residents.

Premier Tolmie's secretary, Jane Eva Denison, recorded the trip in her journal, which she entitled *Caravaning to the Land of the Golden Twilight*. In this she wrote: "This was all very thrilling and the people gave the Caravan a very rousing welcome.... Everyone went to the ball in the evening and had a wonderful time, the only disadvantage being that there were about twenty-five men to each lady. We got home again at daylight." This dance, which 200 attended and for which Gray's Orchestra had been brought in from Smithers, was held at the Omineca Hotel.

The following morning, they toured the local sites — the Hagwilget Canyon, the Gitxsan cemetery, Kispiox, the totem poles and Old Hazelton. The Gitxsan of Kispiox, reported the *Province* newspaper, approved of the highway and looked forward to driving their motor cars northwards. They scattered eagle feathers on the Americans as a mark of great esteem.

Horace jumped at the opportunity. What better way to initiate the new hospital and maintain public interest than by having a sod-turning ceremony! At the designated time, he led the official party from the steps of the hospital across to the spot that would be the southwest corner of the new hospital. First came the Lieutenant Governor, who, as the King's representative, was to have the honour of turning the sod. With him went Miss Mackenzie, his niece and chatelaine of Government House.

After the Lieutenant Governor had made a few introductory words, he handed his jacket to his niece and grasped the long-handled spade. This was not a ceremonial turning over of previously dug soft soil, but hard work on unprepared turf. After some amusement, he finally dug into the soil and managed to turn the sod. Premier Tolmie, Governor Parks, Sawyer and Sands then made a few remarks, all to the effect of congratulations and good luck. Miss Mackenzie was given a souvenir horn spoon carved by First Nations. She smiled as little Leonora Wrinch, Horace's granddaughter, presented her with a bouquet.

Horace, no doubt happy at how well it had gone, thanked all those present. Chief Tom Campbell then stepped forward and presented the Lieutenant Governor with a stone axe. Then, to Campbell's great delight, the Lieutenant Governor gave him his walking stick. The fifteen-man Hazelton Cornet Band under its leader, Abel Oakes, all Gitxsan, provided the musical entertainment.

After the ceremony, the visitors were treated to a drive around the district, then down to Kitseguecla. That evening a banquet, organized by the Ladies Auxiliary of the hospital, with Horace as chairman, was held in the Hudson's Bay Company warehouse. Many of the toasts and speeches boosted the attractiveness of the region for investment and settlement. Sands would have remembered the riotous banquet held when he had last visited Hazelton. This one was probably a little more sedate. Finally, Horace must have thought, as he surveyed the guests in a quiet moment, construction of the new hospital could now start.

Work, in fact, proceeded quickly. Concrete was poured in July. By early August, the walls were half up, and by the end of the month the roof was on. The Hospital board, having enough money, decided to install an elevator, for which Horace and May personally donated a substantial amount. The board met again at the end of October to plan the opening ceremony and to approve the selection and installation of equipment and furnishings. By mid-November, it was almost complete.

The word went out for donors to furnish eight private rooms, each room costing between $200 and $300. Donors were required to buy the standard-issue hospital bed, the swivel table and the metal wardrobe. After that they could furnish the room in any way their taste and desires suggested. The Women's Auxiliary agreed to pay for the furnishing of at least one ward and the Tomlinson family paid for another.

The board set December 29, 1930, as the day for the official opening. By then, the X-ray machine and elevator had been installed in the new building and were working properly. Guests had been invited. Everything was ready. The residents of Hazelton were invited to inspect their new hospital in the afternoon and then to attend the opening ceremony.

A crowd of over 200 Hazelton residents and First Nations gathered in the new hospital for the formal opening. In view of the bad weather, Horace was relieved that so many had been able to come.

Many of the roads were closed. Only one car had managed to get through from Smithers but the driver — probably S.S. Hoskins, who had been a hospital board member for seventeen years — admitted it "was not a joy ride." Many others from Terrace and Smithers had not been able to get through at all. The gathering enjoyed the piano playing of the Misses Dungate and Chappell and the singing of Mrs. Falconer and Miss Burn.

Such an event could not pass without speeches. Mr. Hoskins spoke for Smithers, saying that the hospital was a landmark in the district and that many settlers and travellers owed their lives to it. The Rev. Allen represented the United Church, and he talked of the history of the mission hospitals on the coast. Captain Mortimer, representing the Department of Indian Affairs, spoke about the terrible scourge of tuberculosis and the special efforts being made to eradicate it. But it was Olof Hanson, the new member for the Skeena riding in the federal parliament, who actually opened the hospital.

Hanson spoke about Horace and described him as the pioneer frontier physician of the North. Richard Sargent then recalled that September day in 1900 when Horace and Alice had first arrived in Hazelton. He spoke of the opening of the old hospital in 1904, saying that, other than Horace, only three people present then (excluding Leonard Wrinch, who had been too young to remember) were now present for the opening of the new hospital: himself, William Larkworthy, who had made the hospital possible by surrendering a pre-emption on the land, and Constance Cox (then Constance Hankin), who had been Horace's first assistant even before the first hospital had been built.

In his own words of welcome, Horace expressed special pleasure at seeing so many of the First Nations present. The hospital, he said, was as much theirs as it was for non-Indigenous people. At the request of the Indian Department of Ottawa, a section of the building had been selected for treatment of First Nations only. Their treatment, nursing and ward equipment would be just the same as that of non-Indigenous residents.

In his short history of the hospital, written in 1938, Horace recalled that Duncan Campbell Scott, who was particularly desirous of stamping out tuberculosis among the First Nations, had required that a separate ward be "specially prepared" for tubercular patients. Since the Department of Indian Affairs was paying a third of the costs of the new hospital, his requirements would have carried great weight. In this, Hazelton Hospital was no different from many other hospitals in the province.

After describing the layout of the hospital and its financing, Horace mentioned that a previous speaker had suggested that the hospital might be called the Wrinch Hospital. The *Western Recorder* had also suggested that it should be so named. Horace stated firmly that he would not have the hospital named after him while he was alive, and he wasn't dead yet.

Despite the weather, the patients were moved from the old to the new hospital on the last day of the year. Perhaps it was thought that the risk from fire was greater than the risk of catching pneumonia. "Never was any one more relieved than I," Horace wrote, "when this change was completed and the serious risk of so long-standing was at last a thing of the past."

———

Dr. Simon Fraser Tolmie had the misfortune of assuming office as premier not long before the stock market crash in 1929. For the first year of his premiership, though, the economy prospered, unemployment decreased and Vancouver boomed. In a hopeful, perhaps defiant, headline on Christmas Day that year, the *Herald* had told all its readers, "May You Enjoy Prosperity [and] Happiness in 1930."

The stock market crash on October 29, 1929, ushered in a decade of lost opportunities and hardship. "Stocks at N.Y. Just Escape Complete Rout," the headline of Victoria's *Daily Colonist* shouted on October 30. And again, "Stampede of selling threatened to bring market to condition of complete ruin." The crash helped bring in the

Depression, but was not, though, its cause. It merely detonated the explosions that let out everything that had been undermining the economy for some years.

Hindsight reveals that the signs of impending disaster should have been clear. The boom of the previous years had been a bubble inflated to the breaking point by overconfidence and speculation. The consequences of the collapse included a huge withdrawal of cash from the economy and widespread unemployment which, in some parts of the country, reached a third of the work force.

There was at first denial, an attitude that stayed with many, including the federal and provincial governments, for far too long. Almost every industry now slumped. Suffering and social unrest spread across the land. Food, jobs, in some places water, and money were all in short supply. In having its own farm and water supply, the Hazelton Hospital was fortunate, being largely self-sufficient. Nevertheless, the sick had little money to pay the bills needed to keep the hospital functioning. Later, outside grants were reduced, and this seriously affected hospital finances. Survival was going to be a struggle.

Businesses closed in the Hazeltons. Horace wrote to Premier Tolmie pointing out that as a result of the slump in mining and timber, there was high unemployment in the Skeena district. The men needed work during the winter. The road between Hazelton and Usk, he argued, by way of an example, could well be cleared. This would be suitable for winter work. He invited unemployed workers to write to him so that he could set up an informal registry. By the end of the month, he had received the names of 250 applicants for work during that winter.

It was not as though the government was doing absolutely nothing. In 1930, in and around Hazelton alone it had spent $64,640 on the road to Terrace, $17,700 on the road to Smithers and another $20,569 on the road to Telkwa, as well as $8,500 on maintaining the Hagwilget bridge. These measures had also included eliminating two dangerous railway level crossings. But it was not enough.

In 1931, Horace expressed appreciation for such measures taken to relieve unemployment in the region, but said that the crisis was by no means over. He asked the Ministry of Public Works if more money was available under the federal Unemployment Relief Act. A program of road construction, he recommended, would help open the North, which of itself was a worthy cause.

Horace told the House that he supported the use of national credit to create work of a constructive nature. He suggested extending the roadwork joining Jasper and Banff Parks; fixing of higher farm commodity prices by a provincial board of farmers, consumers and distributors; making drastic reductions in administrative costs; and allowing mild inflation in Canada backed by commodities through the use of new issues of industrial loans. He continued at length:

> Human agencies, and not supernatural, had produced the present economic strain, and human hands would have to remove the tension in a world-wide sense. Like a wash-out on a road, the present crisis held idle factories, idle money and piled-up goods on one side, and workless men, poverty and unsatisfied needs on the other. It was the duty of governments to repair this breach if possible, through use of credit, currency and all legitimate means. The primary task was to start productive work in which willing men could earn money for their needs and to restore money to circulation.

———

The words Horace Wrinch and scandal do not seem to belong together in the same sentence. But in 1931, a political squall came his way like a dark cloud, and it passed just as quickly. The banner headline of the *Daily Colonist* for March 18, 1931, shouted, "Resignations of Two Members Demanded in the House." One of the attacked members was Horace and the other was Alex Manson, Attorney General in the previous government, who at one time had been Horace's lawyer. Both sides disagreed on the facts. Was Horace — perhaps as a result of political naivety — caught doing something wrong? Had Alex Manson done his old friend a favour? Or was W.C.

Shelly, president of the council in the Tolmie government and the outraged accuser, merely playing political games?

This could well have been no more than an attack on Manson. Apart from the fact that there may have been some personal animosity between the two, Manson had been the Liberal Attorney General in the Oliver government and was a political foe of some weight. Shelly might have thought he had clear evidence to bring him down.

Shelly rose to his feet in the House and attacked the honesty of the two members of the opposition. He had done his research. Piled on his desk was a stack of allegedly incriminating papers. He launched into his attack, but took a long time to get to his point. Mr. Manson, he thundered, on the very last day on which the Liberal government was in power had, on behalf of the finance minister, signed an order-in-council authorizing payment to a Mr. Henry of $700 as a tax refund and had taken it to the Lieutenant Governor for ratification.

Mr. Manson, Shelly said, was not authorized to act for the finance minister and Mr. Henry was in fact a straw man for Dr. Wrinch, a member in the House sitting on the opposition bench. Manson, Shelly announced, was the doctor's friend and lawyer. He alleged that the doctor had conspired with Manson to obtain an illegal payment of $700 from the provincial treasury. Somewhere in his allegations, he reported that the tax assessment books in Victoria had been mysteriously changed by some "jugglery." An illegal payment had been made to Horace, he said, and both members had no option but to resign their seats.

If Shelly had been more judicious and had confined his comments to the "jugglery," he might, perhaps, have been more successful. He tried, however, to explain all the details of a complicated real estate transaction and, it seems likely, lost the attention of the House. The real estate in question was the land Horace had bought next to the hospital in 1902. He had sold half of it, then many years later he bought it back. In the process of selling and buying it back, the tax assessment was not changed back to farmland as it should have been, and Horace had been required to pay more tax than he should have. He had been owed a refund. Manson had helped him obtain it.

Mr. Shelly, the *Vancouver Sun* said, had begun his speech with great gusto. Announcing that Mr. Manson would smart before he was through and that if he had a spark of honesty he would resign his seat, Shelly went on, "I will take the smile off his face." When he saw Manson laughing at him from across the aisle, he went on, "There will be silence in the morgue when I am through."

The *Vancouver Sun* noted that Shelley's speech lasted for two long hours "amid alternative roars of laughter and occasional outbursts of recrimination." The *Sun* suggested that members of the House were also wondering what this excessively long speech about a $700 refund was doing holding up debate on the $28 million budget and a proposed super-tax.

Shelly's attack was not helped by the fact that the previous year Mr. Justice MacDonald had ruled that allegations Shelly had made then against the government agent in Prince Rupert had been deemed unfounded. Now, here he was, at it again. His credibility was in doubt. He got some of his facts wrong. He said, for example, that Manson was Horace's lawyer: in fact, Horace had ceased to be his client in 1921, before Manson had become Attorney General. Furthermore, Shelly should have seen that the order-in-council clearly specified that the payment was to be made to H.C. Wrinch, and not to Mr. Henry.

Shelly blundered in focusing his attack on Horace, who was relatively non-partisan and a well-respected member, rather than on the experienced and politically dangerous Manson. Shelly also made the mistake of dealing with the facts chronologically. The facts were indeed confusing, but the most serious allegation — the one that said Manson had improperly had the assessment rolls changed to right the wrong (which was probably true) — came at the end of his story. By the time Shelly reached the end, he had lost his audience, which was by then laughing at him. Laughter can be fatal to a political attack.

Shelly sat down. Horace tried to answer but was prevented by the Speaker who pronounced that the rules of the House laid down who could and who could not speak during a debate on the budget, and Horace could not. The Liberal protest was shouted down by the Conservatives. "The charge is frivolous, anyway, as well as untrue," Pattullo said. Horace was loud in his own protests. "Then a member's character," he said, "may be traduced [attacked maliciously], he may be charged with dishonesty and told he ought to resign his seat and no opportunity is to be given to him to defend himself."

Manson's comment was more pithy. "Twaddle," he said. "It is another case of Mr. Shelly not understanding a comparatively simple matter." This was nothing more, he said, than the Crown in all honesty rectifying a mistake made by the Lands Department in 1905 and refunding to Horace his over-payment of tax. Shelly, he said, had not read the order-in-council well enough, because the supporting details, attached to the application to the Lieutenant Governor, clearly stated that Mr. Henry was acting as Horace's real estate agent. That, he said, was all there was to it.

Both Manson and the press also overlooked the fact that the Executive Council held on August 18, 1928, at which the order-in-council had been signed, had been attended by Premier MacLean as well as by Manson and other members of the cabinet. The presence of the premier accordingly overrode any lack of formal authority of the signing officer. In the premier's presence, Manson had authority to sign. Indeed, Premier MacLean had also signed the order. Nothing seemed amiss in any way.

There the matter appeared to die. Reported in the newspapers for one day, it then disappeared from view. Even the *Herald* merely gave it one short column. Only Shelly seemed worked up by it. From this distance, it appears like one of those little scandals that politicians like to explode every now and then to embarrass someone on the other side of the House. There did not appear to be much substance in Shelly's accusations, except perhaps for the possibility that Manson had arranged for the tax assessment books to be changed without authorization in an attempt to correct an undisputed error by the tax authorities many years previously.

It was the sort of squib that does not upset or disturb a hardened politician who knows how the games are played. If it was intended to injure Manson, it failed. He laughed it off. For Horace, though, who prized his integrity, it must have been a terrible week. Someone had stated in the House, a privileged place, that he was dishonest and corrupt and had obtained a special payment to which he was not entitled. He would have been mortified.

—◦◦◦—

Horace, sixty-five years old in 1931, was showing signs of age. In November 1929, he had travelled to the Mayo Clinic in Rochester, staying at the Damon Hotel. This time, however, he was not there as a student but as a patient. He told Duff Pattullo, the Liberal leader, that he had been "not quite up to the mark for some time." He went to Rochester to get straightened out, he wrote, and he went when he did so as to be fit for duty by the time the legislative session opened. His treatments, he said, would probably take three or four weeks. He wrote later from Hazelton saying he was feeling much better and had benefitted from the trip. In 1932, the *Herald* reported that he was ill, but that "when he had to take a dose of his own medicine he soon got up and returned to work."

Although he played down the extent of his injuries, he did have one serious car accident. He was driving from the hospital to Two Mile one November when his car skidded on a slippery patch of road and turned over. On account of a broken rib and a number of "unbeautiful bruises," Horace, the *Herald* reported, "would not go skating for a few days." Horace made light of it in a reply to a letter of sympathy from Pattullo: "Really the accident was not of a serious character. The papers made more than necessary of it. I am practically over the effects, although I was considerably inconvenienced for a while." This was one more car he had "rolled."

The circle of his old friends and acquaintances was shrinking. In 1932, Robert Tomlinson, who had been the first patient in the old hospital and who had worked as steward at the hospital for the previous eight years, left to go back to New Metlakatla in Alaska. He was one of the oldest pioneers in the district, having come over a grease trail from the Nass with his parents as a child. Richard Loring had left the district in 1921 and would die in Victoria in 1934. Rev. John Field had died many years before. Horace's brother Leonard's wife had died in December 1927, not long after Horace's marriage to May. In March 1930, Mrs. Hogan, Horace's mother-in-law, died. A Welsh girl from Newport, described as a ray of sunshine on her daily visits to the hospital, she had been a stalwart of the Hazelton community since the death of her missionary husband in 1912. During the war she had been honorary chairman of the Hazelton Red Cross. Each death would have brought back memories from the early days and marked the passage of Horace's own steps to what early Methodist literature had called "promotion."

Horace's adult children were finding their own ways in the world. After her training at Victoria's Provincial Royal Jubilee Hospital, Ralphena qualified as a registered nurse. She spent six months nursing in the hospital in Smithers, and then Horace paid for her to take a post-graduate course in obstetrics at New York's Woman's Hospital. She later said she worked so hard that she fell asleep during evenings at the *Ziegfeld Follies* and at the Barnum & Bailey Circus at Madison Square Gardens. In 1932, she joined the staff of the Hazelton Hospital. There she met her future husband, Jock Dunlop, a member of the local Royal Canadian Mounted Police detachment.

Horace's son Leonard married Frances Johnson, the daughter of a prominent Victoria lawyer, at a ceremony in Victoria's Christ Church Cathedral. When they returned from their honeymoon in Alaska, Horace and May gave them an evening reception on the lawns outside the family home on the hospital grounds. The evening was so warm they were able to stay outside, enjoying a bivouac fire and community singing around it afterwards. Leonard began to take on more of the day-to-day duties of running the hospital. He and Frances moved into a house on the hospital grounds. Mary, their daughter, arrived soon, giving Leonora, Horace's older granddaughter, a cousin to play with. Leonard's wife, Frances, though, was not destined for long life, and died of cancer six years later. She was buried next to Alice within the plot on the edge of the bluff overlooking Hazelton.

In 1931, Horace's son Arthur finished the fourth year of his course at the Royal Military College in Kingston, Ontario, after which he went for further studies at Camp Borden. While there he became dangerously ill with typhoid fever which, along with thirteen others, he had contracted after a party in Barrie. For a while his life was in peril, and he was flown to Christie Street Hospital in Toronto for specialist treatment. Horace and May immediately went there to be with him.

While in Toronto visiting him, Horace took the opportunity to attend the American Hospital Association Convention, which was being held in Toronto that year. He had been a member since 1908, but this was the first convention he had actually attended. With 4,000 delegates from all over North America, the convention this year was paying special attention to the problems of smaller hospitals. Horace reported that he had learned a great deal, in particular about modern equipment and procedures.

The *Herald* reported that there had been discussions about Hospital Day and how it was celebrated in the different parts of the continent. The Hazelton Hospital, it said, was mentioned as being among the ten most successful. The first prize was granted to a hospital in Brantford, Ontario. It is not clear exactly what this award was — the only source is the article in the *Herald*. It could possibly have been more of a consensus view than a formal award.

In July 1931, Horace became a Charter Fellow of the Royal College of Surgeons and entitled to add the letters FRCS to the long list of qualifications after his name.

—⁓—

Despite rising unemployment and the increasing hopelessness of people across the land, the routines of the hospital continued. The first Hospital Day festivities at the new hospital were held in May

1931. As usual there were speeches, games, music, a service in St. Peter's Church and celebrations for the graduation of two nurses, Ruth Miller and Edith Bulwar. In his comments, Horace particularly thanked two First Nations for volunteering their musical services: the Hazelton Indian Band in the afternoon and the Kispiox Orchestra in the evening.

At the Hazelton Flower Show in 1932, the Wrinch family again did well, winning eight prizes, including ones for best single rose, best group of roses and best single dahlia. As usual, the day was an occasion for speeches, songs and sports. Moreover, despite the organizers' apprehensions, the show had managed to avoid losing money.

Now finding more time for leisure, Horace took up golf. In the summer of 1931, enthusiasts had pushed for a golf course on the church land on Mission Point and had proceeded to raise the necessary money. Donald McDonald, a professional golfer from Winnipeg, was engaged to lay out the course.

In mid-August, Olof Hanson opened it, describing it as the most northerly golf course on the American continent. The fifth hole, the *Herald* said, was considered to be one of the sportiest holes in Canada. Fees were $10 a year for men, $5 for women and $3 for those under twenty-one. Horace seems to have been enthusiastic. He was a vice-president of the new club and his son Cooper was the secretary-treasurer. In 1932, Harold, with a handicap of twelve, was the favourite for the club prize, but, with a score of eighty-one, came second.

Horace was still active in the community. He donated fifty books from his own collection to form the nucleus of eighty-five books in the new library being set up in what was called the superior school in Old Hazelton. (The superior school was where children of mixed marriages went.) A society called the Hazelton Community Association was formed and a merger with the Hazelton Social Club was approved. Horace was elected vice-president. A new community hall was also planned.

But in truth, as New Hazelton, Terrace and towns in the Bulkley Valley grew, Old Hazelton was becoming quieter. As an indication of its decline, the Royal Bank, after years of losing money at its Old Hazelton branch, closed and moved the business to Smithers. It had been hoped, in vain, that it would stay in the old frontier town for sentimental reasons. The amount of space Old Hazelton took up in the pages of the *Herald* dwindled as New Hazelton, Terrace and Smithers became more important. Old Hazelton was slipping into a backwater.

—◦◦—

The Depression deepened. By the middle of 1931 almost 28 percent of male wage earners in British Columbia were unemployed. Business failures, unemployment, distress and consequent social unrest increased. At the start, few knew how devastating it would turn out to be or how long it would last. Premier Tolmie spent the rest of his mandate wrestling with how to deal with the crisis. He did his best, but his best was not good enough. Provincial and federal government policies in many cases seemed to make the situation worse. Those in power appeared to be bereft of new ideas.

As the months ticked by before the next provincial election, Horace wrestled with whether or not to run for re-election. When reading of his actions in the *Herald*, it is easy to assume that everyone in his riding was happy with his conduct. This paper, though, was Liberal in leaning and friendly to him. Conservatives in the riding were, naturally, not happy with the Liberals. They did not want Tolmie's government to lose power and would not under any circumstances be voting for Horace. That was to be expected. Letters between Pattullo and Horace tell a more nuanced story. Some Liberals along the Skeena also, apparently, wanted a change of their representative. A new generation wanted its chance for political office and thought the old man should not stand again. Was it time for someone younger?

In October 1930, Horace wrote to Pattullo to inform him of his doubts. He also inquired if there was any chance that he might be in the cabinet of a Pattullo government if he was re-elected. He informed the premier that the recent Conservative convention had given some of the Liberals in the Skeena riding the idea that they might hold their own convention and displace him. While not wanting to jeopardize the party's interests in keeping the riding Liberal, he said he was keen on running again and certainly did not like being told to let someone else replace him.

In his letters to Pattullo, he gives the impression of not quite knowing where the rebellion was coming from or how strong was it, and he wanted both information and affirmation. He seems to be thinking that if he let Leonard run the hospital — which he was quite capable of doing by now — he might have more time to spend in Victoria and might have a place in Pattullo's cabinet. Perhaps minister of health? Was that possible?

Pattullo replied soothingly a few days later, saying that he noted what Horace had said regarding the agitation in the riding. He recommended to Horace that he stay in touch with his constituency associations and find out what was happening there. Then he would be able to ensure the associations were guided the way Horace wanted them. "With regard to the future," Pattullo wrote, "there is no question whatever as to your capability for Cabinet position, and your long service and general standing give you a special claim. If it should be in the lap of the gods that I should head a government in this province, I certainly would be delighted to welcome you as a colleague. At the same time, I have not, nor do I intend, to make a definite promise to anyone in the event of our party being successful that he would be taken into the cabinet."

Pattullo later alerted Horace that representations had indeed been made to him from Liberals in Smithers about holding a convention. He asked Horace not to make a decision without checking with him.

In June, Horace told Pattullo that he felt he had been tricked by the Smithers people into not attending an important meeting at which the nomination was discussed. At this meeting, a consensus had developed in favour of a younger and more aggressive candidate.

A short while after, the one-man delegation of John Gray from Smithers called on him and discussed very freely the suggestion that Horace should make way for a younger man.

Horace said he would run if it was in the best interests of the party, but that he wanted to sound out all sections of the Liberal party first and not just be dictated to by one small faction. In fact, he said he had spoken with many in the party and had heard no dissatisfaction with his representation. He told Gray that he would sit back and let the grassroots make the decision.

Horace arrived back in Hazelton in April 1932 after a tiring session in the Legislature. He couldn't get back for the provincial executive meeting in New Westminster on May 30. He had, he said, some critically ill patients on his hands in the hospital and couldn't leave them. In any event, he enclosed his ideas on a list of subjects that could be discussed at the meeting. One of them was that a Liberal government should enforce the Minimum Wage Act that stipulated forty cents an hour. Another was that the government should introduce public health insurance.

By now, it was clear that an election could not be long deferred. In July, Pattullo advised Horace to start preparing for it. In replying, Horace reiterated that it would be a great honour to be selected but the question of who was to run was in the people's hands, not his. He said that he felt he owed that much to them. "I hope," he told the premier, "this meets with your approval." Pattullo replied crisply, "If you desire to run again, you would do well to go out after it to get it. The political arena is often very cold-blooded."

The press soon learned something was in the wind as to whether Horace would stand as the Liberal candidate for Skeena. The *Herald* mentioned there was some unrest in Liberal quarters on the Skeena, but that Pattullo, saying Horace suited him nicely, had been more or less successful in disposing of aspiring candidates. "Whether the boys will stay put," the *Herald* said, "is another matter."

Horace must have pondered his decision through the summer. Perhaps the one-man deputation of John Gray came to see him again. Perhaps he had become too busy in the hospital, and was oc-cupied in dealing with its worsening financial situation. Or perhaps he wanted to spend more time with his children and grand-children.

By August, he had made up his mind. Even though the *Victoria Daily Times* opined that Horace "could be elected in his riding without lifting a finger," he decided not to run for a third term. He informed Pattullo of his decision, giving as a reason that he felt he could not give as much time to the people of the district as he should. He could not, he thought, do that without neglecting his duties in relation to the hospital and his medical practice.

Pattullo replied a few days later, saying he had been sorry to hear of the decision. "You have given long and very faithful service. You never shirked your duty. You were an arduous worker and an intelli-gent worker, and it is a great pity to see men of your capacity unable to longer serve in the Legislature."

Horace announced the decision to his constituents in September. The *Herald* paid him tribute:

Dr. Wrinch has already done a great service to the northern interior country, both as a professional man and a public man. He is, and has always been, one of the outstanding men of the north. When he ac-cepted nomination for the Liberal Party eight years ago, he did so with the idea of serving his fellow man to the utmost of his ability and since he has been the representative of Skeena in the Legislature he has acted as he saw in the best interests of his constituency. No one will deny that. Some there are who disagreed with his views, naturally, but the Doctor could not hope to please all. While a member of the Legislature, he won a high place in the ranks of his party. He was also well thought of by the opposite party. He took his politics seriously and did his best. He is now entitled to relinquish at least that service to the public.

Horace must have thought his public life was over.

CHAPTER 13

Last Years
1933–1939

FREED FROM THE REQUIREMENTS of politics, Horace, now in his sixties, settled down with May in Hazelton. No longer would he have to spend so much time travelling to Victoria for legislative sessions. No longer, though, would he have been in the centre of things. He could have expected a place in any government that Pattullo formed. With his experience and knowledge, he was qualified to serve as either minister of agriculture or minister of health. But did he, when it came right down to it, want to be in government and spend so much time away from Hazelton? Much better now that he stay close to his roots, practise medicine and run the hospital. He was at an age when children — they were all adults now and all active in their careers — and grandchildren might have seemed more important than accepting a new full-time job in Victoria.

Horace's brothers and sisters had all taken their own paths. Mary was living and painting at her home at Wychwood Park in Toronto. With perhaps the most interesting career of all his siblings, she had been a member of the Toronto art community even before Horace had moved to Hazelton. She had a long career of exhibitions of her paintings. In 1901, when still only twenty-four, she was elected the first female member of the Ontario Society of Artists, later becoming its vice-president and treasurer.

In 1918, she became an associate of the Royal Canadian Academy. Group of Seven member A.J. Casson said of her that "she had greater originality in her paintings than almost any of our artists." In 1922, she married the artist and teacher George Reid, being occasionally known thereafter as Mary Wrinch Reid, not to be confused with Mary Hiester Reid, George's first wife, also an artist, who had died in 1921. In May 1937, an exhibition was held in London of work by artists from all over the Empire to celebrate the Coronation of King George VI. Among those representing Canadian artists were all members of the Group of Seven, Emily Carr and Mary Wrinch Reid.

Horace's brother Leonard had sold the family farm in Ontario in 1919 and moved to Chilliwack, in the Fraser Valley near Vancouver. Frank had moved into and then out of academia, first becoming a professor of psychology at the University of Toronto, then at Princeton and later at Berkeley, California. He then changed careers and became a farmer, owning a fruit-dehydration plant in Visalia, California. In August 1934, the news came to Hazelton that he had been murdered by a farmer who disagreed with him over the best time to pick the fruit.

—⁓—

Already by the end of 1931, the Depression had been squeezing the hospital's finances. No one knew how long it would last or when the recovery — if any — would start. Though the hospital had never been busier and at first appeared to be surviving reasonably well, at the end of the year there was a deficit of almost $3,000. The decline in economic activity, the unemployment, the constriction of public finances all meant there was much less cash circulating in the Hazelton district.

Until recently, Horace said, there had been no reason to suspect that the Depression would hit the hospital so hard. But it did. Revenues dropped suddenly because the unemployed could not afford hospital fees and the workmen's compensation board was delaying payment — or not paying — the hospital bills. Furthermore, expenses had increased dramatically.

Part of the problem had been caused by unforeseen expenses with the new hospital. A drying shed had cost $500. A new bungalow had become necessary for the assistant medical superintendent. Horace added pointedly that there were many in the district who owed the hospital money — a perennial problem. If these patients paid their bills the hospital finances would be sound again. But money was scarce and people could not pay.

Mining activity in the district had virtually ceased. The lumber camps were closed. There was little work. People could not afford to be sick. Hard times were calling for hard decisions. The hospital was struggling financially, and this led Horace to cancel the Hospital Day festivities. The financial crisis widened cracks in the hospital's books. "It came, and quite suddenly," the hospital board said of the crisis in December 1931, deciding to cut by ten percent the wages of all staff earning more than $70 a month.

Horace reported that the alternative to reducing wages was to reduce the staff by two graduate nurses. This, he said, he did not want to do, as he had a good staff of faithful and efficient workers. By such a temporary wage reduction, the full staff could be retained and the efficiency of the hospital maintained. Those staff members consulted, he said, had agreed. When the figures were added up, it was discovered that, although receipts had somehow been higher than expected, despite these cuts, expenses had increased even more.

In August 1932, the board made the difficult decision to close the nurses training school. The public was told that after October the hospital would accept only graduate nurses. This, it was estimated, would save $2,000 a year. The closure was not, though, simply the result of financial strain. The nursing profession had thought for some time that small hospitals should not be training nurses because they could not give them a well-rounded experience.

For a number of years, nurses from the Hazelton hospital had taken their last year at Vancouver General Hospital. Miss Doris Robinson, in September 1934, was the last nurse to graduate from the Hazelton nursing school. In his speech of congratulations to her, Horace commented that during its twenty-nine years of existence, the school had graduated twenty-one nurses, five of whom had taken First Class Honours in provincial exams.

Annie Lawrence, the first nurse to graduate in 1908, came back for a visit in August 1934. She said there had been many changes in Hazelton since she had left. "In fact she could hardly tell it was the same country, except for Rocher de Boule mountain and Dr. Wrinch." That was Horace: solid, permanent, prominent, but also not just a little formidable.

The Depression continued unabated, with the federal government still apparently unwilling or unable to take strong measures. In November 1932, the American people elected as president the nephew of Theodore Roosevelt, as the *Herald* put it, barely even mentioning the new president's name. It wasn't yet clear how Franklin Delano Roosevelt would be any different.

By deferring necessary repairs, cutting costs and observing stringent economies, the hospital balanced the budget during 1932, even making a small surplus. Perhaps Horace may have allowed himself to think that the worst of the Depression really was over. It was not.

Much as Horace tried to avoid it, the hospital's finances sank into crisis again at the beginning of 1934. "Hazelton Hospital needs more money to cover the losses of outside grants," the *Herald* said in a January headline. The increasing unemployment and cessation of all mining in the region led to a reduction in the number of patients.

The hospital board agreed to another canvass for funds — but who had any money to spare?

This financial crisis in 1934 was perhaps the most serious the hospital had yet faced. All the cuts they could make in major expenses had been made — closing the nurses training school, reducing salaries, cancelling Hospital Day and postponing needed renovations. In December of 1933, Horace was already alerting Rev. R.B. Cochrane at the Missions Board in Toronto that the hospital was lower in its financial position than it had been all year:

> The situation is somewhat as follows. Between five and six hundred dollars of November accounts are not yet paid. $250 of December accounts are now due. More December accounts will come in immediately after January 1. December salaries, about $1,200, are due at the end of the month. We usually pay them at once. To meet these we have about $350 on hand.

He went on to point out that, although the contribution from the Department of Indian Affairs of $1,018 should arrive in time to pay the salaries, grants overall had been reduced by $4,000. The Missions Board, the Women's Missionary Board, the provincial government and the Department of Indian Affairs of the Dominion government had all cut their grants. He asked the Missions Board to let him increase the hospital's overdraft with the bank. Until then, could they please advance him part of the annual grant for the year? Moreover, the line of credit with the bank would expire if not renewed, for which he needed the Missions Board's authority.

To this appeal, Cochrane replied that, first, the question of the renewal of the line of credit would be put to the Missions Board at the April meeting; second, enclosed was $600, as an advance on the annual grant; third, there was no possibility of an increased grant; and fourth, it was unlikely that the line of credit would be increased.

Horace's feelings on receiving this response may well be imagined. What he did, though, was to send a telegram informing Cochrane that if the line of credit was not renewed, the bank would call on the hospital's notes in full, a sum of $3,000 that the hospital most assuredly did not have. Fortunately, Cochrane understood the implications and took the request for renewal to the Missions Board's executive committee, which was meeting the following day. Cochrane was then able to inform Horace — doubtless to his great relief — that he could renew the line of credit.

Horace wrote that he felt fortunate they had got through the previous year as well as they had in the face of such drastic losses in anticipated income. He also warned he could be coming back to the Missions Board for another advance on its grant soon. As indeed he did. He wrote to Cochrane in March asking for an advance as soon as it could legitimately be sent. Cochrane helped with a small grant. In thanking him, Horace said that this would enable him to pay the March salaries.

This all helped slide the hospital through that crisis, but it did not address the basic problem: the hospital had to have more liquidity to keep it going. Horace returned to the attack. The hospital needed, he wrote to Cochrane, either an increased grant or an increased line of credit. A $1,000 increase would be sufficient. "Our budget for expenditures for this year [1934] is practically equal to our expected income, but we cannot take care, out of current income, of the $2,000 deficit from last year."

Cochrane and the Missions Board finally accepted his arguments and authorized him to increase the overdraft to $4,000. As a result, the hospital's financial situation stabilized. "It is with much satisfaction and profound gratitude to God," he said in his annual report for 1935 "that we report another year of hospital service to the people of Hazelton and the district. We are glad to inform our friends that, in spite of fears to the contrary, every department at the Hospital . . . has been kept open and available for everyone needing any of these services."

―⁓―

By the end of its mandate, Premier Tolmie's government was in disarray. He did try to inveigle Duff Pattullo into a coalition government, but Pattullo, knowing the fate of junior partners in a coalition, would have none of that. With the term of his government running out, Tolmie called an election for November 1933. At this he paid the political price for his inability to deal with the continuing crisis. When the results were announced, the political landscape in Victoria changed. The Conservative majority was replaced by a Liberal majority of a similar size, and Duff Pattullo became premier. The provincial party of the Co-operative Commonwealth Federation — a new left wing party only organized in British Columbia in 1933 — now formed the official opposition.

Premier Pattullo realized that desperate times demanded dramatic measures. In the first session, as well as sponsoring a high-handed and controversial measure that gave him wide executive powers when the Legislature was not in session, he attacked the problems with progressive reforms. These included proposals for minimum wage legislation, maximum working hours, financial assistance to mining and forestry, and new marketing rules. He increased funding for teachers, schools and universities. And, in what would have been of great interest to Horace, he pushed forward the plans to introduce publicly funded health insurance.

Although no longer in the centre of things, Horace did keep up with current affairs. He watched with interest what was happening in Europe, writing that Mussolini had no business in Abyssinia. "It is to be hoped," he wrote to his son Harold, "that the European nations will not allow themselves to be stampeded into fighting too. I don't think they want to, anyway, but they can't let Italy get away with Abyssinia or it would have made too many other complications."

Before Pattullo announced his progressive reforms, Horace had not been impressed by the new government. In March 1934, he was writing to his daughter Ralphena:

> It doesn't appear to be a very exciting session. . . . We are told that the present legislature has more outstanding ability than any previous one, but apparently it is not where it can make itself conspicuous.

They are certainly running along quietly — almost to the point of deadly-dullness, at least from the viewpoint of the onlooker.

The premier had ideas of how Horace could help. It would soon get considerably more lively for him, both provincially and personally.

In February 1934, Premier Pattullo set up an Economic Council. This, being similar to President Roosevelt's Brain Trust, was consequently nicknamed Pattullo's Brain Trust. Under the chairmanship of Professor W.A. Carrothers from the University of British Columbia, it acted as an advisory council to the government on economic matters. In April, Pattullo appointed Horace to be one of its six members, pulling him back into public service.

After his appointment L.B. Warner, the editor of the *Interior News* in Smithers, who had excoriated Horace for supporting the Telkwa Hospital, paid him a gracious tribute:

> Knowing the high respect in which he was held on both sides of the House during his representation of the Skeena, it could not be assumed otherwise than that his appointment will meet with general endorsation throughout the province.... We do not know what the economic council will bring forth for amelioration of our present-day troubles, but we do know that if success depends entirely upon hard work and strict study of prevailing conditions as its own remedy, then the public will get full value from Dr. Wrinch.

Carrothers drew up a list of urgent matters for the Council's immediate attention and the members got to work at once. These included an economic survey of the province's forest resources, a review of employment possibilities for the unemployed and a survey of possible uses for agricultural lands. The Council also acted as a clearing house for the ideas and reports of numerous provincial and federal bodies of research. It started its work amid high expectations and at first met monthly. Over the next two years, the Council produced numerous reports and recommendations. "Under its able chairman," Pattullo's biographer, Robin Fisher, wrote, "the staff of the

Economic Council examined a host of questions: from the potential for the marketing [of] pelts of angora rabbits to the state of the province's major resource industries."

Horace went to Vancouver to attend Council meetings as often as he could. This commitment required a huge amount of travel for him: every trip to Victoria took at least two or three days there and two or three days back. Not being one to waste time, he would likely have briefed himself during these journeys by reading papers, journals and transcripts of evidence delivered to the Council.

He returned to Hazelton in May 1934, after one such meeting, and reported: "We have two chief objects in view as a starter. . . . first is to get the young men out of the unemployment camps and at something which will give them an object in life. The second is to solve the problem of unsuccessful people on land." He later said that the Economic Council was actively looking at ways to train boys recently out of school to fit them for jobs in the mining, fishing and timber industries. It was "no longer enough to have a strong back and a weak head," by which the *Herald*, perhaps quoting Horace, meant someone without training.

Even though Carrothers gave many speeches, the Economic Council was intended as an advisory body and many of its reports were confidential. Much of its work, consequently, was not known to the public. Some of the press coverage of what was public was critical, but also partial. "What the government at Victoria ought really to set on foot is a real and candid enquiry into the possibility of giving us less government rather than more," the *Vancouver Province* said.

While the Council did excellent work and delivered numerous reports to the government, strains soon manifested themselves. Reportedly the government was unhappy that Carrothers was not able to work with industry and actually create employment. By mid-1935, the Brain Trust was already said to be declining from a mysterious cerebral disease. Carrothers was a strong chairman, and this may also have caused problems. Most members of Council — perhaps feeling superfluous as many committee members do when there is a strong chairman, perhaps spending too much time on their own businesses — resigned. By the summer of 1936, Horace was one of the two original members still serving.

Although Pattullo said it would continue, its work was clearly winding down. Carrothers went back to his post at the university that autumn, but remained part-time chairman. The independent existence of the research department came to an end in 1937, when it was merged into the Bureau of Economics and Statistics. Horace would probably have stepped down at the same time that Carrothers went back to academe.

It is hard to assess how much actual influence the Council's reports had on the formation of Government policy. What it did do, though, was to bring the presence of experts into the government and into the civil service, and it was thus at the point of the wedge that dramatically changed the nature of government in modern society.

Pattullo's newly elected and vigorous Liberal government was determined to implement the health insurance reforms that had been debated for more than fifteen years. George M. Weir, a noted reformer, became provincial secretary and minister in charge of the health and welfare portfolio.

Pattullo and Weir hired Harry Morris Cassidy from the University of Toronto to be the province's first director of social welfare. His job was to design and implement a plan of state health insurance. Cassidy came with a reputation as an investigator of social conditions, having also been one of the founders of the Co-operative Commonwealth Federation. As a founding member of the League for Social Reconstruction, he had also helped draft the progressive Regina Manifesto in 1933. This fact, though, was not well publicized at the time, perhaps to avoid alienating the business and professional elites in Vancouver.

Cassidy brought great ideals and enthusiasm to his new job. Had the plan been put into operation, it would have been North America's first scheme of state health insurance. But it was not to be. As the proposals became clearer and more widely known, opposition in the medical community mounted. Despite this opposition, in March 1935 the government presented a draft bill on health insurance to the legislature. Public discussion was spirited.

As Dr. McIntosh had prophesied in 1919, the key was whether the medical profession would accept it. In British Columbia, doctors had seen their average income fall by forty percent between 1929 and 1933. The stock market crash of 1929 had changed the whole debate. By late 1932, a quarter of Canada's workforce was unemployed and one-fifth was receiving some form of government assistance. For doctors, a state insurance scheme could either stabilize their incomes and provide economic security or bind them into a regulatory structure that changed their position from independent professionals to civil servants. If done right, they would accept it; if not, they wouldn't.

Initially, the doctors were prepared to accept state health insurance provided it met certain conditions. It became increasingly clear to them that the Pattullo legislation did not meet those conditions. Doctors were concerned that this legislation excluded groups most in need of medical care, that a commission would have more say in the care given to patients than they would, and that it would have too much control over their incomes. Vigorous disagreement imperiled the legislation.

While this debate raged, the *Herald* reminded its readers that in its ticket scheme, the Hazelton Hospital had had a form of health insurance in place since 1907. "Health Insurance Provided by the Hospital," a headline in February 1935 said. By now, the fee had risen to $1.50 a month or $15 a year. "You never know when you are going to get sick. . . . One accident, or one serious illness, any one of many things over which you have no control, and it would not take long to use up the cost of numerous years of hospital tickets." The annual report for 1935 listed the names of over fifty ticket-holders.

By mid-1935, Cassidy was confiding to a friend that "our modest and essentially conservative plans for health insurance are being fought bitterly by the doctors . . . with the backing of industrial groups." Not only doctors but also most chambers of commerce, boards of trade, professionals and businesses were opposed.

Despite this opposition and after much amendment, the British Columbia Health Insurance Act was given Royal Assent on April 1, 1936. British Columbia was the first jurisdiction in Canada to pass such legislation. Cassidy then started to work immediately on the details of implementation.

In January of 1937, Pattullo announced that health insurance would begin on March 1. Statutory deductions from wages would, he said, also begin on that date. Eligible workers were required to register. The medical profession, opposing even the amended law, then organized a poll of doctors, who, by 622 to 13, voted against it. On February 1, the doctors in Vancouver and Victoria announced they would not work under the new legislation.

By mid-February, Pattullo was already backing down. The *Daily Colonist* reported that the "Provincial Government has given a complete hoist to the British Columbia Health Insurance Act and will not likely move again to impose the levies or commence the benefits until after the forthcoming provincial general election, it was learned yesterday in quarters close to the Ministry and in a position to be well informed."

Pattullo postponed the implementation of the Act until after a referendum on the health insurance legislation, to be held at the same time as the election that summer. Pattullo did win this election albeit with a reduced majority. The referendum passed with fifty-nine percent approval. He knew, however, that without the co-operation of the doctors, which he did not have, he would not be able to make the Act work.

Sensing that the public appetite for health insurance had waned, Pattullo quietly let the legislation lapse. An editorial in the *Daily Colonist* in December 1937 bluntly stated that "the Health Insurance Act on the statutes of British Columbia is a dead letter." And there the matter remained until after the Second World War. Nevertheless, long before the reforms in the years following the war, in British Columbia there had been two major commissions that had investigated and recommended publicly funded health insurance. There had been broad and substantial public support for it. An election had in part been fought and won on it. The electorate had approved a referendum, and there had been legally effective legislation, albeit withdrawn. In this, British Columbia laid the foundations on which succeeding generations would build publicly funded health care in Canada.

When Horace left Hazelton in October 1936, he would have had the satisfaction of seeing the legislation that he had been advocating for the last twenty years become law. He would, though, have been deeply disappointed at its suspension. In any event, in Hazelton, ticking like a weekly clock, the advertisement again appeared in the *Herald* stating that by buying a hospital ticket for $1.50 a month, medical benefits could be obtained at the Hazelton Hospital. He at least had that accomplishment.

———~~~———

On Christmas Day 1935, Horace wrote to Harold, then working in Ocean Falls, saying:

> Merry Christmas! Today we have said this so many times it becomes a habit. This is at five p.m. and I am just going down with the mail. I want to get this note in the mail to tell you how pleased May and I are with your nice presents. But if we could have had you with us for this day instead of the presents, we would have been very much more pleased. We have had the usual round of events today. Had Leonard and Cooper and their families for turkey dinner at 1 p.m. Then some Christmas singing in the hospital preliminary to the visit of Santa Claus. . . . The ground was quite bare for days and people had given up hope expecting snow for Christmas. But last night it snowed two or three inches and just covered the ground nicely. So we have a white Christmas after all.

A few days later, on January 6, Horace celebrated his seventieth birthday. This would have been a time for reflection. By now, he had been in Hazelton almost thirty-six years. His beloved wife Alice had died many years ago. He may well have passed much of the day-to-day management of the hospital and surgery to Leonard while he himself remained as a practising physician. Leonard would be well qualified to take over the position of superintendent when Horace eventually retired.

The country itself remained deep in the Depression. Signs of it were everywhere, including the still-increasing financial pressure on hospital finances. And, deepest cut of all, his beloved God was increasingly slipping out of people's minds and hearts. This was a new age with new ideas and with what must to him have seemed a distressing erosion in moral standards.

A petulant note on occasion creeps into his letters about how he would like to have his children visit more often. Then, of course, being a parent, he made excuses for their not doing so. Like many fathers, he followed his children's progress closely, rejoicing in their successes and commiserating with their failures. "We were a little disappointed," he wrote to Harold, "that you did not get the rumoured promotion." And of course he offered good advice. "It was certainly good news to hear that you are likely to get the position of drugstore manager. . . . It's a good thing to listen to suggestions from your subordinates if you can. Of course, you can't always carry them out." Later in the year, Harold became engaged and brought his fiancée, Ersul McKay, to Hazelton to meet her prospective parents-in-law, a daunting event for any young girl. Nevertheless, she charmed them and they enjoyed her visit.

In 1936, for the first time in several years, Horace tried to revive Hospital Day celebrations. He planned a small, modest reception and was able to add some sports, but it was not the same as it had been. The 1930s had lost the exuberance of the 1920s.

In 1936, Horace decided to retire and make a clean break from Hazelton by returning to Ontario. Having been dropping hints in his recent letters, he confirmed it in July, writing to Harold:

> I don't think I told you definitely that May and I expect to leave Hazelton for good when we go east in October. I have decided that it's not wise to try to keep up the full time work I have had here for so long. And it does not seem feasible under present conditions to slow down on the work enough to make a sufficient difference that would warrant my trying to keep on. As long as I am here, it will not be convenient to slow down as much as I would like. So I have decided to pull out after the end of September.

Knowing that he would not be able to refrain from interfering, he possibly did not want to linger around Hazelton when Leonard took over the hospital as superintendent. Having spent almost twenty years of his life in Ontario before coming to Hazelton in 1900, he may have cherished a dream of returning there when he retired.

The first week of October was actually when it all happened. Although he was a private person and would perhaps have preferred just to slip away, he had to make arrangements. The hospital board and patrons, the Missions Board, colleagues and staff — they all had to be told. The whole community would then quickly have known about it. His last hospital board meeting was on October 2, 1936, and here his formal resignation was accepted. "Dr. Wrinch has filled so large a place in the life and work of both church and state in British Columbia that it would be difficult to think of the Skeena River valley without him," the Missions Board recorded in a motion of thanks. The fuss was grand and, it seems, genuine.

The old doctor was leaving. For residents in the Hazelton district, he was their link to the pioneer days. He could tell stories of Pierce, Cataline and Gunanoot, of the steamers arriving after their long and treacherous haul upriver from Port Essington and of the days of no cars, no railway — just horses, mules and pack dogs. How long ago it all must have seemed!

The entire front and back pages of the *Herald* for October 8, 1936, were devoted to his departure. "Dr. H.C. Wrinch, accompanied by Mrs. Wrinch," the *Herald* said, "leave tomorrow . . . for the east to make their future home." There was an auction of their household furniture and possessions "at 1.00 p.m. sharp at the residence. . . ." The list of goods offered for sale included wicker chairs, oak tables, kitchen utensils, pictures, the hall clock, bedsteads and "many other articles too numerous to mention." What must Horace have thought as he watched thirty-six years of his life sold all around him, all the tables and chairs and other furniture he had himself made, all those memories? He sold his car to Father Dean, the priest at Hagwilget, for $350. "I had the fender straightened when the brakes were fixed," he told Harold. "So it is in splendid shape."

Retirement gifts were given. Farewell tributes poured in. The *Herald*, noting that he had arrived thirty-six years previously, said that his arrival and departure were as his life in the district — quiet, unassuming but always with a purpose, which he carried out with quiet efficiency and without thought of turning back. "No man has accomplished so much. It is indeed doubtful if another will ever have the privilege of doing the combination of works which fell to the lot of Dr. H.C. Wrinch. Certainly no one could have fulfilled his mission better." He had very decided opinions, the *Herald* said, on what were and what were not pleasures, and he adhered strictly to these ideals. That is, he disapproved strongly of alcohol, swearing, gambling, irreligion, working on Sunday and loose living. Although Hazelton was still in many ways a frontier town and many seemed to enjoy these sins, Horace was still beloved.

In a speech accompanying the presentation of a gold watch by the citizens of Hazelton, it was said:

We have called upon you at any hour of the day or night and have always had instant response, whether in a storm and darkness, or in the depth of winter, and your hopeful word and kind touch have soothed and comforted us and allayed our fears, thus paving the way for your unnumbered cures of our many ills. We also greatly appreciate and remember your great services to us in our social problems. We have always looked upon you as our sheet anchor in any movement which was put afoot to enlarge the social life of our community, and you have never failed us. You have taken time from your always busy days to give us service and in doing so have not spared your purse. Your home has been thrown open to us upon so many occasions when fun, frolic and feasting were the order of the day. Upon such occasions you have been the fun leader and never allowed a dull moment.

One may be allowed a slight frisson of surprise at hearing Horace described as a "fun leader," and wonder in what ways he allowed "fun, frolic and feasting" to be the order of the day in his home. Nonetheless, this was the opinion of the citizens of Hazelton. Horace surprises us often.

———

We know little about Horace's movements after his departure from Hazelton. No longer is the *Herald* reporting every time he left town or returned. No longer is he acting as chairman of meetings or societies. No longer is he making speeches. On his way to Ontario he visited Harold at Ocean Falls, Ralphena, who was nursing at the Tranquille tuberculosis hospital in Kamloops, and other family members in Vancouver. The October weather was so hot, it was said, that "at times the men had to remove their jackets." Writing soon after that he had begun to feel the relief of having no professional cares, he and May settled into an apartment on Jarvis Street in Toronto.

In December 1936, he wrote of his plans to have Christmas festivities with his brother Warwick. The letter seems to confirm that he and May were planning to live in Toronto and were not merely visiting. "We are quite comfortable here," he wrote to Harold:

We have a dining-sitting room, two bedrooms, bathroom and kitchen. All on the ground floor, with south and east windows for the sitting room, which makes it very nice for winter as we get all the sunshine there is, which is not too much anyway this time of year. We are fairly close to the downtown store district but on a quiet street. . . . It is not a balmy climate and I think BC has it well beaten. Of course one must not tell these people that. . . . We expect to have a family gathering for Christmas dinner at your Uncle Warwick's, which no doubt will be quite a pleasant time.

Horace was living in Toronto in February 1937 when Frances, his son Leonard's wife, died. Not long after, Leonard decided he did not want to stay in Hazelton, with all its associations, and he moved to Trail, where he later remarried. When Leonard left Hazelton, the Gitxsan sent him an address of thanks and expressed deep regret that the Wrinch relationship, so helpful to their people, had now been severed:

> In consideration of these facts, we, the people of Kitsecugkla, wish to assure Dr. L.B. Wrinch that we are sorry he must leave us. Although we cannot express all our feelings, we want him to know that we appreciate what he has done for us, we thank him for his services and we thank his father, Dr. H.C. Wrinch, through him, for all they have both done for our people. . . . We would assure him that he will find no more loyal friends than those of the Indian people.

After his departure from the familiar surroundings of Hazelton, Horace appears to have been unsettled, rootless. He tried living in Toronto but didn't like that. In June 1937, he spoke to a group at St. Andrew's Memorial House there about his missionary work on the Skeena. He and May went to Ottawa for the wedding of his son Arthur to Madalene Wightman at Glebe United Church on August 28th.

Soon after, they returned to Vancouver. The climate in Toronto, it was later said, was not suitable for Horace and so he and May had not stayed. "We had a good time in the East and could live there again if things pointed that way," he told the Smithers *Interior News* diplomatically in October. "In the meantime, however, they seem to point to BC. So here we are — and feeling very fit."

He attended Canadian Memorial Church in Vancouver, where he became an elder. In June 1938, he gave an account of his work at Hazelton to a meeting of the Myrtle Wheeler Auxiliary of the Church at Mrs. Tate's home on West 14th Avenue. In July, he wrote to congratulate George Reid, his brother-in-law, on his completion of a large mural for the east wing of the Royal Ontario Museum and to try to persuade George and Mary to come to Vancouver for a visit.

In Vancouver, Horace and May moved numerous times. In November, he was writing from 1325 West 10th Avenue, but they soon moved again to 1545 West 13th Avenue. The following June he wrote to Harold:

> May and I are planning to move again. We will probably take a room at Mrs. Hugh Harris's and not look after housekeeping ourselves. . . . I suppose the truth is we are getting no younger as time passes and so feel like taking things easier.

In July 1939, he was writing from their new lodgings at 2116 West 21st Avenue. "My Dear Harold," he wrote:

> Note our new address. We moved here from 13th Avenue the day before yesterday and are getting settled in now. . . . May and I are paying guests and don't have anything to do with domestic affairs except to come to dinner when the bell rings. This suits us very well as we are feeling not quite equal to attending to all the details of shopping and getting meals. And it suits Mrs. Harris very well too. We have had a wash basin and toilet put into the corner of our room — partitioned off in the regular way of course, and with a suitable window. So we are not having to divide such facilities with others in the house. It's like a small apartment without a kitchen or dining-room. . . . This is a quiet section and close to some wild land. So it is almost like country air and really quite different from where we were, although it is only a few blocks (about ten) away from it.

Horace wrote to Ralphena in August that quite a few northern people were dropping in to see him from time to time, but apart from a visit to see to Dr. Hambleton once a week for a treatment, he was not going out much. Among his visitors was Constance Cox, his nurse assistant in the days when he had first arrived on the Skeena, and she kept him informed about happenings in Hazelton. That summer, with his friend Robert Peers who was visiting from Colfax, Horace drove out to Chilliwack to visit his brother Leonard. Peers later wrote that Horace, although mentioning his health worries, at that time had "no definite diagnosis of his cancer."

These could well have been sad days for Horace, with the walls closing in. His brother Alfred, the one who had come out to help at the hospital for two years when it had been first built, had died in hospital in 1938. In September 1939, the Second World War started and was already casting its shadow over the last days of Horace's life. He would have remembered the previous war and what it had done to men of fighting age and their families.

With four sons, one already in the army, he would naturally have been fearful for their futures. Arthur, a professional soldier with the Signalling Corps in Halifax, was drawn quickly into the war machine. Ralphena's policeman husband Jock was busy rounding up Germans living in the province.

In these last months of his life, Horace knew he was seriously ill. In his mind, he may have strayed back to his childhood, to those days running along the reedy banks of the marshes of his native Essex or standing on the deck of SS *Sarmation* watching England fade into the mists, wondering what he would make of his life in Canada. He may have retraced his steps on the eight-mile journey from Kispiox to Hazelton, with his Newfoundland dog beside him carrying his medical supplies, or wandered again through Old Hazelton when letters came from the outside world twice a winter. He may also have recalled pacing over the cleared ground on the bench above Hazelton for that first hospital in the wilderness, wondering how he would raise the money to build it.

Horace died of prostate cancer at his lodgings in Vancouver on October 19, 1939. For some time, his health had not been good. But being a very private person, he had kept this to himself and to close family members. An obituary in the *Herald* said that he had maintained a brave front and had not gone to his bed until the last few days. There were many memorials, obituaries and testaments. "I feel deeply grieved," Premier Pattullo said when he heard of Horace's death. "He was a very able man and most painstaking and thorough in all that he did, and he had the most complete confidence and regard for every member of the House."

"Dr. Wrinch, Horse [and] Buggy Doctor Dies," the *Vancouver Sun* reported, saying that he was "for forty years perhaps the best known and most beloved man in Northern British Columbia, especially among the early settlers and the Indians to whom he devoted his skill and kindly services when there was no other doctor within two hundred miles." The enormity of another war, though, dwarfed the death of one individual. The Vancouver newspapers briefly reported his death, and then moved on to report that Nazi planes had appeared again over the Firth of Forth in Scotland.

The funeral service in Vancouver was held in the Canadian Memorial United Church. The Rev. S.S. Osterhout, who had travelled with Horace to Port Essington and the Nass in 1900, conducted the service. Alex Manson, a judge since 1935, was one of the pallbearers. As a Mason, Horace was buried in the Masonic Cemetery in Burnaby. At the same time, a well-attended memorial service was held for him in Hazelton.

The Gitxsan of Kispiox held their own memorial service. The entire population of the village attended. The village band was out and played hymns. The Rev. D.W. More conducted the service and invited two of the oldest men present to stand and tell their stories of Horace's arrival in their community thirty-nine years before. They were, they said, very proud of the fact that it was to their village that he came first.

"He was," the *Herald* said, "a leader in many movements for the welfare of the district and Hazelton in particular, and never tired of well-doing" and continued:

Dr. Wrinch was probably the most influential man, and the best liked man that ever blessed the district with his presence. He won the love of his fellow citizens by his service, his kindness and an outstanding ability as a leader, administrator and as a real friend in time of need. The district profited greatly from his life spent here and no monument to his memory is needed so long as the youngest resident remains. . . . Dr. Wrinch was appreciated by the people as was proven by their loyalty to him over the years. He never made an appeal that was not heartily responded to. He was given every position of trust and honour in the gift of the people.

His long journey had ended. During his lifetime Horace had travelled from the peaceful pastures of Essex to the wilds of northern British Columbia. On his journey, he had been a farmer, missionary, doctor and surgeon, hospital builder, politician and early standard-bearer for state health insurance. His belief in God gave him his inspiration; his practicality, born from his farming, gave him his tools. His sense of public service to the community was profound. His motivation was worthy, his execution efficient and his results beneficent. His contribution to the welfare of the peoples of the Skeena River and the Province of British Columbia endures.

Afterword

HORACE HAD REFUSED to allow the new hospital in Hazelton to be named after him when it opened. The year after he died, however, it was renamed the Wrinch Memorial Hospital. State of the art in 1931, it grew old and was replaced. The new hospital, also named Wrinch Memorial Hospital, was officially opened on May 28, 1977. Dr. J.E. Whiting, administrator of the hospital from 1955 to 1976, gave the dedication. The Honourable R.H. McClelland, minister of health for British Columbia, cut the ribbon and Major-General Arthur Wrinch officially unveiled the plaque. To this day, the hospital compound remains a community with numerous health care facilities — including a child-care facility, a doctors residence and a Wrinch Residence for visiting employees — as well as a modern hospital. It remains an important part of the Hazeltons.

Horace would have been pleased by the re-introduction of health care insurance proposals after the war, which led incrementally to the Canada Health Act of 1984. In British Columbia in 1948, Premier Boss Johnson introduced a medical insurance and financial aid plan that was to be paid for by mandatory payroll deductions and directly collected premiums. Because the administration of this was poorly thought out and did not work well, the plan became unpopular and did not last for long after the 1952 election. But it was a step forward and provided lessons on what to do and what not to do.

The Co-operative Commonwealth Federation government in Saskatchewan introduced the Hospitalization Act in 1946, providing a measure of free health care in that province. In 1950, Alberta's Social Credit government introduced its health plan. Later steps included the expansion by Tommy Douglas of Saskatchewan's health care coverage, although this was actually implemented in 1962 by his successor premier, Woodrow Lloyd. The Royal Commission on Health Services chaired by Justice Emmett Hall led to the introduction by Prime Minister Lester B. Pearson of Medicare nationwide.

Horace's second wife, May, died in Vancouver in 1946. Leonard remained a doctor all his life. Cooper was a pharmacist, and Ralphena a nurse. Arthur had a distinguished career in the Canadian Army and, after retirement as a major-general, became national commissioner of the Canadian Red Cross (1963–1975). Harold became an accountant in Nanaimo, Port Alberni and Victoria.

Today the approximate population of Old Hazelton remains what it has been since the 1920s — about 300 — whereas the population of New Hazelton, astride the railway and main road, has increased to between 600 and 700.

On April 1, 2016, the United Church Health Services Society transferred Wrinch Memorial Hospital to Northern Health, thus severing the link with the Church that began at the turn of the previous century when Horace and Alice arrived on the Skeena River. Horace may well have approved of this. Certainly he anticipated it. In 1925 — at the time the three churches merged to become the United Church — he wrote that, when "medical service through ordinary channels is available and is within the reach of any who may require it . . . it is a fair assumption that the Church does well to withdraw her competition from regularly organized medical service."

He predicted that in a few years it would be reasonable for churches to expect local communities to assume responsibility for medical services. There again we have Horace — far-seeing, ahead of his times, committed to medical care for the population and, above all, practical.

Author's Note

FROM THE 1860S UNTIL the arrival of the railway in 1912, Hazelton was the most important town in the interior of northern British Columbia. At a time when there were no roads, it derived its importance as the highest navigable place on the Skeena River. It was accessible — with difficulty — primarily by river steamer and then only in the five or six months each year when the river was navigable. When Horace Wrinch arrived in 1900, it was an isolated settlement of little more than forty settlers, lying on the point where the Bulkley River joins the Skeena River, set deep in a forested, mountainous wilderness.

Two peoples live in the Hazelton district: non-Indigenous people, mainly but not entirely of European origin, and the Gitxsan and the Wet'suwet'en First Nations. The relationship between non-Indigenous people and the First Nations has not been uniformly happy over the years. On one hand was possession of the instruments of power and an all-pervasive sense of racial superiority, and on the other was a lasting and deep awareness of injustice and loss. There has been a continuing claim by the First Nations for legal recognition of territory and rights, and there have been occasional flashpoints. This claim led, eventually, to the historic decision in 1997 of the Supreme Court of Canada on Gitxsan and Wet'suwet'en rights in *Delgamuukw v. British Columbia*.

This biography is not a history of the First Nations living in the Hazelton district, nor is it a story of the relationship between them and the non-Indigenous settlers. It is certainly not a discussion of First Nations claims to land or to the minerals beneath them. The values of those early times — with its paternalism, racial superiority, assimilationist tendencies and gendered outlooks — are not today's values. These issues have all been well documented and discussed elsewhere. I have touched on First Nations matters only where they thread through Horace's life. In his actions, he was a doctor and a surgeon, and as such he brought healing to everyone regardless of racial background.

Horace was sent to the Upper Skeena as a medical missionary by the Methodist Missions Board in Ontario. Missionaries in British Columbia have been much criticized. Many of them, William Duncan and Thomas Crosby, in particular, were controversial at the time and remain so today. By 1900, though, it was being seen — and said — that the day of the missionary was over. Horace may possibly have realized this. As the years passed, he became more of a doctor and less of a missionary. While never losing his deeply held faith, he embraced the twentieth century with its modern medicine, electricity, railways and automobiles.

Many of the statements made by writers at the time would be considered unacceptable today. In most cases, I have let their words speak for themselves rather than add unnecessary comment.

The present road down into Old Hazelton, past 'Ksan Historical Village did not exist in Horace's time. This road, built in the 1950s, runs straight down the hill. In early days, the hill was considered too steep for wagon trains, and the track into town ran below the bluff. In the 1960s, the 'Ksan Historical Village was built on the banks of the Skeena opposite Mission Point (now Anderson Flats Provincial Park). Beside it is a large campground and park.

With very few speculative exceptions, all the incidents and scenes described in this biography happened. All the words in quotations are taken from letters, speeches, newspaper reports and books, almost all of which are contemporaneous. On a few occasions, I have converted indirect speech into direct speech. I have endeavoured to be careful of the distinctions among facts that are supported by evidence, facts that must necessarily be so, facts that are probable and facts that are only possibilities. The proven facts come from personal papers, letters, newspaper reports and archival materials. That Horace was on the scene of the 1906 murders before the police and was examining the bodies when they arrived, for example, is shown by the evidence at trial. Other statements are appropriately qualified.

I have used imperial measures rather than metric, because that is what the people of the time used.

Other than when used in quotations, I have used modern spellings for place names. The Gitxsan did not have a written language. Settlers wrote down the names as they heard them, and the result is a bewildering variety of spellings, complicated by the fact that the Gitxsan have a different language from the Wet'suwet'en. Moricetown, for example, was known as Lach-al-sap by the Gitxsan and as Witset by the Wet'suwet'en. The name has recently been changed back to Witset. There was also a settlement of the Nisga'a people on the Nass River with the very similar name of Laxgalts'ap, which, given the varieties of spelling in those days, was also sometimes spelled Lach-al-sap.

The word Git (or Kit) means "people of" and is a prefix to many local names. Gitxsan (alternatively spelled Gitksan) therefore means "people of the Skeena." Skeena (Xsan) itself means "river of mist." Gitanyow is Kitwancool; and Ghitwangah, or Gitwangak, is Kitwanga.

Kishpyax, where Horace went first, is clearly Kispiox, though the local Gitxsan name is An'spa'yaxw. The Nass River was at the time often spelled Naas. Rocher de Boule, the mountain that presides over Hazelton so majestically, is variously written as Stekyooden, Stekyawden or Stegawden. In one letter, Horace calls it Skedanden — although possibly the transcriber in Toronto at the time misread his "u" for an "n". The Widzin Kwah or Watsonquah River was renamed the Bulkley River after Colonel Bulkley, who was in charge of the aborted attempt to build a telegraph line to Europe through British Columbia via a connecting line in Siberia.

The Gitxsan village of Gitanmaax is known by many as Hazelton, although the settler village of Hazelton is actually located on the riverbank encircled by the Gitanmaax Reserve and was, and is, a separate place. Hazelton itself became a settlement thirty years before the Gitanmaax First Nations reserve was created around it, leaving it effectively an island of about thirteen acres of non-Indigenous habitation surrounded by the reserve.

Today there are three Hazeltons. The first is the original settlement, which I call either Hazelton or Old Hazelton, depending on the context. The second is New Hazelton, which lies across the Bulkley River on the south side of the Hagwilget Canyon. The third, South Hazelton, a few miles to the southwest, was originally the railway town. Each has a part to play in the history of the district. Collectively I refer to them as the Hazeltons.

Dr. Wrinch's Maiden Speech in the British Columbia Legislature, as Reported by the *Omineca Herald* on November 14 and 21, 1924

The following is taken from a transcript of the speech made by Dr. H.C. Wrinch, MLA for Skeena, in seconding the adoption of the King's Speech before the Legislature last week. After a brief introduction, the speaker continued:

I would like to digress for a few moments to speak of certain matters not mentioned in the Speech from the Throne. In the first place I would like to say a few words on public health. Looking over the health situation of the province we find that in three years the government has spent on public hospitals no less than $1,380,000. It is true that if this amount is divided by the number of hospitals in existence and again by the number of months in the period the amount is, perhaps, not very large. But let us compare the amount spent by the government on hospitals with the amount spent by the governments of the neighbouring prairie provinces and we shall find ample room for pride.

In British Columbia the government's contribution to hospitals is eighty-eight cents per head of the population; in Alberta forty-four cents; in Saskatchewan thirty-four and a half cents; in Manitoba thirty-eight cents. Thus it is seen that our government spends on hospitals twice the amount spent by the governments of the prairie provinces.

But in addition to the ordinary hospitals to which these payments are made, we have other institutions, such as Tranquille Sanatorium for tubercular patients at Kamloops. I desire to express the opinion that this is an ideally-managed institution and, if possible, the government should provide other hospitals of a similar character for those suffering from mental diseases, where patients who have money can pay as much as they can afford and the rest can be made up by the government. Under the present system we are more liberal in this regard than the neighbouring provinces.

Outside of these institutions we have a Department of Health which is working to prevent disease, maintain sanitary conditions and attending to all other health matters. Altogether our government spent in 1923 $1,750,000 on health, a goodly amount surely.

Dr. Wrinch then referred to the work being carried on at Tranquille [a hospital at Kamloops], where patients are enabled to stay long enough to effect a real recovery. He then lauded the philanthropic work of the government in providing mother's pensions.

Referring to the recent work of consolidating the provincial statutes, he noted that the Speaker compared its cost to that of previous revisions, and found it to have been only about half of former costs. Dr. Wrinch then turned to the building of WBC at the new campus in Point Grey:

Turning from the physical side of the questions under consideration, we find that the Speech from the Throne refers to the work on the new University of British Columbia buildings and these buildings will be ready for occupancy in September 1925. May I be permitted to go back to the time ten years ago when in the flood tide of our prosperity, someone conceived the idea of building a university at Point Grey. Plans were drawn and some of the buildings are still on paper but others have been completed. The new Science building, in our good British Columbia granite, is almost ready, and two more

buildings are on their way to completion while some semi-permanent
structures are being built. Why, it may be asked, are buildings of
stucco being erected? The answer is that while the building scheme
was in abeyance the student body increased to a number over 14,000.
These had to be accommodated, so instead of waiting until we could
build all these new structures of stone, we are making cheaper buildings as permanent in character as possible. Contracts have been let
for $2,250,000, but we still have a balance. We want our young people
educated and I do not believe that many will criticize these expenditures.

Dr. Wrinch then made reference to the race-track measure to be
brought down this session in the House.

Speaking in regard to the mining industry of the province, Dr.
Wrinch pointed out that whereas two years ago the revenue from
this source amounted to $28,000, the returns for the past year were
$41,000 and would probably exceed $50,000 this year. He noted the
decreasing number of accidents in the mines as a result of safety legislation, and spoke of the laws passed to prevent overstatement of
facts in mine promotion literature.

We note from reports published from time to time that the great
salmon fisheries of the Fraser River are being depleted. The Skeena
River, however, has come to the forefront now as one of the biggest
salmon fishing streams on the continent and perhaps in the world. . . .

Let us now pass, then, to another division of matters and discussion — what the government may do in the future. The government,
I feel, should not only take care of our natural resources, but should
help the people to bring these resources to market. Let me touch for
a few moments on the resources of the Skeena district. I believe that
in that district there are all the resources found in other parts of the
province. Indeed, so varied is the agriculture possible in that district
that I have heard it called the "banana belt." Although I have not seen
that fruit growing in our district, the range of our agricultural possibilities is enormous.

In minerals, too, our resources cover a wide range. Gold is found both in placer forms and quartz. We have also silver, copper, zinc, lead and coal. Oil has not yet been found but our enthusiasts tell us that the surface indications indicate oil beneath.

Our timber resources, too, are great. We have pulp, timber, ties and other forest products.

Dairying finds ideal conditions in our district. The growth of crops there is succulent and vigorous and ideal forage is produced. Dairying thus will be one of our leading industries in the future. Fruit, too, grows admirably. The small fruit industry is developing rapidly and we are now shipping our berries to the Edmonton market and supplying our own fruit requirements.

Conditions in my riding are excellent for the production of beef and mutton. We can turn out our stock in the spring and, after grazing in the open range about our farms, the animals are fat by the time they are ready for slaughtering. We also produce mutton in a small way. Hay grows well, and our potatoes and other vegetables will be in competition with those of the older districts in fairs this year and we hope we will not be ashamed of them.

The fur, fisheries and water power resources of Skeena were then reviewed and last but not least the value of the scenery was considered by Dr. Wrinch, who continued:

The development of our resources, Mr. Speaker, may be considered logically under two headings: capital and transportation. I used to think we should go out and get capital to develop our resources. Lately, however, I have come to the conclusion that it is a mistake to chase capital in this way. In the past many capitalists have come to this country, looked over our resources, pronounced them excellent and then gone away again without investing here. What is the reason? What do we need to do to keep capital here? The great need, the first need, I believe, is transportation to open resources and then to deliver the products of these resources to markets, local and overseas.

The wise policy for the government, it seems to me, is not to attempt to chase capital, but to make the resources of the country available for capital. How can this be done? First, by the construction of roads and bridges for automobile and horse traffic and, secondly, the opening up of railways for longer hauls.

It is not in this connection, Mr. Speaker, that mention has been made of the Transprovincial Highway. The construction of a road link from Hope to Lytton is often regarded, I think, as the completion of a highway eastward and westward across the province. That, however, is a wrong conception of the new highway, for it will also be a road north and south — an extension of the Pacific Highway, indeed, to the most northern districts of the province. I would like to see Victoria tied up by road connection with Hazelton, and this, in effect, will be the result of the construction of this new road. Let us look over the distances covered by roads in the province. The distance by water from Vancouver to Victoria is, I am informed, 73 miles. Now, the distance from Vancouver to Hope is 92 miles — a total of 165 miles. Then at Hope comes a dead stop — a gap and 70 miles to Lytton, which, however, we hope to see covered next summer.

I wonder if the House realises the vast area north of Lytton which will be opened in this way? From Lytton to Clinton is 80 miles and on to Prince George, 255 miles — a total of 611 miles from Victoria to Prince George. When another section of the road is built to connect the two points there will be a connection between Victoria and Endako, 799 miles. I would urge the completion of the 43 miles of road required between Endako and Burns Lake. Fine work has been done on this section and I hope that it will be completed next year. This would make a total of 987 miles from Victoria northward.

The future of British Columbia then came to the attention of Dr. Wrinch, who stated that while it was admitted that Vancouver was destined to become the rival of Liverpool, yet even Liverpool was but one of many large ports in Britain. In the East, there were other large ports besides New York and Montreal.

Now what do we find in connection with these big ports? We find that they have vast areas of land tributary to them. Am I to believe, sir, that the resources of the north of this province are any less than the resources of other places where big ports have been built up? Or that one port will be sufficient to carry the products of British Columbia to the world's markets? Certainly not.

If you are interested, take a tape measure, as I did, and a map of Canada and find the centre of the Dominion. You will find that the centre lies somewhere in Ontario, slightly to the east of the boundary of Manitoba. This calculation, however, takes in a large part of the Atlantic Coast. Perhaps a more significant measurement would define the centre between Montreal and Vancouver. This point lies west of Winnipeg so that the western section directly tributary to our ports — and this is giving the East the benefit of a very generous measurement — includes all the three western provinces and a large part of Manitoba. That vast area should be tributary to our ports, other things being equal.

While I admit that it is a fair and reasonable prediction that Vancouver will be the Liverpool of Western Canada, I believe also that there will be ports and important ones at such places as Victoria, New Westminster and Prince Rupert, each carrying on the business naturally tributary to it.

May I suggest also a glance at the map of British Columbia? Look for a second at the northern districts. You will find that in the five northern ridings is included more than one-half the total area of British Columbia. You will find, too, that they are served by a great transcontinental railway system terminating in a city of the Pacific Coast. This, gentlemen, is an area capable of producing more wheat than all Canada. This is a big conception. It takes time to appreciate it and understand it.

In conclusion, I would point out that all those five ridings are represented in this House by supporters of the government. This government has started and is carrying on a great fight for lower transportation rates and we in the north have felt that in lining up behind the government we can make no mistake, for we believe that in the direction in which the government is working lies the prosperity, success and happiness of our people.

Recollections of Harold Wrinch: Notes on the Hospital Farm

MAINTAINING AN AMPLE food supply at the hospital during the winter months when there were no means of transportation to bring in supplies from outside sources was a problem of considerable proportions. In the spring, the boats commenced coming up the Skeena after the river was clear of ice and the spring floods were over, usually sometime in May. And in the autumn navigation ceased when ice started forming in October or November. The remainder of the year, the only transportation was by dog team from Port Essington at the mouth of the Skeena or by dog team from the Naas River, which apparently was an easier route to the coast. Mail was the only item brought in by this method and even this was limited to letters. No junk mail! As a result of this limited means of transportation and to supply the hospital with food on a very limited source of income, means had to be developed to grow vegetables and fruit and keep them all winter.

The long daylight hours in the summer, the fertile soil and the keen agricultural skills of Dr. Wrinch combined to result in excellent crops of vegetables, grains, hay and small fruits. But the long winters with temperatures at times of −40 F presented problems of storing the crops till spring. But the doctor was a most resourceful person and always had a solution to any problem. There was never any fuss or furor — things were always done calmly and easily. I expect that the numerous problems that he faced were anticipated long before they arose and solutions were sought and found during his long and lonely trips by horseback, dog team, horse and buggy or on foot to visit patients.

The permanent staff of the hospital farm consisted of two men — a farm man and a general helper. The agricultural area consisted of two main plots — a flower, fruit and vegetable garden behind the hospital about two acres in extent and the farm itself consisting of about twenty acres.

The smaller garden produced the following vegetables: peas, beans, carrots, beets, spinach, lettuce, celery, radishes, broad beans, cucumber, marrow, squash, cabbages, cauliflower, Brussels sprouts, turnips. And these fruits (the climate was not suitable for tree fruits): black, red and white currants (profusely), gooseberries, raspberries, strawberries and rhubarb. Producing all these fruits and vegetables was achieved without a great deal of labour. No spraying or fertilizing was done, other than the application of manure from the stables in the spring. As boys we were paid ten cents a dozen for eliminating cutworms. Also some watering had to be done by pulling water from the twenty-foot well by a pail on a rope. This was also done by my brother and me. I do not remember any payment but we were happy to assist.

The fields provided the following crops: hay for the cattle and horses, alfalfa (three crops a year), oats, field corn and sunflowers for ensilage, potatoes, swedes, turnips, mangels and pastureland kept for grazing the cattle.

Growing all the above produce was one job and preserving and storing the products for winter was another phase of work and a most important one. In those early years, the paid staff at the hospital was very small — a housekeeper, cook, and two helpers in the kitchen. I mention this so it will be obvious that so few paid staff would not be able to preserve or can all the small fruits and vegetables. So other sources of help had to be found. The doctor's family was always a good source of help. Schools or universities were out for vacations at the time most of the crops were ready for attention — so this was the first supply of help. Also a hospital serving such a large area — central and northern BC — required obstetrical cases to come to hospital in plenty of time before their due date and surgical cases to remain in hospital until completely "ready for the trail" again. So this situation meant that many patients enjoyed work to fill in otherwise idle time, such as picking berries, peas, beans and preparing them for canning. So much work was accomplished, all in a happy atmosphere.

Originally small fruit and vegetables were preserved in two-quart "economy jars." After these were packed, shelled etc., they were put in the jars and the lids clamped on them. Then they were placed in larger, specially made square boilers, which held sixteen two-quart jars. These boilers were put on the large wood stove in the hospital laundry and boiled the required length of time. Later when "home" canning devices were developed the jars were replaced by cans. Of course, jams, jellies and pickles were also made and processed in methods prescribed in the Boston Cook Book. These preserved fruits and vegetables were stored in the hospital basement. This same basement had bins along one wall in which potatoes were stored. These potatoes were the first ones used. Other potatoes, stored in cooler areas, were used later in winter and spring.

An underground root cellar was located conveniently under a building partly used as a granary and partly as storage for buggies in the winter and cutters and sleighs in the summer. The root cellar was dark and dingy. It had double doors. The ceiling consisted of heavy planks supported by beams held up by cedar posts. The planks were covered by about three feet of earth. The interior consisted of a workway, on either side of which were bins for vegetables. In here were stored carrots, beets, turnips, cabbages (hung from the ceiling beams) — these were for human consumption. For the cattle [there] were turnips and mangels, which were sliced on a chopping machine as required. A coal oil lantern was always left at the door of the cellar and provided light when necessary.

The hay and alfalfa were brought in from the fields and hoisted up into the large hayloft above the barn (horses and cattle lived in the lower floor). In about 1924 a silo was constructed. It was the first such thing in the district, and for it fodder, corn and sunflowers were grown and chopped up. After having [been] "worked," this provided excellent fodder for the cattle.

I mentioned earlier that potatoes were stored in bins in the hospital cellar. In addition to these, more were stored in pits dug in the ground and lined with planks. These were about four-by-six-by-six feet deep. When these were filled they were covered with planks and then covered with dirt to a depth that would prevent the frost from penetrating. Usually three pits were used. These kept the potatoes in excellent condition for use in late winter and spring until the new crop was available.

So many were the ways of providing food for the patients, nurses and staff of the Hazelton Hospital during the long winter months when lack of transportation forced everyone to supply their own requirements.

APPENDIX 3

Receipts and Disbursements
of Hazelton Hospital

The figures in this table are taken from the financial statements of the Hazelton Hospital in the hospital annual reports, and from the *Omineca Herald* and *Omineca Miner*. They are not presented in accordance with generally accepted accounting principles. Since the accounting presentation changed over the years, comparisons are misleading. For instance, the year-end for 1906–1908 was March 31. At the end of each financial year, there were always uncollected accounts, undistributed government grants and bills still unpaid. The figures are stated in absolute dollars, and not thousands. The figures for 1929 are approximate.

YEAR	RECEIPTS	DISBURSEMENTS	TOTAL
1901	$ 300	$ 281	$ 19
1906			2,072
1907	9,678	9,632	46
1908	5,736	5,747	(11)
1909	7,343	7,733	390
1910	13,828	13,493	335
1911	13,772	13,823	(52)
1912	14,077	14,993	(916)
1913	16,115	12,874	3,241

YEAR	RECEIPTS	DISBURSEMENTS	TOTAL
1914	22,895	23,156	(261)
1915	13,272	12,728	544
1916	14,345	13,923	422
1917	13,371	14,624	(892)
1918	20,109	20,332	(223)
1919	19,284	20,645	(1,361)
1920	23,435	24,217	(783)
1921	21,555	22,871	(1,361)
1922	21,841	21,706	165
1923	19,143	27,716	(3,573)
1924	27,342	26,492	400
1925	25,335	24,638	697
1926	25,494	24,458	1,036
1927	28,763	29,355	(592)
1928	29,430	30,040	(610)
1929	27,000	30,000	3,000
1930	31,820	28,888	2,932
1931	36,737	39,683	(2,943)
1932	28,920	28,213	715
1933	25,294	26,794	(1,500)
1934	23,324	26,310	(2,986)
1935	22,848	23,897	(1,049)
1936	23,051	22,657	394
1938	28,047	28,000	47
1941	43,400	42,135	1,265

Acquisition of Land
for the Hospital in 1902

IT IS EASY TO CONSTRUCT a picture of Horace pacing in the brush between Hazelton and Two Mile Creek, inspirationally pushing apart the hazel bushes and turning to Alice to proclaim, "Here! This is the place. Here we will build the hospital." Then of him deciding how much land he needed for the hospital compound, acquiring it and starting to build. The acquisition of the land was, in fact, much more complicated, and it leaves us with unanswered questions.

■ How Land Was Acquired

In the first years of the twentieth century, much land in British Columbia was acquired from the provincial government by means of pre-emption followed by a Crown grant. (This process disregarded issues of underlying First Nations ownership of the land. The First Nations reserves in the Hazelton district had been laid out in the 1890s.) A prospective buyer selected a site, filed a pre-emption request and was then awarded pre-emption rights. Since the purpose of the pre-emption procedure was to develop the land, the pre-emptor had to survey the land, show evidence of development and pay the required taxes. If he or she didn't develop the land, the government cancelled the rights. If he or she did, the government would issue a Crown grant.

A holder could relinquish the pre-emption rights to the government, but not transfer them to another person. Following receipt of a Crown grant, the owner could sell or transfer land in the ordinary way.

Once awarded pre-emption rights, a buyer paid for the land either with cash or with what was called "war scrip." The government issued to veterans from the South African War (1899–1902) a document — war scrip — that gave them the right to select a parcel of land and then apply for a Crown grant for it at no cost. Since many veterans did not want to farm and these rights were transferable, there was a brisk secondary market in war scrip. Much of the land around Hazelton and in the Bulkley Valley was acquired in this way. It is possible — but entirely conjectural — that some patients at Hazelton paid their medical bills with war scrip. This might explain how Horace acquired many pieces of such otherwise disparate land.

■ The Choice of Land for the Hospital

In July 1900, before Horace had even arrived on the Skeena, Richard Loring, the Indian Agent in Hazelton, wrote to Dr. Bolton saying there were a couple of sites around Hazelton that would be suitable for a hospital. Neither Kispiox nor the Methodist land on Mission Point would be suitable, he said, because of the need to cross a river over which there were no serviceable bridges at that time. There was the elegant Indian cantilevered bridge at Hagwilget, of course, but that swung in the breeze and unnerved many. One "lovely and ideal building site" was near Two Mile, "two miles south of here [Hazelton] and on common land." This sounds like the land between the Gitanmaax Reserve at Hazelton and Two Mile, land on which the hospital was in fact eventually built. Loring wrote to A.W. Vowell, superintendent of Indian Affairs for the province, on December 13, 1901, saying he had attended a meeting of thirteen Hazelton residents, not including himself and Dr. Wrinch, to deliberate upon the ways and means of establishing a hospital. It would be built, he wrote, "in a splendid locality on the Two Mile Creek, to the south-east, at the distance indicated . . . readily accessible to the Kit-Ksan of the Skeena below and above here and to the Hagwilget to the south-west a little."

Despite Loring's certainty, Horace was still considering various sites in the Hazelton district during the winter of 1902, although it appears he had made up his mind before April of that year. In a 1909 letter to Dr. Sutherland, Horace wrote:

> It was found at the inception of the work that the hospital must either be built at a little distance from our two mission villages, and more centrally placed in relation to all the Indian villages as well as to the few whites then in the country or we would not be able to draw any of the available grants that would make the work self-sustaining. If located in our own mission village [Kispiox], the hospital work would have been very limited and much less remunerative and consequently much more costly to the Society.

He appears to have decided that one piece of land, District Lot 105 (which is where the hospital was soon to be built) met his criteria, but he had to move quickly to take preparatory steps before the Missions Board in Toronto had finished its bureaucratic procedures and approved it. Head offices, then as now, were often seen as being too slow and too far away. This land, on the other side of the Gitanmaax reserve land, was as close to the town of Hazelton as it could be and yet would still be convenient for Gitxsan First Nations coming from surrounding villages and Wet'suwet'en First Nations coming over the Hagwilget Canyon, as well as for settlers starting to come into the Bulkley Valley.

There were, however, two problems. First, William Larkworthy from Hazelton had already acquired pre-emption rights to the land, and, second, there appeared to be no water on it. Larkworthy, who soon became a leading merchant in Hazelton, had been a clerk in the Hudson's Bay Company store there, but in 1904 was recorded by Henderson's Directory as a telegraph linesman.

■ A 1908 Letter

On April 18, 1908, Horace wrote a letter to Rev. Alexander Sutherland at the Missions Board in Toronto about an application for a right-of-way over hospital land, and he attached a map he had drawn.

On this map he identified that the hospital and his home were clearly on District Lot 105 and also that the Gitanmaax First Nations band had donated thirty acres of their reserve for hospital purposes.

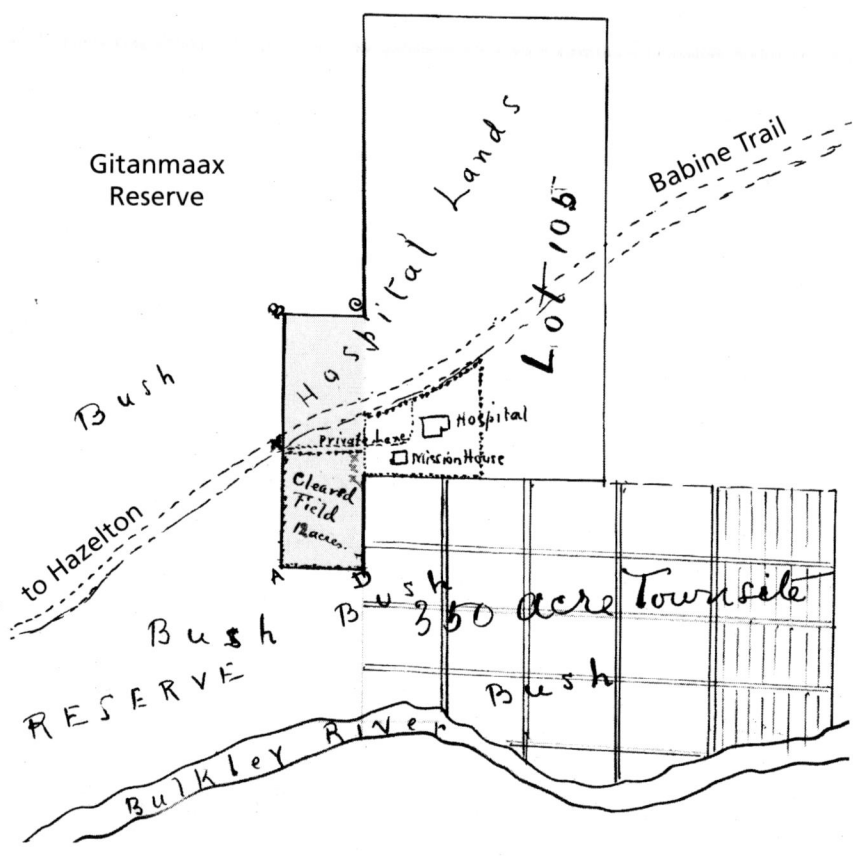

The shaded area represents 30 acres of land alienated to the Hospital from the Gitanmaax Reserve. Detail from a map drawn by Horace Wrinch in his April 1908 letter. Courtesy United Church Archives (printed words added).

■ Acquisition of District Lot 105

In a letter he wrote on April 14, 1909, Horace summarized for Sutherland and for new members of the Missions Board in Toronto how the hospital land had been acquired. What happened may be seen as a four-step transaction.

First, Horace persuaded Larkworthy to give up his pre-emption rights on District Lot 105 in return for good and valuable consideration. In a letter to Horace of September 9, 1904, Sutherland noted that Larkworthy, who was in Ontario at the time, had been to see him about the agreement that he and the church had signed in August relating to the surrender back to the Crown of his pre-emption on the 320 acres (DL 105) in exchange for about twenty acres.

Second, Horace and Whittington, Horace's Methodist colleague in Victoria, acquired District Lot 105 for the Methodist Church. They were helped in this by a prominent Methodist named Victor Spencer. He was the son of the wealthy Victoria department store owner David Spencer, who was also a lay preacher and Sunday school teacher. The senior Spencer was head of one of the leading Methodist families in the province and well-known for giving financial and other help to church causes. His wife was active in the Women's Missionary Society, which, perhaps not coincidentally, was an active supporter of Hazelton Hospital by paying the salaries of the nurses.

Victor Spencer acquired war scrip from two sources. Wilfrid Fraser served in Lord Strathcona's Horse in the South African War from February 1900 to March 1901, and the grateful government gave him war scrip so that he could acquire land for free. For whatever reason, Fraser did not want land, and so on May 10, 1902, he sold this war scrip for $115 to Victor Spencer. On October 4, 1902, Harold Daly, a law student, also sold war scrip (probably acquired from a veteran specifically for the transaction) to Victor Spencer for $1. On October 11, 1902, Victor Spencer transferred both items of war scrip, each for 160 acres, to the Methodist Church for $1. (The dollar amounts in the transfer documents were not necessarily the full consideration.)

The Methodist Church applied for a Crown grant for District Lot 105 on September 10, 1902. In October 1902, Horace later wrote that Whittington had negotiated the purchase of 320 acres for the hospital from the British Columbia government with war scrip acquired for about $500, although he said he never knew the exact amount. In October, a surveyor working for David Spencer (Victor's

father) surveyed District Lot 105 and reported directly to Whittington. The Missions Board formally approved the acquisition of the
land on November 3, 1902. The Province executed the Crown grant
two days later, on November 5, 1902. So now the Church had legal
title to the land.

Third, to compensate Larkworthy for relinquishing his pre-
emption rights, the Methodist Church deeded to him twenty acres
of that land. Larkworthy shortly sold that parcel of twenty acres to
Edward Charleson.

Fourth, there was still one problem to be solved. The highway ran
over both the church land and the twenty-acre parcel, and this was
inconvenient to all parties. To tidy this up, in 1906 Charleson and the
church entered into an adjustment agreement as a result of which the
road went between their two properties and not over both of them.
In 1906, therefore, the hospital transferred four-and-a-half acres to
Charleson, who then transferred half an acre to the hospital and paid
an additional $132.

■ McCoskrie — District Lots 103 and 42

This does not explain the whole story. In a letter published in the
Missionary Outlook in 1903, Horace wrote that "A good building site,
about one mile east of Hazelton, has been donated for the hospital by
Captain McCoskrie and Mr. A.C. Murray." He repeated this information in the Annual Report of the Methodist Missions Board.

Here then was the consequence of those conversations with Captain McCoskrie on board the *Queen City* on their journey up the
coast in 1900. Manifestly, the explanations are inconsistent: in the
one, the Methodist Church acquired a Crown grant with war scrip
acquired from unrelated third parties after Larkworthy had given up
his pre-emption rights; in the other, the land was donated by
McCoskrie and Murray. The simplest explanation is that Horace
merely made a mistake or that Whittington, who handled the legal
details of the acquisition in Vancouver, did not tell him the whole
story. Horace, however, was not one to make such mistakes.

McCoskrie's role, therefore, remains unclear. One possibility is that the original plan was to build the hospital on District Lot 103, which McCoskrie and his partner Murray, an old Hudson's Bay Company trader, owned. They had applied for this land on November 15, 1901. McCoskrie himself also owned District Lot 42. These lots, between the hospital land and the Bulkley River, stretched from the First Nations land in Hazelton to the First Nations land at Hagwilget. On this land McCoskrie and Murray had plans to establish a town-site, surveyed by J.W. Vaughan and shown on an October 1905 map.

This possibility is supported by Horace's 1903 letter in the *Missionary Outlook*, and by a letter from Loring dated September 13, 1902, when the Gitanmaax Band donated land for hospital purposes. In his letter, Loring tells Vowell that the hospital was "to be built on Captain McCoskrie's and Mr. Murray's land," south of the Larkworthy land. The possibility is also supported by a statement by David Spencer's surveyor that he had also surveyed another piece of land, this one being for Captain McCoskrie and Dr. Wrinch, which adjoined the Larkworthy land he had surveyed. If this is true, then clearly something happened to change the situation. By September 1902, the Methodist Church was well into its acquisition of District Lot 105 (the Larkworthy land).

By 1905, Captain McCoskrie and Murray appear to have transferred District Lot 103 to the Hazelton Townsite Syndicate, which had filed a subdivision plan for a 350-acre town site, with streets laid out and named. Full-page advertisements in the *Vancouver Daily World* in January 1906 described Hazelton as "The Premier City in Northern British Columbia.... Hazelton like Winnipeg, another old Hudson's Bay centre, will boom with the coming of the Railway.... The townsite is being placed on the market for the first time — a $10,000 hospital, physician's house etc. are already built. Six sites for hotels and stores will be given free. Large numbers of the streets are being cleared."

Clearly the promoters believed that the town of Hazelton would grow fast and spread out along the bank north of the Bulkley River.

They were wrong, and the land remains mostly forest and brush to this day. They did, however, sell or lease one five-acre lot to Rev. Price, land that the Methodist Church later owned. It is at least possible that McCoskrie and Murray donated this lot on District Lot 103 to the Methodist Church. On July 11, 1906, the *Vancouver Daily World* described Captain McCoskrie as the man who made Hazelton known. His role in both the hospital and the development of a Hazelton that never happened remains unclear.

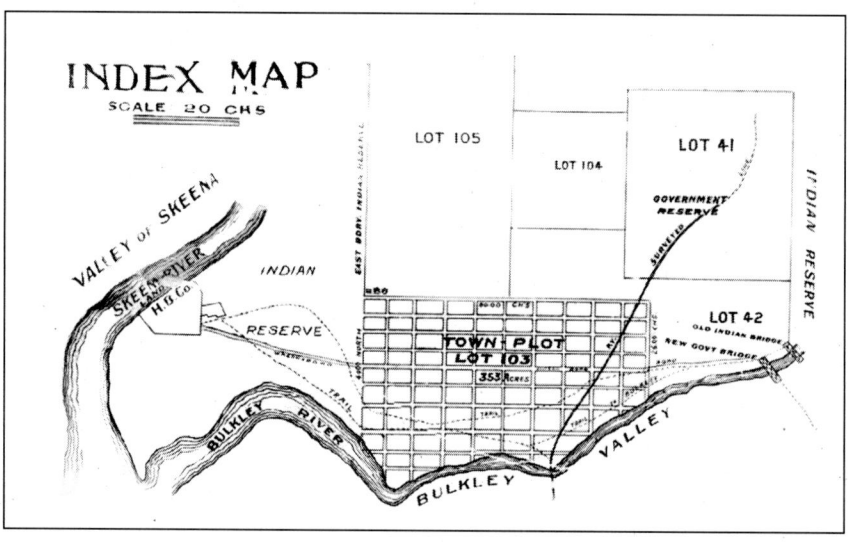

Map of the proposed Hazelton townsite promoted by Williams, Hoare & Co., General Agents on District Lot 103. *Vancouver Daily World.* January 13, 1906, p.10.

■ The Gitxsan Donation

The map that Horace drew in 1908 for Dr. Sutherland clearly delineates District Lot 105 and the hospital on it. Alongside it to the west is the thirty-acre plot of land that was donated for hospital purposes by the Gitanmaax Band in Hazelton.

On September 13, 1902, five chiefs of the Gitanmaax Band passed the following resolution:

We, the undersigned Chiefs and representatives of the Gitanmaax Indians of Hazelton, B.C. agree and herewith do set aside thirty (30) acres of land situated on the reserve line, intersecting from north to south its trail to the Two Mile Creek . . . one and a quarter miles east of Hazelton. . . . Upon the hospital ceasing to be operated as such, the aforesaid designated land of thirty acres shall revert to the Gitanmaax Band of Indians, together with all improvements thereon made up to such time, providing the whole of the transaction meets with the approbation of the Department of Indian Affairs.

Names:

Get-dam-gal-don	Head Chief
John G (illegible)	Deputy Chief
Get-dam-gal-don	Deputy Chief
Alexander Moat	Deputy Chief
Ma-de-gam-get	Deputy Chief.

Loring, the Indian Agent, wrote to A.W. Vowell the superintendent of Indian Affairs in British Columbia, based in Victoria, saying that the hospital would be invaluable to the First Nations and settlers in the district. He recommended, the approval of the donation of the thirty acres. On November 21, Vowell confirmed the donation was acceptable and authorized the drawing up of an agreement to implement the resolution, conditional on the Department of Indian Affair's final ratification.

The agreement was prepared, executed and sent to Vowell for approval on December 31, 1902. Vowell confirmed on May 8, 1903 that he was sending it on for approval by the department, which replied on May 28 authorizing the Methodist Church to occupy the land for "mission purposes during the pleasure of the Superintendent General of Indian Affairs." Loring sent the agreement, which Horace had signed for the Methodist Church, to Vowell on December 11, 1903. The hospital itself was not, though, built on this donated land, which was used by the hospital farm for hay fields.

■ Interest in Adjacent Lots

Horace and Whittington, principals of the Methodist Church, owned or had a clear interest in four adjacent district lots immediately to the east of the hospital site. These were DL 104, DL 38, DL 39 and DL 43. These were separate from the hospital site on DL 105. These lots ran east from DL 105 across to Four Mile Creek, which ran into the Bulkley River in the Hagwilget Canyon, where DL 43 was riverbank property.

District Lot 105

The hospital was built in the south-west corner of DL 105. District Lot 103 to the south was, on paper, subdivided for a townsite. District Lot 41 was government reserve land.

District Lot 104

Horace applied for District Lot 104 on March 16, 1902. In September of that year, he was awarded it by way of Crown grant, and for it he paid $300. This 160-acre lot was immediately to the east of Lot 105 and almost reached Two Mile Creek.

District Lot 38

Whittington himself acquired District Lot 38, which lay immediately to the east of District Lot 104 on both sides of Two Mile Creek. Victor Spencer also assisted Whittington in this acquisition by buying the necessary war scrip and transferring it to Whittington on October 21, 1902. The Crown grant was issued in 1904.

District Lot 39

Whittington also filed an application for District Lot 39. Victor Spencer again assisted him in this acquisition by buying the necessary war scrip on October 10, 1902, and transferring it to Whittington a few days later, on October 21. The Crown grant was issued in 1904.

District Lot 43

Whittington had an undefined interest in District Lot 43, but no rights as such. In 1903, he was helping Laing Stocks, of Nelson, British Columbia, acquire the land with war scrip and indeed selected the land for the pre-emption for Stocks and acted as his agent in acquiring it. This lot went along the Babine trail as far as Four Mile Creek.

These acquisitions raise the interesting question. Why would principals of the Methodist Church be assembling land in that area? Speculation suggests two possible reasons.

The first is that as soon as Horace decided that the hospital should be at Hazelton, he would have seen that available land was disappearing fast. Did he perhaps acquire District Lot 104 as insurance in case he couldn't strike a deal with Larkworthy or, even if he could, in case he couldn't find water on that site?

On the same logic, perhaps Whittington acquired District Lot 38 across Two Mile Creek as insurance in case they didn't find a reliable water supply? With so much war scrip being bought and sold and with so many pre-emptions being made, Horace might have realized he had to act without waiting for formal authorization. Bureaucratic wheels turn slowly. It took a long time to get replies from Toronto — the various committees and boards had to meet and deliberate, and then send their reply.

Horace and Whittington would have understood that they could not formally acquire the land in the name of the Methodist Church because they would not yet be able to show their authorization. Consequently, they had to purchase it in their own names. If they needed extra money, then perhaps the wealthy Spencers could help.

They also would have realized that a reliable source of water was imperative. At this time, 1902, Horace had not yet found water on the hospital land, and he could not be sure of its reliability even if he did find it. It is true that there was a lake at the northern end of the hospital property, but the hospital lacked the necessary power to pump water from that distance. If the supply of water from a well on District Lot 105 did turn out to be unreliable, Horace would have needed to use water from Two Mile Creek, which ran through Whittington's land, or even locate the hospital closer to that water supply. When he was satisfied with the water supply on the hospital site

(D.L. 105), he and Whittington would have disposed of their interest in the other lots. Horace sold half his land in 1905 and tried to sell the other half, but, to his chagrin, missed the market. Whittington had probably sold his land long before June 1906, because he would not for one moment have tolerated the notorious hotel that was then located in the hamlet of Two Mile either on or very close to his property.

The second possible explanation is that Horace and Whittington were trying to establish a stream of income to support the hospital. McCoskrie had staked out and believed in the townsite. If a town were to grow there, any land adjacent to his land — such as the Wrinch and Whittington land — would increase in value. It could be let out as farmland or sold for building purposes, all of which could have provided cash to run the hospital. Perhaps Horace needed some insurance that they could in fact afford to keep the hospital running. By 1904, though, it was becoming more evident that the much-talked-of railway would not come north of the river and that no town would ever grow on the McCoskrie land.

It is always possible that Horace and Whittington were buying the land for their personal accounts. As far as Horace was concerned, what could be easier? It was already in his name. All he would have had to do was to make a payment to the Methodist Church. He had a growing family to provide for, so his personal expenses were increasing, and he was certainly not averse to buying land for himself. In any event, in 1905 or 1906, Horace sold half of District Lot 104 to five purchasers, who subdivided it into eighteen parcels. Much later, he bought this same land back for his own personal use. This was the land that would give him some personal trouble in the provincial legislature in the 1930s.

Bridges across the Skeena and Bulkley Rivers

THE STORY OF OLD HAZELTON is in part a story of bridges. Hazelton could not have survived into the twentieth century at all without bridges across the Skeena and Bulkley rivers. It could easily have followed the fate of Aldermere, isolated from the railway and the developing road system, and withered away. Bridges saved it.

Old Hazelton is on the point where the two rivers meet. Up the northern arm are bridges crossing first the Skeena and then the Kispiox rivers. Up the southern arm are bridges crossing the Bulkley. When transportation was by water, travel was relatively simple: you went by the shortest route by canoe, ferry or, in later years, launch, paying the levied fee. In winter, you went over the ice on foot using snowshoes or dog-sled. If, on the other hand, you wanted to go by land, you had to cross whatever bridge was available. When Dr. Horace Wrinch arrived in the district as a medical missionary in 1900, other than a small number of First Nations cantilever bridges, the most famous one being at Hagwilget about four miles up the Bulkley River, there weren't any bridges.

■ Skeena and Kispiox Rivers

The Skeena River is joined by the Kispiox River at Kispiox and then flows south to Hazelton, where it is joined by the Bulkley River. The

Gitxsan village of Kispiox is on the point where the Kispiox and Skeena Rivers merge. When Horace arrived in Kispiox in 1900, he used to walk the eight miles or so to Hazelton. To do that, he would have had to cross at least one river — the Skeena — or, depending on which route he took, two — the Kispiox and then the Skeena. Presumably he crossed by canoe, paying the customary toll. (He could of course have gone all the way by canoe, but that would have been more expensive.) He would have walked past Simon Gunanoot's farm at Anlaw, across the river from Glen Vowell. Here there was a ford for the packers to take pack trains across, but it was a deep one and the animals had to swim part of the way.

Mule-train packers, missionaries, miners, fur trappers and farmers wanted bridges and roads over the Skeena and Kispiox rivers. Farmers had been working on their farms in the Kispiox Valley for years and now needed ways to get their products to market. Surveys for a bridge and wagon road had been made in 1908, and these surveys made the construction of bridges more achievable. Settlers in the Kispiox Valley formed the Kispiox Settlers' Association in 1909 to persuade Premier McBride to authorize the construction of bridges.

By August, the government had announced that it would build two bridges. Despite determined opposition from the Gitxsan in Kispiox, construction of the Kispiox Bridge was under way by June 1910 and was almost finished by the end of July. The bridge across the Skeena above Hazelton was finished by the end of the year. By 1912, therefore, when travelling to Kispiox, Dr. Wrinch could have crossed one bridge across the Skeena and then another one across the Kispiox.

■ Bulkley River

The Bulkley River was a formidable obstacle. For one thing, it was wide. Close to where it met the Skeena at Hazelton, the banks were low. A bridge over to Mission Point here would always be susceptible to high water and ice jams. Upstream the cliffs very quickly grew higher, and the river flowed rapidly through the Hagwilget Canyon, which had steep and, in many places, unstable sides. Building a bridge over the canyon was a challenge for engineers.

First Nations Bridges

When Horace arrived in 1900, the only way he could cross the Bulkley River, except by canoe or by going thirty miles upstream on the Babine trail to Witset (Moricetown) and using the First Nations bridge there, was to use the First Nations bridge at the Hagwilget Canyon, approximately four miles from Hazelton. Not that the bridges were always usable. Richard Loring, the Indian Agent, reported in December 1893 that one faction of the First Nations at Witset had torn down the bridge and were stopping others from rebuilding it. He made a special trip to try to settle the dispute.

The First Nations bridge across the Bulkley at the Hagwilget Canyon was the last in a number of bridges that had been built there, being one of a number of First Nations bridges in the district. Built without nails or screws by people without engineering training, these bridges cantilevered over streams and rivers with elegance and beauty. The ones across the Hagwilget Canyon were the highest and longest.

Five statements can be made about the First Nations bridges at Hagwilget.

First, high waters tended to destroy or damage them. The First Nations then repaired or rebuilt them, it being difficult to distinguish between repairs and new constructions. It is perhaps, therefore, a little simplistic to refer to the series of bridges across the Bulkley as first, second or third bridges. It is reasonable to assume that there have been numerous bridges at Hagwilget for many hundreds of years.

Second, even within history recorded by the settler and travellers, there have been numerous bridges across the canyon. In June 1833, Simon McGillivray, the Hudson's Bay Company trader, recorded crossing a bridge at Hagwilget. The map he drew clearly shows two bridges across the canyon: one thirty miles east at Witset, and another about four miles upstream from where the Bulkley joined the Skeena at what was then known as the Forks and at what is now Hazelton. His map showed trails leading to both bridges. (This map reportedly lay unnoticed in the Hudson's Bay Company Archives in Manitoba until researcher Alan Pickard, who has done very valuable research on the early bridges, brought it to light.) This bridge across the canyon may have been the one that the engineers for the Collins Overland Telegraph found when they came in 1866 to lay cables, or it may have been a successor to it.

When the Gitxsan or Wet'suwet'en refused to let the engineers build another bridge there, the engineers strengthened the existing one with cables being used to build the telegraph. (Another account has the bridge being strengthened by First Nations with cable left behind when the telegraph line was abandoned.)

Third, there is evidence for the belief that in the 1890s at least once, perhaps more, a low-level bridge at the Hagwilget Canyon had been swept away by high water. In one account, Deputy Chief Charles of the Wet'suwet'en brought the Wet'suwet'en and the Gitxsan together to rebuild this bridge in about 1890–1893. In November 1895, Loring noted that the bridge at the Lower Hagwilget was under repair. In April 1896, he was reporting that the bridge there was unsafe and that he had to cross the river by canoe. By approximately 1898–1899, it appears that high water may have severely damaged or swept away the existing bridge at the Canyon, and that a new bridge would have to be built. When George Dorsey visited the district in 1898, he saw First Nations re-building a bridge at the Canyon.

In his monthly report of occurrences in the Babine Agency for June 1897, Loring reported that, as a result of extremely high water, "Not a single bridge was left standing: of the principal ones carried away . . . are the one at Kis-ge-gas, suspended thirty-eight feet above ordinary stages of water and . . . the one at Tsitsk at Hagwilget" where the water was twenty-nine feet above average in the Canyon. In his report for the following month, Loring reported that a new bridge was already being built. There is further support in an article on the First Nations bridges at Hagwilget in the *Herald* in November 1913. There had been three bridges, it said, since (and including) the one built about twenty years before: the first, which would have been in 1890–1893, the second completed in about 1895 (the one that Loring reported as coming down in the high waters of 1897), and the third completed in about 1900.

Fourth, it could well be that there have been two places at the Hagwilget Canyon where a bridge was built. Immediately to the west of the current high-level bridge, there is a short kidney-shaped stretch of lower land where the canyon is wider. Here is a stony river-bank and a narrow strip of habitable land. Within photographed history there was a First Nations village there. The river tumbles through a low choke point at each end of this lower land. The First Nations bridge which collapsed in 1917 was built at the eastern end, close to the current high-level bridge.

Some evidence indicates earlier bridges had been built at the western end. In November 1913, the *Herald* reported that, after the 1897 washout, Deputy Chief Charles had "proposed that they build across the eastern end of the canyon and at a height which would protect them from the high waters." The bridge was then rebuilt closer to the Hagwilget village and closer to where the Craddock high-level bridge would be built in 1913. This is the First Nations bridge that was much-photographed and much-admired.

Fifth, it is probable that there were other bridges across the Bulkley River between Hagwilget and Witset (Moricetown), notably at Six Mile Creek. Loring mentions crossing one at Six Mile Creek in the 1890s. Since these probably would have been low-level bridges, they too would have been vulnerable to being swept away by high water, which they probably were.

For the first five or six years after Horace Wrinch arrived in the district, the only way to cross the Bulkley River at Hagwilget was on the First Nations bridge. Six-feet wide, made of logs and ropes, and without nails, it could allegedly take 300 pounds of weight. Although it could take horse and mule traffic — one at a time, one would imagine — it swayed in the slightest breeze and was not for the faint of heart. Sperry Cline, no timorous soul, wrote that he was not ashamed to dismount and lead his horse across. Father Morice, who sounds as though he did not have a head for heights, confessed to having attempted to crawl across it on hands and knees, with perspiration on his brow and swearing that he would never cross it. He gave up the attempt and chose to make the long detour around.

By 1913, this bridge needed repairing. Neither it nor the low-level government bridge built in 1906 was in any way able to support the increasing amount of mining and farming traffic among Hazelton, Kispiox, New Hazelton and the Bulkley Valley. By then, though, the Craddock high-level bridge had been built. A meeting was held in 1913 to consider ways of repairing the First Nations bridge. "Steps should be taken at once," the *Herald* recommended, "to secure permission to repair the structure and retain it for its historic value." To no avail. It was allowed to decay. On the morning of Sunday, August 19, 1917, the First Nations bridge at Hagwilget collapsed into the Bulkley River.

The 1905–1906 Bridge

In 1905–1906, the government built a mid-level bridge across the canyon approximately three miles from Hazelton. The Victoria *Daily Colonist* in December 1905 stated that "the government bridge across the Bulkley River at the mouth of Two Mile Creek was being pushed forward by Mr. Williscroft." The Ministry of Public Works stated in its annual report that in the year ended on June 30, 1906, it had built a bridge across the Bulkley at a point three miles from Hazelton. This was a suspension bridge, 144 feet long and six feet wide, designed for pack trains and pedestrian traffic only. No one liked it. The steep approaches made it difficult to use, and when there was ice on the hill it was dangerous for horses and pack trains.

In an article on October 17, 1913, headed "Three Bulkley River Bridges Within Ten Miles of Hazelton," the *Herald* reported that years after the First Nations bridge had been built "the provincial government built a pack-train bridge about a mile farther down the river. Why the site was selected is hard to imagine, unless it was to impose upon the pioneers the greatest possible hardship." Sperry Cline wrote that it was built farther down the Bulkley River, and that its approach was too steep, rendering it difficult or useless for freight. It was so narrow, he wrote, that a team of horses could not get over. The *Herald* complained about this bridge, saying it should never have been built for general traffic. "It is in the wrong place altogether and it is a regular death trap and horse-killer." The sides of the bridge were light boards and the bridge itself was good only for pedestrians and mules. A new high-level bridge, it said, was badly needed. The 1906 bridge lasted until May 1924, when, the *Herald* reported, it was dismantled.

The Craddock Bridge

By the time the railway was being planned, it was clear that the increasing traffic between Hazelton and new town across the river necessitated a new bridge. The need for a stronger, wider bridge to handle the shipments of ore from mines north of the river to the railway was becoming imperative. The location of the bridge would influence where the new townsite would be built. There were numerous competing sites. Robert Kelly, who owned real estate south of the river, across the Hagwilget Canyon, decided to build a bridge privately to try to ensure that the railway station would be built near his land, which is where the town would then grow, causing his land values to increase. In July 1912, the *Herald* announced that the new high-level bridge was assured and that the contract to build it had been awarded to George Craddock & Company from England. It would be 450 feet long, 240 feet above water and regulation width for wagon traffic.

Contractors were hired. Construction started and continued apace. Concrete was poured, cables were strung. By September 1913, this high-level bridge was almost finished and people were crossing it with great excitement. But there was a problem. Dr. Wrinch wrote to the minister of public works about the lack of access roads. As the *Herald* said:

> Unfortunately there is no road connecting it with the government road on each side of the river. This has, however, been applied for and there is no reason to believe that the provincial government will not

grant the request. With the road built, New Hazelton district enters upon a new era of progress.

By the end of 1913, therefore, there were three bridges across the Bulkley River at the Hagwilget Canyon: the First Nations bridge, the horse-killer government bridge of 1906 and the Craddock high-level bridge. The government reportedly purchased the Craddock bridge for $12,000 in 1920.

The Hazelton Bridge

At first glance, the most convenient place for a bridge across the Bulkley River from Hazelton was a hundred yards or so upstream from where the Bulkley merged into the Skeena. Here, at Mission Point, the riverbanks were low and flat. The Bulkley River, however, was powerful. A bridge there would always be in danger of destruction from ice in winter and from high waters in summer. One already had been destroyed. In December 1912, the *Herald* reported that a bridge, built at considerable expense by the government to replace a ferry then out of commission, had been washed away by high water after heavy rains.

When Premier Bowser visited Hazelton in June 1916, he announced that he would be giving orders — immediately, he said — for the construction of a new bridge. This bridge, built to connect Old Hazelton with the railway at South Hazelton, was opened in early 1917, replacing the ferry. By 1932, however, it had been condemned as unsafe by the chief engineer of the province. Some short-term repairs were made that would extend its life for about two years, but that was it. It was increasingly likely to come down when hit by ice or high water. On May 19, 1942, when the river was "on a rampage" high water carried away one pier and one 140-foot truss of the bridge. When attempts were made to dynamite a log jam, the rest of the bridge came down. Part of the iron was salvaged, but the balance of the bridge was then dismantled.

The High-Level Bridge

By the mid-1930s, the Craddock bridge was coming to the end of its useful life. Government engineers condemned it, and proposed building another bridge 900 feet farther upriver, necessitating a mile or so of additional roads. In the early stages of the ensuing controversy about where the new bridge would be built, Dr. Wrinch, the local member in the Legislature, was caught uncomfortably between his constituents and the plans of the government he represented in Victoria.

The location for the replacement bridge caused great consternation in the community. A new bridge at the existing location would surely be more convenient for some, but for others moving the bridge to a new location would mean a new railway station and new town. Those who had invested in land and buildings in New Hazelton saw a real risk that their investments would suffer. The new bridge would have a steep slope down to it, thus repeating the mistakes of the 1906 bridge. Moreover, it was to be a two-lane bridge, something that Sawle, the *Herald*'s publisher, claimed loudly was an unjustified and unnecessary extravagance. This, he proclaimed, the community could not allow.

Dr. Wrinch spoke to the minister of public works, who told him that there could be no question of a new bridge on the existing site. The engineers had said that the rocks supporting the foundations for the Craddock bridge were crumbling. It had to be replaced at a different site. Government engineers did agree, though, to study it further. In November, they reported back and said they had found a new site, one between the existing bridge and the low-level bridge from Mission Point to Hazelton, both of which they proposed to take down.

This did not satisfy Sawle and his friends. The *Herald* excoriated the government and its representatives. Sawle blasted the new proposal in December 1927. Under the headline "Why Move Bridge to Low Site," his editorial thundered. "Why destroy the whole town?" It went on to say, "There are already three Hazeltons now and surely that is enough."

Where did Dr. Wrinch sit in all this? As the representative of both the government, which was planning the new bridge, and the community, which, if you believed the *Herald*, was dead set against it, he was deeply conflicted. A group, led by Sawle, wrote an open letter to him that he published in his paper:

> "You have not yet taken a stand on this matter. . . . Are you, Sir, going to permit the town of New Hazelton to be destroyed and financial ruination brought to all those people who own property in New Hazelton and have their all invested there? Are you going to forget the noble support the people of New Hazelton have given you and your institution for the last fifteen years? Are you going to forget the splendid majority New Hazelton gave you at the last election, the largest majority the government got in any poll in any riding? We do not believe, Sir, that you can show your appreciation of the above support by permitting such havoc be wrought on your supporters and your constituents. We ask you, Sir, to make a public declaration opposing any move of the bridge from the present site crossing the Bulkley River at Hagwilget."

In other words, if you support the government's plan, don't bother trying to run for office again and don't ask for more support for the hospital. An election was coming up in 1928, and this threat was probably a real one.

Wrinch was not, though, going to take this lying down. He replied that if this were merely a matter for the future, he would favour the new middle site being proposed. But people were too set in their ways — and it was here that he came off the fence. He wrote in a letter to the *Herald*:

> I believe that now too many people have become too deeply rooted (financially) to warrant being asked to change their location, and, since they have decided not to do so voluntarily, I shall give my support and do all I can to have the bridges maintained at their present location.

Accordingly, he pressed the minister for public works during Question Period in the House, and in February he was informed that the government had decided to replace the old bridge with a suspension bridge at much the same place. Soon, though, the government would change and the Conservatives would be in power. Although Wrinch won back his own seat, the Liberal Party lost the election, and he was now sitting on the opposition benches. His influence on decision-makers in Victoria was consequently reduced.

Nevertheless, the newly elected Tolmie government announced in May 1929 that it would build a new suspension bridge to replace the Craddock bridge. Editorials were written. Petitions circulated. Meetings held. In one such public meeting that he chaired, Wrinch pointed out that the grade down to and up from the bridge the government engineers were proposing, at six percent, was too great. He said the problem could be solved by building the bridge at a greater height above the river than the government had proposed. This proposal was accepted and the design work commenced. The new bridge was to be 650 feet end to end and 262 feet above the river. Married men were given priority in the hiring. While it was being built, traffic — including mining and logging vehicles — had to cross the Bulkley over the Hazelton bridge.

Dr. Wrinch and Dr. Bamford, the Conservative candidate who had stepped in for the minister of public works, opened the new bridge on August 21, 1931. An arch at the Hagwilget end was decorated with bunting, flags and a banner of welcome. Little Patsy Russell handed Horace a pair of scissors and he cut the ribbon. In his words opening the bridge, Wrinch thanked those who had to be thanked, politely regretted the absence of those who could not be there and expressed the enthusiasm and relief of those who were.

The bridge, he said, would connect the northern half of the province with the southern half. (This was at a time when the road to Alaska was still being proposed to go up the Kispiox Valley.) It settled for good, he said, the transportation question. Those investors who had held back could now come forward. After cutting the ribbon, he and other dignitaries got into a car and drove across the new bridge, and then back again.

The Wet'suwet'en First Nations paraded over and back and were reported to say how happy they were. Then everyone progressed to the New Hazelton sports ground and watched New Hazelton beat Smithers 13 to 11 at a celebratory game of baseball. In the evening, there was a dance in New Hazelton.

This bridge remains today as the principal way into Old Hazelton and as a spectacular place from which to view the Hagwilget Canyon.

Three Hazeltons and Two Railway Stations

THE RAILWAY FROM Prince Rupert to Winnipeg was always going to come through the Hazelton district south of the river. Where it passed Hazelton, though, only one new town and only one railway station were needed. But where would the new town be located? When the dust settled and the Last Spike driven, the Hazelton district was left, more by accident than by design, with three towns and two railway stations. How did this come about?

The question of where the railway station would be built consumed the attention of the residents of Hazelton for several years. Several facts were clear. First, the railway line would come south of the Skeena and Bulkley Rivers. Second, a new town would grow where the railway station was built. Third, anyone who owned land there could earn a fortune. Fourth, the old town of Hazelton would probably wither, and could die altogether as more and more of its residents moved to the new town. Fifth, the location of a bridge across the Bulkley River was critical to the mining companies north of the river, which needed to get their ore as economically as possible to a railway station south of the river. The geography of the area — hence reference to maps — is critical to the complicated story of what happened next.

When the residents of Hazelton heard the whistle of the first train from across the river, they still did not know where the station and new townsite would be. There was fierce competition about its location. Speculators bought land, well aware of the monetary potential of being the first owners on a new townsite.

At least seven sites were promoted — New Hazelton, South Hazelton, Larkford (owned in part by William Larkworthy), Ellison, Sealey, Bulkley City and Taylor. Two quickly emerged as the favourites. The first was across the Hagwilget Canyon, where New Hazelton absorbed both Taylor and Larkford. The second was across the Bulkley near Mission Point, at what was to become South Hazelton. Bridges were critical. By 1910, the only two bridges across the Bulkley River were the First Nations bridge and an unsatisfactory pack-train bridge, built in 1906. Both bridges fed traffic towards the New Hazelton site. There was no bridge at that time from Hazelton to Mission Point. There was a ferry, but it could not operate when the water was too low. The government had, reportedly, already built one bridge that had been swept away by the river after heavy rains.

Robert Kelly, a Vancouver man and the owner of land south of the Hagwilget Canyon, was the first to establish a town, which became known as New Hazelton. As early as 1911, he was laying out this townsite and naming streets. He then commissioned a high-level bridge across the Hagwilget Canyon in an attempt to make his site the only logical location for a railway station. With this new bridge he believed his site would be more attractive to the residents of Old Hazelton, to the settlers up the Kispiox Valley and, perhaps more importantly, to the mining concerns in the hinterland north of the river.

Although Kelly and the Grand Trunk Pacific reportedly did try to work out some sort of compromise at various times, they could not — or would not — agree. The Grand Trunk Pacific promoted the site it called South Hazelton, just south of Mission Point. The railway lines there would be running on higher ground, minimizing significant grade problems, and would also be within easy reach of unloading points on the river. The promoters of South Hazelton townsite promised a bridge, this one across the Bulkley River a little to the east of Hazelton, 150 feet above the river.

Horace himself supported the South Hazelton proposal. "As a member of the Board of Trade of Hazelton," he wrote in May 1912, "I have given active support to the South Hazelton point. On the two occasions, upon which we made presentations to the [Railway] Commission, I was either the mover or the seconder of the resolution which was passed by the Board and in each case was the author of the resolution."

While the rail tracks were moving out from Prince Rupert, proponents of the two proposed townsites fought hard: Kelly for New Hazelton on the one hand and the Grand Trunk Pacific for South Hazelton on the other. Competition between the two factions was fierce and increasingly bitter. In the autumn of 1911, full-page advertisements started to appear in both local and Vancouver newspapers.

Kelly, boosting New Hazelton, was enthusiastic in promoting his coming city. Describing it as the new Spokane of Canada, his advertisements listed all its advantages in glowing terms. "New Hazelton . . . is attracting the attention of the whole world. . . . The Most Important Town-site. . . . The Most Talked of Town-site along the line of the Grand Trunk Pacific Railway." A full page advertisement in the *Vancouver Daily Province* described Hazelton district as the Pittsburgh of Western Canada on account of its abundant coal deposits. Investors in land were exhorted to hurry.

Although the Grand Trunk Pacific had by now built a station and was developing a townsite at South Hazelton and declared the competition over, as early as 1911 many residents in Old Hazelton were already moving to New Hazelton. The Ingenika Hotel relocated. The *Herald* itself, which supported the New Hazelton site, moved in 1912 and remained there for several decades. The MacLeans moved and built a Presbyterian Church and manse. Horace opened a drugstore there. With several hundred residents now living there, New Hazelton already was a bustling town. The railway station, though, was at South Hazelton, a much quieter place a few miles away.

The location of the townsite was taken to arbitration. In December 1911, the Board of Railway Commissioners delivered a decision in favour of New Hazelton. Judge Mabee, in ordering the Grand Trunk Pacific to build a station at New Hazelton, was severely critical of the company, saying that if any private individual had done what the Grand Trunk Pacific had attempted to do, he would be sent to the penitentiary. This was appealed to the Governor-General in Council, who ordered a re-hearing by the Railway Commissioners on the basis that this was not merely a simple contract matter and that the voices of the local citizens and businesses had not been sufficiently taken into account.

In June, the Railway Commissioners rescinded their earlier decision and allowed the Grand Trunk Pacific to build a station at South Hazelton. It gave additional approval to the South Hazelton station in November but also authorized an extension to New Hazelton. It appeared that the Grand Trunk Pacific had won. The *Miner*, which supported the South Hazelton site in its articles and editorials, was understandably triumphant.

Then, towards the end of 1912 and perhaps faced with the reality of the existing town at New Hazelton, the Grand Trunk Pacific changed its position. The cost of building the promised bridge, together with a disappointingly low number of sales of its lots in South Hazelton, led them to give in. Furthermore, the Railway Commissioners had started to give warnings to the company about the need for full compliance with some conditions they had specified about levelling out a grade. In addition, mine owners were not prepared to accept the higher costs of shipping ore to the South Hazelton station.

The deciding factor, though, may well have been that construction of the bridge across the Hagwilget Canyon was well under way. In October, when the South Hazelton bridge had been no more than a vague promise reported in the *Miner* (later withdrawn), bridge contractors in New Hazelton had been given the building plans and had started ground preparation. The representative of the Craddock firm, which was building Kelly's bridge, arrived on site to supervise construction. The *Herald* reported in the last week of October 1912 that the New Hazelton Bridge and Power Company had been incorporated to build the bridge and ancillary projects. The Grand Trunk Pacific, faced with what looked like a *fait accompli*, agreed to build a station at New Hazelton. The first passenger train arrived there on January 17, 1913.

The managers of the Grand Trunk Pacific did not accept defeat gracefully. In his book, *A Thousand Blunders: The Grand Trunk Pacific Railway and Northern British Columbia*, Frank Leonard suggests that the managers of the company did what they could to make life difficult for New Hazelton, even going so far as to stop four carloads of lumber for construction of the Craddock bridge. More significantly, they increased freight rates for mines in the district, which led to increased shipping costs and to reduced revenue for the railway. "Only in the context of this townsite dispute," Leonard wrote, "does the series of GTP actions after 1912 that hindered development and eventually closed local mines become comprehensible."

Old Hazelton refused to die and both New and South Hazelton survived. All three towns continue to exist and together are known as the Hazeltons.

Notes

I have had the benefit of access to Dr. Wrinch's surviving letters and photographs, and most of the photographs that appear in the book are from this collection, unless otherwise stated. Dr. Wrinch, though, was a private person and was not one to keep papers for posterity. He probably destroyed most of them when he left Hazelton in 1936. He did write a short history of the hospital in 1938, one that is frustratingly short on personal details. Having married Dr. Wrinch's granddaughter Alice, I also knew her father Harold Wrinch well and have visited Hazelton with him.

I have referred to reports in the *Omineca Herald*, which was the weekly newspaper that started to record events in Hazelton in 1908 and also the *Omineca Miner*, for a short time its rival. I have also researched material in the British Columbia Archives in Victoria and on microfilm reels online with Library and Archives Canada.

In the notes below, UCCA (Vancouver) means the United Church of Canada Archives (BC Conference), and UCCA (Toronto) means the United Church of Canada Board of Home Missions Fonds in Toronto.

Introduction

PAGE 1 ... "for forty years": *Vancouver Sun*, October 20, 1939, p. 21.

PAGE 2 ... "Mr. Speaker, the necessity of health": Dr. Wrinch's speech was reported in the *Vancouver Daily Province* on February 8, 1927, p. 22, and in Victoria's *Daily Colonist* on February 8, 1927, p. 3.

Chapter 1: The Farmer's Boy

PAGE 7 ... Leonard and Elizabeth Wrinch had a large Victorian family. Their children were: Georgina (Gina) Elizabeth (born October 30, 1861, died November 9, 1954); Leonard Edward (born December 24, 1862, died June 12, 1944); Marion Agnes (born September 18, 1864, died August 10, 1949); Horace Cooper (born January 6, 1866, died October 19, 1939); Walter Godfrey (born January 13, 1867, died April 23, 1939); Frank Sydney (born September 17, 1868, died August 28, 1934); Warwick (born November 17, 1870, died November 4, 1944); John Alfred (born August 28, 1872, died January 21, 1938); Charles (born July 20, 1874, died November 6, 1951); Mary Evelyn (born May 12, 1877, died 18 September 1969). Horace is a distant cousin of the distinguished mathematician and biochemist Dorothy Maud Wrinch (1894–1974).

PAGE 8 ... Kirby-le-Soken: E.R. Kelly, editor. *Kelly's Directory of Essex, 1882.* UK: Kelly & Co., 1882, pp. 176, 188.

PAGE 9 ... "never to join in any undertaking": *Ipswich Journal*, December 31, 1878, p. 4.

PAGE 9 ... "The greatest single event of the 'seventies": G.M. Trevelyan, *English Social History*. London, UK: Longman Group Limited, 1978, p. 491.

PAGE 10 ... "In the present depressed condition": *Essex Standard*, September 6, 1879, p. 2. Issue 2543.

PAGE 11 ... "The reports received of good": *Manchester Courier and Lancashire General Advertiser*, October 3, 1879, p. 5. Issue 7141.

Chapter 2: Farmer, Missionary and Medic

PAGE 13 ... Information on St. Francis Agricultural School comes from the Annual Report of St. Francis Agricultural School and its Catalogue. Toronto Reference Library, Ontario.

PAGE 15 ... "he had inquired of farmers": *Ipswich Journal*, September 20, 1881, p. 4. Issue 7985.

PAGE 15 ... "As a mark of respect": *Essex Standard*, April 15, 1882, p. 8.

PAGE 16 ... Currency: In 1880, £1 was equivalent to C$4.87. Therefore, £2,317 was $11,283.79. A guinea was one pound and one shilling, when there were twenty shillings to one pound.

PAGE 16 ... "all the valuable household furniture": *Ipswich Journal*, April 18, 1885, p. 3.

PAGE 17 ... "for there are few paupers": *Emigration: The British Farmer's and Farm Labourer's Guide to Ontario, the Premier Province of the Dominion of Canada*, issued by the Government of Ontario. Toronto, Ontario: C. Blackett Robinson, 1880, p. 3. Toronto Reference Library, Ontario.

PAGE 17 ... Leonard and Horace Wrinch's farm in Halton County was on SDS 53, Lot 35.

PAGE 18 ... "thriving city": *Canada: Its History, Productions and Natural Resources*. Prepared by the Canadian Department of Agriculture for the Colonial and Indian Exhibition in London in 1886, p. 113. Toronto Reference Library, Ontario.

PAGE 20 ... "No one will ever understand Victorian England": Sir Robert Ensor. *Oxford History of England: 1870–1914*. Oxford: Clarendon Press, 1966, p. 137.

PAGE 21 ... "Brother Horice C. Wrinch": *Palermo Parish Minutes*, July 5, 1894. UCCA (Toronto), Nelson-Palermo Pastoral Charge (Ont.) Fonds, 1321, Accession No. 77-100L, Box 1.

PAGE 21 ... "Dr. Wrinch was converted at twenty-two": *Missionary Outlook*, XIX, No. 8. August, 1900, p. 180.

PAGE 22 ... "great enthusiasm prevails": *Acton Free Press*, January 26, 1893, p. 3.

PAGE 23 ... The Reverend Dr. Alexander Sutherland (1833–1910) was the General Secretary of the Methodist Missionary Society from 1878 until his death. He was most likely the one who chose Horace to be the medical missionary to go to the Upper Skeena. He was also the one who held down the Toronto end of the project of building the Hazelton Hospital and obtained the grants for it.

PAGE 23 ... "I believe missionary work": H.C. Wrinch, undated application form to be a student volunteer. UCCA (Toronto). F.C. Stephenson Family Fonds, 1978.091C, Box 6. Young People's Forward Movement for Missions, List of Campaigners, 1898–1899.

PAGE 24 ... "Preliminary Examinations for the Methodist Church": *Albert College Times*, Belleville, Ontario, March 1, 1889.

PAGE 24 ... "From January 1894 to July 1895": *Missionary Outlook*, XIX, August 1, 1900, p. 180.

PAGE 24 ... "thus giving them a hearty welcome": Undated and unsigned paper in H.C. Wrinch's biographical file. UCCA (Toronto), Biographical File collection, file of Rev. Dr. Wrinch.

PAGE 25 ... "to a missionary movement": A.C. Sutherland, *Missionary Campaigner*, Vol. 1, No. 1, May 1896, p. 2.

PAGE 26 ... "Campaigners. Please Read this": H.C. Wrinch, *Missionary Campaigner*, Vol. 1, No. 1, May 1896, p. 7.

PAGE 26 ... "at least as thoroughly prepared": *Missionary Campaigner*, Vol. 3, No. 7, November 1898, p. 3.

PAGE 27 ... Mary E. Wrinch exhibited a picture she called "Old Time Vanities" in the Sixteenth Annual Exhibition of the Royal Canadian Academy of Arts in Toronto in 1895. RCAA Catalogue, 1895, p. 13.

PAGE 27 ... "My mother and family backed": Mary E. Wrinch, quoted in Muriel Miller, *Famous Canadian Artists*, Peterborough, Ontario: Woodland Publishing, 1984, p. 101.

PAGE 27 ... "our Methodist Church": *Missionary Campaigner*, Vol. 3, No. 7, November 1898, p. 2.

PAGE 28 ... Visits to Congregations: H.C. Wrinch filed reports about his visits to congregations. UCCA (Toronto). F.C. Stephenson Family Fonds, 1978.091C, Box 6. Young People's Forward Movement for Missions, List of Campaigners, 1898–1899.

PAGE 28 ... H.C. Wrinch was now writing for medical journals. In the *Canada Lancet* of January 1900 he wrote an article entitled "A Case of Interstitial Emphysema": *Canada Lancet*, Vol. 32, No. 5, January 1900, p. 241. In the August edition there is a note by him on "A Case of Incarcerated Ovary": *Canada Lancet*, Vol. 33, No. 12, August 1900, p. 665.

PAGE 28 ... H.C. Wrinch graduated as a doctor and surgeon: *The Globe*, June 5, 1900; *Canada Lancet*, Vol. 31, No. 10, 1899.

PAGE 28 ... That H.C. Wrinch turned down good offers in Toronto is related in an undated and unsigned biographical sketch. UCCA (Toronto), Biographical File collection, file of Rev. Dr. Wrinch.

PAGE 29 ... "a very thorough study of a case of interstitial emphysema": H.C. Wrinch, *The Canadian Practitioner and Review*, Vol. 24, No. 12, December 1899, p. 707.

PAGE 30 ... "Owing to the thorough training received": *Acton Free Press*, December 30, 1886, p. 2.

PAGE 30 ... Alice spoke at the Christian Endeavour meeting: *The Globe*, July 14, 1894, p. 20.

PAGE 30 ... Alice shared the platform with Albert Carman at the Methodist

Young People's Association of Ontario: *The Globe*, February 27, 1895, p. 2.

PAGE 30 ... Visiting and Relief pamphlet: *The Palm Branch*, Vol. 2, No. 3, March 1895, p. 8; also *Methodist Magazine and Review*, Vol. 43, No. 5, May 1896 (Advertisements).

PAGE 30 ... Grace Homeopathic Hospital was established in 1893 at the corner of Huron and College streets. Alice Breckon (Wrinch) attended the nurses training school at this hospital.

PAGE 31 ... "About twenty-five years ago": Obituary of Alice Wrinch, *Christian Guardian*, Vol. 94, No. 18, May 2, 1923, p. 7.

PAGE 32 ... "infectious laughter": Obituary of Alice Wrinch, *Christian Guardian*, Vol. 94, No. 18, May 2, 1923, p. 7.

PAGE 33 ... "Contact with whites": A.E. Bolton, *Medical Work Among the Indians*. Women's Missionary Society of the Methodist Church, 1896. Also see *Missionary Outlook*, No. 9, September 1900, p. 202.

PAGE 33 ... Messrs. Field, Stephenson and Clifford, residents of Hazelton, had applied to the Indian Department for a doctor in early 1888. This was referred to in a letter from the Department of Indian Affairs to Lieutenant Colonel J.W. Powell. Library and Archives Canada, Microfilm reel C-7683, Image 593.

PAGE 34 ... "No medical man has yet": R.E. Loring, letter to A.W. Vowell, May 14, 1896. Library and Archives Canada, Microfilm reel C-14856, Image 88.

PAGE 34 ... "Transportation from the coast": H.C. Wrinch, *History of Hazelton Hospital*, p. 3. 1938. Unpublished document in the author's possession. The original is in UCCA (Vancouver). Archive Reference Collection. H.C. Wrinch, Biographical File, Box 2093.

PAGE 35 ... "Dr. Wrinch was then preparing": W. Pierce, *From Potlatch to Pulpit: Being the Autobiography of the Rev. William Henry Pierce, Native Missionary to the Indian Tribes of the Northwest Coast of British Columbia*. Vancouver, BC: Vancouver Bindery Limited, 1933, p. 57.

PAGE 35 ... "When attending General Conference": Thomas Crosby, *Up and Down the North Pacific Coast by Canoe and Mission Ship*. Toronto, Ontario: Missionary Society of the Methodist Church, 1914, p. 299.

PAGE 35 ... The Methodist Missions Board was considering sending a missionary to the Upper Skeena. Methodist Missions Board minutes for Saturday, October 14, 1899. UCCA (Toronto). Fonds 14, Series 2, Subseries 2. Correspondence of Alexander Sutherland, 78.081C, Box 1, File 4.

PAGE 36 ... "For some time we have been thinking of Dr. Wrinch": Dr. A. Sutherland, Letter of November 10, 1899. UCCA (Toronto). Correspondence of Alexander Sutherland Fonds. Fonds, 14 Series 2, Subseries 2. AC 78.083C, Box 14. (Letterbooks, Dr. Sutherland.)

PAGE 36 ... "As the undertaking will involve": Dr. A. Sutherland, Letter to R. Loring of November 9, 1899. BC Archives, GR-0429, Box 5, File 04, Attorney-General's Correspondence Inward.

PAGE 37 ... "He was accepted by the Toronto Conference": *Missionary Outlook*, Vol. XIX No. 8. August 1900, p. 180.

PAGE 37 ... "We are sending you": H.C. Wrinch, Letter to the Missions Board, April 12, 1912. UCCA (Toronto). Fonds 14, Series 2 Shore Papers, Indian Missions: B.C. Correspondence re Hazelton. II, 1911–1912.

PAGE 38 ... "Dr. Wrinch, who is going to British Columbia": Dr. A. Sutherland, Letter to the Reverend E.R. Doxsee, Belleville, June 1, 1900. UCCA (Toronto). Correspondence of Alexander Sutherland Fonds. Fonds 14, Series 2, Subseries 2, 78.083C Box 14. (Letterbooks, Dr. Sutherland.)

PAGE 38 ... "pretty house wedding": *Canadian Champion*, Milton, Ontario, June 21, 1900, p. 3.

PAGE 39 ... "We will want to read": Undated and unsigned notes of the farewell meeting held at the Holloway Street Church in Belleville. UCCA (Toronto). Biographical File collection, file of Rev. Dr. Wrinch.

PAGE 39 ... "Dr. H.C. Wrinch (Trin '99) of last year's House Staff": *Canada Lancet*, Vol. 33, No. 11, July 1900, p. 651.

Chapter 3: Up the Skeena River to Kispiox

PAGE 43 ... "wet and disagreeable": *Western Methodist Recorder*, August 1900, Vol. 2, No. 11, p. 4.

PAGE 43 ... The Reverend Robert Whittington in 1900 had been president of the British Columbia Methodist Conference for two years. He was now in charge of the missionary work for the First Nations of the province. Based in Vancouver, he was one of the key players in the establishment of the Hazelton Hospital. He held down the Vancouver end while Dr. Sutherland, Whittington's superior, held down the Toronto end. Whittington handled the negotiations with the provincial government and the Vancouver lawyers for the real estate transactions.

PAGE 43 ... "Nor have we heard anywhere among the ship's crew": Letter to Captain McCoskrie, dated August 14, 1900; *Daily Colonist*, August 23, 1900, p. 8. Also in photocopied manuscript in the author's possession.

PAGE 44 ... "I have only followed": Letter to Captain McCoskrie, dated August 14, 1900; *Daily Colonist*, August 23, 1900, p. 8. Also in photocopied manuscript in the author's possession.

PAGE 45 ... "To have changed your appointment": Dr. A. Sutherland, Letter of August 15, 1900, to H.C. Wrinch. UCCA (Toronto). Correspondence of Alexander Sutherland Fonds. Fonds 14, Series 2, Subseries 2. AC 78.083C, Box 14. (Letterbooks, Dr. Sutherland.)

PAGE 45 ... Whittington's visit to the Nass River. Although I have found no hard evidence to prove it, I think Horace accompanied Whittington on his visit to Ketchikan, Alaska. We know that he went with Whittington (and Rev. S. Osterhout) to the Nass, where they left the *Queen City*, because Dr. Sutherland comments on it in a letter to Horace; we know that Whittington did not go back to Port Essington before going on to Ketchikan; and we also know that the only reason that Whittington went to Ketchikan was to catch the MV *Tees* back to Port Essington. It is therefore reasonably safe to assume that Horace went with Whittington for the whole of the tour, including the visit to Alaska, where the three missionaries buried the desperado. It was not, furthermore, in Horace's nature merely to hang around in Port Essington for Whittington to visit the missions on the Nass. The question is, did Alice go with him? My guess is that she would have, but we have no evidence of it. The report of the murder in Ketchikan is set out in the *Daily Colonist*, August 23, 1900, p. 8; in the *Seattle Times*, August 24, 1900; and in the *Alaska Morning News*, August 22, 1900. Whittington describes this incident in his report of the tour in the *Western Methodist Recorder*, Vol. 2, No. 4, October 1900, p. 10.

PAGE 46 ... William Duncan (1832–1918) was the Anglican missionary who set up strict Christian communities at Metlakatla, near Port Simpson, and then at New Metlakatla, near Ketchikan, Alaska. He quarrelled with many, including Bishop Ridley.

PAGE 47 ... "a flock of sheep on the rampage": Wiggs O'Neill, *Steamboat Days on the Skeena River, British Columbia*. Smithers, BC: Self-published, 1961, p. 4.

PAGE 48 ... "On Monday, Bro. Jennings, Dr. and Mrs. Wrinch": Rev. R.

Whittington, Report on his Inspection of the Northern Missions. *Western Methodist Recorder*, Vol 2, No. 4, October 1900, p. 10.

PAGE 49 ... "My first journey from Port Essington": Whittington, p. 10.

PAGE 49 ... Could Horace have reached Kispiox by steamer? Possibly. On August 22, 1900, the *Victoria Daily Times* reported on page 5 that the *Monte Cristo* on its previous voyage had reached thirty miles up the river beyond Hazelton, being the "first steamer to attempt this part of the voyage." Kispiox was likely not on the regular steamer run. The *Skeena District News* of July 18, 1904, noted that although Hazelton was the head of navigation, "Kispiox has on occasion been reached by steamer." The same paper, on August 8, 1904, recorded a visit by the *Hazelton* to Kispiox, where it picked up 35,000 feet of lumber from the sawmill for the new hotel in Hazelton.

PAGE 53 ... "This Indian village": William Pierce, *Missionary Outlook*, Vol. XIX, No. 9, September 1900, p. 202.

PAGE 53 ... "congratulating herself": H.C. Wrinch, *Albert College Times*, Vol. XIII, No. 1, November 1900, p. 9.

PAGE 53 ... "My travelling company consisted of a guide": *Albert College Times*, Vol. XIII, No. 1, November 1900, p. 8.

PAGE 56 ... "He treated us like people": *Interior News*, Smithers, BC, December 13, 1951, p. 5.

PAGE 57 ... "much more could be accomplished": W.H. Pierce and H.C. Wrinch, Report, *Missionary Outlook*, February 1901, Vol. 20, No. 2, p. 34.

PAGE 57 ... "To give my present geographical position": H.C. Wrinch, Letter, *Missionary Outlook*, Vol. 19, No. 12, December 1900, p. 274.

PAGE 58 ... In August 2017, Robert Wilson's grandson, Clifford Wilson, showed Horace's granddaughter, Alice Wrinch, where the site of the village at Kispiox had been on the banks of the Skeena before the floods in 1936 led to moving the village to higher and safer ground.

PAGE 58 ... "Thus far we have not supplied": Dr. Sutherland, Letter to H.C. Wrinch, August 15, 1900. UCCA (Toronto). Correspondence of Alexander Sutherland Fonds. Fonds 14, Series 2, Subseries 2, AC 78.083C, Box 14. (Letterbooks, Dr. Sutherland.)

PAGE 59 ... "Our Christmas passed off very well": Rev. W.H. Pierce, *Western Methodist Recorder*, Vol. 11, No. 9, January 5, 1901, p. 12. *Missionary Outlook*, XX, No. 1, April 1901, p. 78.

PAGE 59 ... "The girls she taught various kinds of needlework": W. Pierce, *From Potlatch to Pulpit*, p. 74.

PAGE 59 ... "Dr. W. came down over the trail": *Western Methodist Recorder*, Vol. 2, No. 10, April 1901 p. 4.

PAGE 60 ... "successfully passed the examination": H.C. Wrinch, *Missionary Outlook*, May 1901.

PAGE 60 ... "They are each made out of one log": H.C. Wrinch, Report, *Missionary Outlook*, Vol. 20, No. 7, July 1901, p. 136.

PAGE 61 ... "during the spare moments from his arduous duties": Annual Report of the Department of Indian Affairs for the year ended on June 30, 1902. Library and Archives Canada, p. 209.

PAGE 61 ... "In winter, when the rivers are frozen": H.C. Wrinch, Letter, *Missionary Outlook*, Vol. 20, No. 7, July 1901, p. 136.

PAGE 61 ... "Weather conditions were not always favourable": W. Pierce, *From Potlatch to Pulpit*, p. 74.

PAGE 61 ... "We were fortunate in having with us": Dr. A.E. Bolton, Letter of November 11, 1901, published in the *Missionary Outlook*, January 1902, p. 6.

PAGE 62 ... "rather larger than a goose egg": H.C. Wrinch and Dr. Bolton, "Two Cases of Extra-Uterine Gestation, Operation, Recovery." *Canada Lancet*, Vol. 35, No 3, November 1901, p. 139.

PAGE 62 ... "the second operation of the kind": Arthur Barmer, *Surgeon of the Skeena*, Hazelton, BC: Committee on Missionary Education, Woman's Missionary Society and the United Church of Canada, undated, p. 9.

PAGE 62 ... "The smallpox outbreak at Port Essington": H.C. Wrinch, Letter, *Missionary Outlook*, September 1902, p. 199.

PAGE 62 ... "After the fishing is done": W.H. Pierce, Letter to Dr. Sutherland, June 18, 1901. UCCA (Toronto). Correspondence of Alexander Sutherland Fonds. Fond 14, Series 2, Subseries 2, AC 78.083C, Box 14. (Letterbooks, Dr. Sutherland.)

PAGE 63 ... "I was very much pleased to hear": Dr. Sutherland, Letter of November 29, 1901, to H.C. Wrinch. UCCA (Toronto).

PAGE 63 ... "Admittedly, medical work loses much of its efficiency": UCCA (Vancouver) Methodist Missionary Society Reports. Microfilm reel No. 7. H.C. Wrinch, Annual Report to the Methodist Board, 1900–1901, p. xxxviii.

PAGE 64 ... "the acquisition of a doctor": Richard Ernest Loring, Monthly Report to A.W. Vowell, September 29, 1900. Library and Archives Canada, Microfilm reel, Babine Agency, C-14856, Image 832.

PAGE 64 ... "services are invaluable": R.E. Loring, Letter to A.W. Vowell of July 3, 1902. Library and Archives Canada, Microfilm reel, Babine Agency, C-14856, Image 1198.

PAGE 65 ... Constance Cox (Hankin) (1880–1949) described assisting Horace in his operation, and his methods and procedures, in an interview conducted on March 29, 1940. UCCA (Vancouver). Archives Reference Collection, Box 2147, Prince Rupert Presbytery–Hazelton (2).

PAGE 65 ... "A human life is placed in our hands": Constance Cox, quoted in Arthur Barmer, *Surgeon of the Skeena*, p. 22.

PAGE 65 ... "In conclusion, I here must not omit": R.E. Loring, Letter, October 26, 1901. Library and Archives Canada, Microfilm reel, Babine Agency, C-14857, Image 30.

PAGE 65 ... "Dr. Wrinch himself really did most of the nursing": Constance Cox, interview conducted on March 29, 1940. UCCA (Vancouver). Archives Reference Collection, Box 2147, Prince Rupert Presbytery–Hazelton (2).

PAGE 65 ... "bringing herself down before him": Constance Cox, interview conducted on March 29, 1940. UCCA (Vancouver). Archives Reference Collection. Box 2147, Prince Rupert Presbytery–Hazelton (2).

PAGE 65 ... "He had just a door with two trestles": Constance Cox, Aural Interview. BC Archives, Item AAAB0360, Component T 0313:0002.

PAGE 66 ... "The doctor was a wonderful carpenter": Constance Cox, interview conducted on March 29, 1940. UCCA (Vancouver). Box 2147, Prince Rupert Presbytery–Hazelton (2).

PAGE 66 ... "Dr. Wrinch was sent out as a medical missionary": Dr. Sutherland, Letter of January 31, 1902, to Rev. R. Whittington. UCCA (Toronto). Correspondence of Alexander Sutherland Fonds. Fond 14, Series 2, Subseries 2, AC 78.083C, Box 14. (Letterbooks, Dr. Sutherland).

PAGE 66 ... "On the Skeena you and Dr. Wrinch will require the wisdom of the serpent": Dr. Sutherland, Letter of January 31, 1902, to Rev. R. Whittington. UCCA (Toronto). Correspondence of Alexander Sutherland Fonds. Fond 14, Series 2, Subseries 2, 78.083C, Box 14. (Letterbooks, Dr. Sutherland.) The original source for this quotation is St. Matthew, 10.16 (*King James Bible*): "Be ye therefore wise as serpents and harmless as doves." Mark Twain obviously used it before 1902, but the earliest reference I can find is in a 1906 letter in which Twain states, "Be wise as a serpent and wary as a dove."

PAGE 66 ... "Incidentally, I learned that it had been decreed": R.E. Loring, Letter to Dr. Bolton dated July 21, 1900. Library and Archives Canada, Microfilm reel, Babine Agency, C-14856, Image 743.

PAGE 67 ... "It has been fully deliberated": R.E. Loring, Monthly Report to A.M. Vowell, September 29, 1900. Library and Archives Canada, Microfilm reel, Babine Agency, C-14856, Image 832.

PAGE 67 ... "bright, capable": A description of Richard Sargent in his personnel file with Hudson's Bay Company Archives at the Manitoba Archives.

PAGE 68 ... The Loring–Sargent feud is well-documented. For example, Sargent wrote to the attorney general on January 19, 1900, complaining about Loring ("Loring's high-handed and over-ruling ways of doing things") that followed a petition of his friends sent in an attempt to forestall a petition by Loring's friends. Continuing the feud, Loring wrote to the attorney general on February 11, 1902 ("though opposed at every possible opportunity by Mr. R.S. Sargent"), asking that he be replaced as a magistrate. BC Archives, Attorney General's Files, Incoming Correspondence, GR-0429, Box 3, Files 4 & 5, Reel BO9320.

PAGE 68 ... "not on speaking terms": R.E. Loring, Letter of April 18, 1901 to the Deputy Commissioner of Lands and Works, Victoria, BC. Library and Archives Canada, Microfilm reel, Babine Agency, C-14856, Image 897.

PAGE 68 ... Loring correspondence: Letters to A.W. Vowell, November 14 & 15, 1902, and January 21, 1903. Department's letters of March 9, 1903, and cheque of July 18, 1904. Library and Archives Canada, Microfilm reel, Babine Agency, C-14857, Image 959.

PAGE 69 ... "in a splendid locality on the Two Mile Creek": R.E. Loring, Letter to A.M. Vowell, December 12, 1901. Library and Archives Canada, Babine Agency, Microfilm reel, C-14856, Image 1038.

PAGE 70 ... "Respecting a permanent location": Dr. Sutherland, Letter to H.C. Wrinch, 22 March 1901. UCCA (Toronto). Correspondence of Alexander Sutherland Fonds. Fonds 14, Series 2, Subseries 2, AC 78.083C, Box 14. (Letterbooks, Dr. Sutherland.)

PAGE 70 ... "The first important question confronting us": H.C. Wrinch, *History of Hazelton Hospital*, p. 6. Unpublished document in the author's possession. The original is in UCCA, Archives Reference Collection, (Vancouver) Hazelton Hospital File, Box 2118.

PAGE 71 ... "The growing white population": H.C. Wrinch, Report, *Missionary Outlook*, September 1902, p. 199.

Chapter 4: Building Home and Hospital

PAGE 72 ... The description of Hazelton was set out in a letter by H.C. Wrinch. "Our surroundings now are somewhat different": H.C. Wrinch, Letter of October 5, 1902, *Missionary Bulletin*, Vol. 1, 1903–4, p. 101.

PAGE 72 ... For the inhabitants of Hazelton in 1903 see *Henderson's BC Gazetteer and Directory*. Victoria, BC: Henderson Publishing Company, 1903.

PAGE 74 ... The provincial government appointed Horace the Resident Physician for Hazelton, *BC Gazette*, April 2, 1903, p. 640 and on January 1, 1903, a Justice of the Peace, *BC Gazette*, March 19, 1903, p. 508.

PAGE 77 ... "going over as carefully": Dr. A. Sutherland, Letter of July 28, 1902, to Rev. Whittington. UCCA (Toronto). Correspondence of Alexander Sutherland. Fonds 14, Series 2, Subseries 2, AC 78.083C, Box 14. (Letterbooks, Dr. Sutherland.)

PAGE 77 ... "Among the guests at the Angel hotel": *Daily Colonist*, April 17, 1902, p. 5.

PAGE 78 ... "We confidently hope": H.C. Wrinch, Report, *Missionary Outlook*, September 1903, p. 204.

PAGE 79 ... "the Department may consider": Library and Archives Canada. Department of Indian Affairs, Letter to H.C. Wrinch of January 15, 1903, Microfilm reel C-8568, Image 168.

PAGE 79 ... "We have medical men in different parts": Prime Minister Wilfrid Laurier, House of Commons, Debate on the Estimates, October 12, 1903, p. 13785.

PAGE 79 ... "To me it seems hardly possible": Anne Sherwood, Letter of January 19, 1903, *Missionary Outlook*, April 1903, pp. 94–95.

PAGE 80 ... "whenever it is possible": Anne Sherwood, pp. 94–95.

PAGE 80 ... "You took your life in your hands": Helen Dean, Aural Interview. BC Archives, Item AAAB0096, Component T0093:0001.

PAGE 81 ... "You will be glad to learn that the building": Miss Sherwood, Letter to Mrs. Strachan, *Missionary Outlook*, September 1903, p. 214.

PAGE 82 ... "He then built the house": Herman J. Ferrier, Report on Hazelton Hospital, circa 1919–1920. UCCA (Toronto). Board of Home Missions Fonds, Series 2, Subseries 2, AC 83-050C, File 128-1. British Columbia Conference, Prince Rupert Presbytery, Box 128.

PAGE 82 ... "I can imagine that": Harold Wrinch, Recollections in author's possession. See also an aural interview in the BC Archives, Item AAAB2943, Component T 2693:0001.

PAGE 82 ... "As soon as we found": H.C. Wrinch, Letter of September 17, 1903, *Missionary Bulletin*, Vol. 3, 1903–4, p. 284.

PAGE 83 ... The patients Horace and Alice Wrinch took into their own home before the hospital was built are listed in the Hazelton Hospital Register. UCCA (Vancouver). Wrinch Memorial Hospital Fonds, Box 2393, File 19; *Missionary Outlook*, May, 1904, p. 99.

PAGE 83 ... "I cannot tell [you] what a help Dr. Wrinch": Anne Sherwood, undated letter but probably written in February or March, 1904, *Missionary Outlook*, July 6, 1904, p. 166.

PAGE 83 ... "She is now sitting up": H.C. Wrinch, Letter of January 26, 1904, *Missionary Outlook*, Vol. 4, 1904, p. 433.

PAGE 84 ... "We were able to remove": H.C. Wrinch, Letter of January 26, 1904, *Missionary Bulletin*, Vol. 4, 1904, p. 433.

PAGE 85 ... "We were sent for in haste": H.C. Wrinch, Letter of May 7, 1904, *Missionary Bulletin*, 1904, pp. 187 & 190.

PAGE 86 ... "The undertaking is being pushed": Library and Archives Canada, Annual Report of the Department of Indian Affairs for the year ended June 30, 1903.

PAGE 86 ... "Thus far the work has been accomplished": H.C. Wrinch, quoted in a Report, *Missionary Outlook*, May 1904, p. 98.

PAGE 86 ... "Your report of progress": Dr. Sutherland, Letter to H.C. Wrinch of February 26, 1904. UCCA (Toronto). Correspondence of Alexander Sutherland Fonds. Fonds 14, Series 2, Subseries 2, AC 78.083C, Box 14. (Letterbooks, Dr. Sutherland.)

PAGE 86 ... "It will cost considerably more": H.C. Wrinch, Letter, *Missionary Bulletin*, May 7, 1904, p. 192.

PAGE 87 ... "When first planning for the building": H.C. Wrinch, Letter, *Missionary Outlook*, July 14, 1904, p. 285.

PAGE 87 ... "At present": Anne Sherwood, Letter, *Missionary Outlook*, October 1904, p. 239.

PAGE 88 ... The first patient in the new hospital was Robert Tomlinson: Hazelton Hospital Register, 1903–1919. UCCA (Vancouver). Wrinch Memorial Hospital Fonds, Box 2393, File 19.

PAGE 88 ... "very pleased. It would be difficult": Rev R. Whittington, *Western Methodist Recorder*, Vol. 6, No. 4, November 1904, p. 1.

PAGE 89 ... "absolutely prohibited": H.C. Wrinch, Rules of the Hospital, in a letter to Dr. T. Egerton Shore, June 29, 1910. UCCA (Toronto). Correspondence of the General Secretaries 1868–1923. Fonds 14, Series 2, File 5. Correspondence with T.E. Egerton Shore, 1907–1912, File 118. Indian Missions: British Columbia, re Hazelton Mission, 1, 1907–1910.

PAGE 89 ... "there ought to be no more drumming": H.C. Wrinch, Letter, *Missionary Outlook*, July 14, 1904, p. 291.

PAGE 89 ... "Father always seemed to find out": Harold Wrinch, Recollections, based on family conversations and his written notes and in part from an aural interview in the BC Archives, Item AAAB2943, Component T 2693:0001.

PAGE 89 ... This was probably the first telephone in Hazelton. The first telephones in British Columbia were installed in Victoria as early as 1878. A telephone exchange — Victoria and Esquimalt Telephone Directory for 1881 ("profanity and vulgarity over the wires is prohibited") — was set up in 1880. The first telephone on the mainland of the province seems to have been set up by the missionary William Duncan in 1881. See John Arctander, *The Apostle of Alaska: The Story of William Duncan, of Metlakahtla*. New York: Fleming H. Revell Co., c. 1909, p. 196. When Dr. Wrinch built the Hazelton hospital, he installed a telephone that ran from the hospital to the offices of Edward Hicks Beach, the magistrate and coroner. There had been a donation of $26 for this installation when the hospital was being built. Since Hazelton did not have electricity at the time, it appears that the power must have been generated locally and the line was a one-to-one line. That telephones were coming to Hazelton soon was clear. The *Herald* records in July 1910 that a telephone system was being put in between Hazelton and the Foley, Welch & Stewart construction camp (*Omineca Herald*, October 21, 1911). And in December 1912 a public telephone service was being advertised connecting Hazelton, New Hazelton and Sealey (*Omineca Herald*, December 6, 1912).

PAGE 90 ... "particularly fond of music": Alice Wrinch, Letter, *Missionary Outlook*, June 1905, p. 142.

PAGE 91 ... "Last summer in our new garden": H.C. Wrinch, Letter, *Missionary Bulletin*, April 11, 1905, p. 832.

PAGE 92 ... "The whole-souled energy which these young ladies": Hospital Annual Report, 1907–1908, p. 2. From the author's collection. A selection of these annual reports is also held by each of the BC Archives, UCCA (Toronto) and UCCA (Vancouver).

PAGE 92 ... "Nursing is an art, the importance": Clara Weeks-Shaw, *A Text-Book of Nursing*. Third edition. New York: D. Appleton & Company, 1905, p. 122.

PAGE 93 ... The information on nurses comes from the Hazelton Hospital Training School Register. UCCA (Vancouver). Wrinch Memorial Hospital Fonds, Series Administrative Records, Box 2391, File 6.

PAGE 93 ... "wooden building, prettily painted": *Canadian Nurse*, Vol. 3, March 1907, p. 122.

PAGE 93 ... Health Insurance in Germany: John Mitchell, "How the German Government Insures the Workingman." *Daily Colonist*, October 9, 1904, p. 10.

PAGE 94 ... "Hazelton is today probably": *Daily Colonist*, November 19, 1911, Sunday Magazine Section, p. 25. It reported that between them Charley Barrett and Cataline owned 300 horses and 100 mules.

PAGE 95 ... "He could speak three languages": A.C. Milliken, *Canadian West Magazine*, Vol. 6, No. 4, 1990, p. 142.

PAGE 96 ... "a little insida, a little outsida": Sperry Cline, "Cataline," pp. 96–103 (at p. 101) in Art Downs, editor, *Pioneer Days in British Columbia*. Vol. 1, 1973.

PAGE 96 ... "He was ... the best packer": Sperry Cline, p. 98. In 1866, Cataline hired Joseph Guichon as a packer. Guichon, who had himself left France in 1866, was soon managing one of Cataline's pack trains and stayed with him for two years before branching out as a rancher and family patriarch. In 2012, Judith Guichon, a descendant, was appointed the 29th Lieutenant Governor of British Columbia.

PAGE 97 ... "To occupy a field of any considerable": Dr. A. Sutherland, Letter to H.C. Wrinch of March 22, 1901. UCCA (Toronto). Correspondence of Alexander Sutherland, Fonds 14, Series 2, Subseries 2. AC 78.083C, Box 14. (Letterbooks, Dr. Sutherland.)

PAGE 97 ... "The loose lives of many of the white people": H.C. Wrinch, Letter, October 5, 1902, *Missionary Outlook*, Vol. 1, No. 1. March, 1903, p. 276.

PAGE 98 ... "The splendid hospital, lately constructed": *Daily Colonist*, August 18, 1905, p. 2.

PAGE 98 ... "It is hard to contemplate": Order-in-Council, 1906-0770, RG2, Privy Council Office, May 10, 1906. Library and Archives Canada. RG2, Privy Council Office, Series A-1-a. For Order-in-Council, see Vol. 908, Access Code 90.

Chapter 5: New York Interlude

PAGE 99 ... "Our staff has been recently reinforced": H.C. Wrinch, Letter, July 20, 1905, *Missionary Bulletin*, p. 69.

PAGE 100 ... Alice was seriously ill: *Annual Report of the Methodist Missions Board*. UCCA (Vancouver). Methodist Missionary Society Reports, 1905–1906, Microfilm reel No. 9, p. lvii.

PAGE 100 ... "Dr. F.C. Wrench": *Vancouver Daily Province*, October 11, 1905, p. 10.

PAGE 101 ... "For some little time Mrs. Wrinch": H.C. Wrinch, Letter, October 23, 1905, *Missionary Bulletin*, p. 70.

PAGE 101 ... "to show people here he does not": *The Globe*, October 27, 1905, p. 6.

PAGE 102 ... "when I considered that he engineered": Dr. Rolls, Letter of November 2, 1905, *Missionary Outlook*, February 1906, p. 30.

PAGE 102 ... "who are in the thin red line": *Canadian Statesman*, Bowmanville, Ontario, January 31, 1906, p. 4.

PAGE 103 ... "Throughout the world, ... this is the pioneer": New York Post-Graduate Medical School and Hospital, Twenty-Fifth Annual Announcement, 1906–7, p. 4.

PAGE 104 ... "What I have paid for": H.C. Wrinch, Letter dated February 13, 1906. Original in possession of the author.

PAGE 104 ... "You can see how a simple analysis": H.C. Wrinch, Letter dated February 11, 1906. Original in possession of the author.

PAGE 104 ... "I am getting down to steady work": H.C. Wrinch, Letter dated February 17, 1906. Original in possession of the author.

PAGE 106 ... "The swellest since I have been": H.C. Wrinch, Letter dated February 18, 1906. Original in possession of the author.

PAGE 106 ... New York Entertainment. The references to entertainment available to Horace in New York are all taken from the *New York Times* for the second week of March 1906.

PAGE 107 ... "You are indeed putting me in the shade": H.C. Wrinch, Letter dated March 3, 1906. Original in possession of the author.

PAGE 107 ... Letters of February 25 and March 9, 1906, are in the author's possession.

PAGE 108 ... "Then I took a walk": H.C. Wrinch, Letter dated February 18, 1906. Original in possession of the author.

PAGE 108 ... "And the following week": H.C. Wrinch, Letter dated February 13, 1906. Original in possession of the author.

PAGE 109 ... "I want as far as is possible to consult": H.C. Wrinch, Letter dated March 9, 1906. Original in possession of the author.

PAGE 109 ... Horace described his journey home: H.C. Wrinch, Letter of September 16, 1906, *Missionary Bulletin*, p. 813. Although this letter was written in September, they travelled back home in the first week of May 1906. See also *Annual Report of the Methodist Missions Board*. UCCA (Vancouver). Methodist Missionary Society Reports, 1905–1906, Microfilm reel No. 9, p. lvii.

PAGE 109 ... "ordained for special purposes": *Western Methodist Recorder*, Vol. 7, No. 12, June 1906, p. 1.

PAGE 109 ... "Mrs. Wrinch is still under instruction": H.C. Wrinch, Annual Report of the Methodist Missions Board. UCCA (Vancouver). Methodist Missionary Society Reports. 1905–1906, Microfilm reel No. 9, p. lvii.

PAGE 109 ... "has within the last few weeks": H.C. Wrinch, Letter to Dr. Sutherland, July 20, 1906. UCCA (Toronto). Correspondence of General Secretaries (1868–1923). Fonds 14, Series 2, Subseries 2, File 2, Correspondence of Alexander Sutherland 1875–1910.

PAGE 110 ... "And usually the little boys": Flora Martin, Aural Interview. BC Archives, Item AAAB1349, Component T 1220:0001.

PAGE 110 ... "Even the dogs got excited": Wiggs O'Neil, "Dog Days in Hazelton," in Art Downs, editor, *Pioneer Days in British Columbia*, Vol. 2, 1975, p. 90.

PAGE 110 ... The story of the journey of George MacKenzie is related in the *Vancouver Daily Province*, May 8, 1906, p. 5. His epic story is one of bad luck, of the humanity of a passing First Nations trapper to someone suffering from scurvy and of a terrible journey through the mountains to the Hazelton Hospital, where, after losing a few of his toes, he was treated and released at the end of May.

Chapter 6: Murder, Missionaries and Medicine

PAGE 112 ... "At about 9 o'clock in the morning": H.C. Wrinch, Testimony, BC Archives, Attorney General's Papers Re Gun-an-Noot, GR-0419, 102/1919 and MS-0618.

PAGE 113 ... "The ground floor was topsy-turvy": James Kirby, Testimony, BC Archives, MS-1572, Attorney General's Papers Re Gun-an-Noot, GR-0419, 102/1919 and MS-0618.

PAGE 114 ... "disreputable caravanserai": David Ricardo Williams, *Trapline Outlaw*. Victoria, BC: Sono Nis Press, 1982, p. 35. This is the most reliable account of the Gunanoot affair. Williams was a lawyer who reviewed the evidence carefully. I have also relied on the testimony in the British Columbia Archives taken at the time of the murder and the testimony at the trial, including Gunanoot's defense lawyer's papers. Neil Sterritt's book, *Mapping My Way Home: A Gitxsan History*, Smithers, BC: Creekstone Press, 2016, also contains useful information. There have also been many other accounts of the Gunanoot affair.

PAGE 116 ... "Life was extinct": H.C. Wrinch, Testimony, BC Archives, MS-1572, Attorney General's Papers Re Gun-an-Noot, GR-0419, 102/1919 and MS-0618.

PAGE 118 ... "Peter and Simon Believed to Have Perished": *Port Essington Sun*, May 18, 1907; also *Daily Colonist*, May 18, 1907, p. 8.

PAGE 119 ... The story of Gunanoot's visit to Rev. Lee and Dr. Wrinch's involvement is set out in a letter in the *Daily Colonist* of February 27, 1945, p. 4.

PAGE 120 ... The story of Gunanoot slipping into Hazelton to watch movies is related by David Ricardo Williams in *Trapline Outlaw*, p. 142.

PAGE 121 ... The story of the fumigation of the steamer *Hazelton* was related in R.E. Loring's letter of October 19, 1907. Library and Archives Canada, Microfilm reel C-14856, Image 1937.

PAGE 121 ... "We now have 'almost' modern": Hospital Annual Report, 1906–1907, p. 1. From the author's collection. A selection of these annual reports is held by each of the BC Archives (GR-1549), UCCA (Toronto) and UCCA (Vancouver).

PAGE 121 ... "It is next to impossible": H.C. Wrinch, Letter, *Missionary Outlook*, March 22, 1907, p. 219.

PAGE 122 ... "Fortunately, the steamer *Mount Royal*": *Daily Colonist*, August 10, 1906, p. 5.

PAGE 122 ... "An accident happens": H.C. Wrinch, Letter, September 16, 1909, *Missionary Bulletin*, 1909, p. 355.

PAGE 123 ... "He'll get up some day soon": H.C. Wrinch, quoted in the *Daily Colonist*, May 18, 1907, p. 8. Michell's name is listed in the Hospital Register. UCCA (Vancouver). Wrinch Memorial Hospital Fonds, Box 2391, File 19, Patient Register 1904–1918.

PAGE 123 ... "A very severe injury, almost resulting in death": *Daily Colonist*, May 18, 1907, p. 8.

PAGE 123 ... "an emergency call for a hundred mile journey": H.C. Wrinch, Letter dated July 25, 1907, *Missionary Bulletin*, p. 541.

PAGE 124 ... "an urgent call came for me to attend": H.C. Wrinch, Letter dated September 16, 1909, *Missionary Bulletin*, p. 356.

PAGE 125 ... "The response to our appeal": H.C. Wrinch, Letter dated March 22, 1907, *Missionary Outlook*, p. 220.

PAGE 126 ... "stranded on a gravel bar": H.C. Wrinch, Letter reported in the *Missionary Outlook*, November 1907, p. 246.

PAGE 127 ... "Famine prices prevail in Hazelton": *Daily Colonist*, October 2, 1907, p. 5.

PAGE 127 ... "was a very good horticulturalist": Harold Wrinch, Recollections. Based on family conversations and his written notes, and in part from an aural interview in the BC Archives, Item AAAB2943, Component T 2693:0001. See Appendix 2.

PAGE 128 ... "a record yield of wheat": *Vancouver Daily World*, November 29, 1907, p. 21

PAGE 128 ... "The head officer is Dr. Wrinch": *Daily Colonist*, August 8, 1907, p. 8.

PAGE 129 ... "My own opinion, . . . if I may express it": H.C. Wrinch, Letter to Rev. A.C. Farrell at the Missions Board, February 3, 1912. UCCA (Toronto). Correspondence of the General Secretaries, 1868–1923. Fonds 14, Series 2, File 6. Correspondence with Allan C. Farrell, 1910–1912.

PAGE 129 ... "There were a certain number": *Vancouver Daily Province*, October 11, 1905, p. 10.

PAGE 129 ... "I think he adapted": Harold Wrinch, in conversation with Grant Edwards, 1996. In the author's possession.

PAGE 130 ... "The special grievance at present": H.C. Wrinch, Letter dated September 16, 1906, *Missionary Bulletin*, 1906, p. 815.

PAGE 132 ... "Reflecting beliefs about the harmonious interaction": L.M. Johnson Gottesfeld and B. Anderson, "Gitksan Traditional Medicine: Herbs and Healing." *Journal of Ethnobiology*, Vol. 8, No. 1, Summer 1988, p. 15.

PAGE 133 ... "As long as any tribe remains in heathenism": A.E. Bolton, *Medical Work Among the Indians*. Women's Missionary Society of the Methodist Church, 1896, p. 2. Also see *Missionary Outlook*, September 1900, p. 202. (These texts are not exactly the same)

PAGE 134 ... "Just before administering the anesthetic": H.C. Wrinch, Letter dated September 17, 1903, *Missionary Bulletin*, Vol 3, 1903–1904, p. 285.

PAGE 134 ... "At the root of the high rate of mortality": H.C. Wrinch, Letter, *Missionary Bulletin*, March 22, 1907, p. 215.

PAGE 135 ... "Indian Proves His Magic": *Daily Colonist*, August 2, 1931, Supplement, p. 2.

PAGE 135 ... "Medicine men drummed": Harold Wrinch, Recollections, based on family conversations and his written notes, and in part from an aural interview in the BC Archives, Item AAAB2943, Component T 2693:0001.

PAGE 136 ... "Our work is settling down": H.C. Wrinch, Letter, March 22, 1907, *Missionary Bulletin*, p. 217. The competition was real. Horace and the halayts did compete to heal the bodies and souls of patients. Horace rejoiced when he was successful and Gitxsan converted or came to him for medical help. However, he was nothing if not practical. There is an unverified story that when Horace was stumped by an ailment of a First Nations patient he would consult with First Nations healers. In her excellent and nuanced 2018 study of the convergence of First Nations medical practices and the modern medical practices of the Methodist medical missions on the coast, Alice Huang notes numerous instances where First Nations adopted modern medicine into their culture alongside their own traditional practices. She also noted instances where Drs. Spencer and Large of those missions stood back and did not interfere in the application of First Nations medicine. It seems probable that this practical accommodation to the realities of co-existence would have appealed to Horace.

PAGE 136 ... Joe Coyle's main claim to fame was as the inventor of the egg carton. He died in 1972, at age 100.

PAGE 137 ... "A hospital ticket . . . is a form of insurance": *Omineca Herald*, October 31, 1908.

PAGE 137 ... "When you carry a hospital ticket": *Omineca Herald*, February 6, 1935.

PAGE 138 ... "nearly all those having business in the wilds": *Daily Colonist*, August 8, 1907, p. 8.

PAGE 140 ... For an informative article on the history of Friendly Societies see the article by Lynne Bowen, "Friendly Societies in Nanaimo," *BC Studies*, No. 118, Summer 1998, pp. 67–92.

PAGE 140 ... The ticket scheme at the Kootenay Lake General Hospital is mentioned by A.S. Monro, "The Medical History of British Columbia," *Canadian Medical Association Journal*, Vol. 26, No. 6, June 1932, p. 725. This is also discussing the contracts between companies and doctors: employees had a dollar (or some such sum) deducted from their wages and doctors were placed on a retainer. The reference to the scheme at Fort Steele is mentioned in the *Fort Steele Prospector* of January 14, 1899. The reference to the scheme at Atlin is mentioned in the *Atlin Claim* of December 9, 1905.

PAGE 140 ... The use of hospital tickets by hospitals in British Columbia at the beginning of the twentieth century was not uncommon. When St. Paul's Hospital opened in Vancouver in 1894, "its sisters were well-known visitors in the logging and mining camps of the Coast and the men working in these places used to buy hospital tickets for ten dollars a year, which entitled them to care when they were sick" (*The Bulletin of the Vancouver Medical Society*, Vol. 20, No. 8, May 1944, p. 201). Other examples include Sandon, with Dr. J.E. Browse at the Slocan Hospital (*The Paystreak*, September 17, 1898, p. 3.); Greenwood, with Dr. Jakes at $2 a month (*Boundary Creek Times*, April 23, 1898); Rossland (*Industrial World*, August 11, 1900); Ferguson, at a proposed hospital (*Lardeau Eagle*, January

25, 1901); Hedley, at a proposed hospital (*Hedley Gazette*, February 23, 1905, p. 1.); Revelstoke (*Mail-Herald*, October 19, 1907). In Enderby, "It is proposed to run the hospital on a system similar to those of other small towns in the province, i.e., issue hospital tickets monthly or yearly at $1 or $1.50 per month or $10 or $12 a year, these tickets to entitle the holder to medical and hospital treatment in case of sickness." The proposal went on to recommend that every church set apart a special Sunday service for hospitals. The proposal also recommended putting collection boxes in stores and having fundraising concerts, all of which Horace did at Hazelton (*Walker's Weekly*, December 2, 1908). In Prince Rupert the hospital board wrestled with the issue of whether or not to implement a hospital ticket system in 1911 (*Daily News*, May 11, 1911; *Prince Rupert Journal*, Saturday May 13, 1915).

Chapter 7: Community, Cars and the Coming of the Railroad

PAGE 142 ... The description of Hazelton in 1909 is taken from one of Horace's letters. H.C. Wrinch, Letter dated September 16, 1909, *Missionary Bulletin*, 1909, p. 354.

PAGE 144 ... "a regular taxi service": Frank Chettleburgh, Aural Interview. BC Archives, Item AAAB, Component T 1206:0001.

PAGE 145 ... "The saloons which previously": Pinkerton's Agent No. 28, Report dated September 29, 1909. BC Archives, Attorney General Correspondence, GR-0429, Box 17.

PAGE 145 ... "Everything was paid for in gold dust": Mrs. Vicky Simms, Aural Interview. BC Archives, Item AAAB0355, T 0311:0001.

PAGE 146 ... "Just in small amounts": Mrs. Vicky Simms, Aural Interview.

PAGE 146 ... "performed his duties": *Omineca Herald*, February 12, 1910.

PAGE 148 ... Information about missionary wives: Jan Hare and Jean Barman, *Good Intentions Gone Awry: Emma Crosby and the Methodist Mission on the Northwest Coast*, Vancouver, BC: UBC Press, 2006.

PAGE 148 ... "I know how awfully difficult it is to relax": Mary E. Wrinch, Letter of November 6, 1964, to Horace's daughter, Ralphena Dunlop. In the author's possession.

PAGE 150 ... "It is expected ... that many profitable": *Omineca Herald*, October 21, 1911.

PAGE 150 ... "Taking umbrage at the implication": *Omineca Miner*, December 2, 1911.

PAGE 151 ... "Another cow is needed": H.C. Wrinch, reported in the *Omineca Herald*, January 30, 1909.

PAGE 152 ... "Besides the aspect of simple utility": H.C. Wrinch, Report in the Hazelton Hospital Annual Report for 1908; also noted in the *Omineca Herald*, January 30, 1909.

PAGE 152 ... "Its nearest neighbouring hospitals": *Omineca Herald*, January 1, 1910.

PAGE 153 ... "decided increase in all departments": Hospital Annual Report, 1911, quoted in *Omineca Herald*, January 26, 1912.

PAGE 153 ... "To his skill as a practitioner, Dr. Wrinch": *Omineca Miner*, January 27, 1912.

PAGE 153 ... "One would not expect to find": R.O. Jennings, Letter in *Omineca Herald*, December 18, 1909.

PAGE 154 ... "The quiet, simple life that has": H.C. Wrinch, Letter to Dr. Sutherland, dated April 7, 1910. UCCA (Toronto). Correspondence of the General Secretaries, 1868–1923. Fonds 14, Series 2, File 2, Correspondence of Alexander Sutherland 1900–1910.

PAGE 154 ... "It seems impossible to operate": Hazelton Hospital Annual Report, 1911, p. 11. In the author's collection. A selection of these annual reports is also held by each of the BC Archives, UCCA (Toronto and Vancouver).

PAGE 155 ... "Personally I have no interest (financial)": H.C. Wrinch, Letter to William Manson, February 25, 1911. BC Archives, Hospital Programs Administration Files–Hazelton, GR-1549, Box 3, File 19.

PAGE 155 ... "This . . . has left us nothing": H.C. Wrinch, quoted in *Omineca Herald*, January 26, 1912.

PAGE 156 ... "a point further north": *Daily Colonist*, September 10, 1911, p. 3 of Supplement. The first automobile in Alaska was built there in 1905 by Robert (Bobby) Sheldon who, reportedly, to win a young lady's affections away from a rival who sported a horse and buggy, built an automobile of his own to impress her. He lost the girl, but kept the car.

PAGE 156 ... "bent on securing": P.E. Sands, *First to Hazelton in a Flanders 20: A Story of a Pathfinding Expedition that Made Its Own Path*, p. 1. Compiled by Paul Hale Bruske from the log of the trip by P.E. Sands. Studebaker Corporation, Detroit, Michigan. (Accessible at https://www.yumpu.com/en/document/view/25736682/first-to-hazelton-flanders-20-the-revs-institute.)

PAGE 157 ... "At both places were profitable dispensaries": Brab Hoops, *Blazing the Motor Trail, Bulkley Valley Stories: Collected from Old Timers Who Remember*, Heritage Club Smithers, BC: See-Moore Print: 1973, p. 9; also *Omineca Herald*, June 3, 1911.

PAGE 158 ... "One of the finest roads": P.E. Sands, *First to Hazelton in a Flanders 20*, p. 9.

PAGE 158 ... "The Flanders No. 20 automobile arrived in Hazelton": *Omineca Herald*, October 7, 1911.

PAGE 158 ... "When the muffled beat": P.E. Sands, *First to Hazelton in a Flanders 20*, p. 16.

PAGE 159 ... "I feel sure . . . that Seattle": *Omineca Herald*, October 7, 1911.

PAGE 159 ... "Sands chronicled in his log": P.E. Sands, *First to Hazelton in a Flanders 20*, p. 16.

PAGE 159 ... "Mr. P. Sands and his friends": *Omineca Herald*, October 7, 1911.

PAGE 160 ... Alvin Kingsley relates the story of Bob Montgomery in "First Car to Hazelton: 1911." *Pioneer Days in British Columbia*, Vol. 3, Surrey, BC: Heritage House Publishing, 1977, p. 100 Art Downs, editor.

PAGE 160 ... The only contemporaneous evidence of Sands's confession at this banquet I could find is in the *Fort George Herald* of October 28, 1911, which records that "the fact has just come to light that that auto was dismantled and packed for a distance of about 100 miles between Fraser Lake and the Bulkley Valley." Sadly, it does appear likely that Sands did not comply with the terms of the prize. Eva MacLean repeats the story in her memoir *The Far Land*. Prince George, BC: Caitlin Press, 1993.

PAGE 161 ... "full connexion": UCCA (Vancouver). Minutes of the British Columbia Methodist Conference, 1910, p. 383. Compilation by Rev W.T. Blunt, August 1969.

PAGE 161 ... "A patient in a poor home": H.C. Wrinch, reported in the *Omineca Herald*, December 15, 1911.

PAGE 162 ... "vocal and instrumental music": *Omineca Miner*, August 10, 1912.

PAGE 162 ... Donald and Eva MacLean: Eva MacLean, *The Far Land*. The reference to the Presbyterian Club is from the *Omineca Herald*, July 29, 1911.

PAGE 163 ... "added considerably to the success": *Omineca Herald*, November 1, 1912.

PAGE 165 ... "is not on the railway line": *Omineca Herald*, March 18, 1911.

PAGE 166 ... "In railway construction": H.C. Wrinch, Letter dated June 25, 1908 to Dr. Sutherland. UCCA (Toronto). Sutherland Papers, 1908/1909, 101. Fonds 14, Series 2, File 2, Correspondence of Alexander Sutherland, 1900–1910. British Columbia: Indian Missions Correspondence re Hazelton Hospital.

PAGE 167 ... Mission Point: Since the property was owned by the Methodist Church, Horace would not rent to any establishment that sold liquor or facilitated prostitution. Horace wrote to Dr. Sutherland on September 15, 1909: "Even if we keep the subletting in our own hands, etc, it will be most difficult to select tenants who will all be above reproach. And in accepting some and refusing others, your representatives here will make many enemies." H.C. Wrinch, Letter dated September 15, 1909, to Dr. Sutherland. UCCA (Toronto). Sutherland Papers, 1908/1909, 101. Fonds 14, Series 2, File 2, Correspondence of Alexander Sutherland, 1900–1910. British Columbia: Indian Missions Correspondence re Hazelton Hospital.

PAGE 168 ... "which will be ... better for all concerned": *Omineca Herald*, June 27, 1913.

PAGE 168 ... This first train's journey along the Skeena River is reported in the *Omineca Miner*, June 15, 1912.

PAGE 169 ... "The whistle of the locomotive": *Omineca Miner*, August 17, 1912.

PAGE 170 ... "Last Steamer Has Gone Below": *Omineca Herald*, September 13, 1912.

Chapter 8: Mining, X-rays and Daylight Robbery

PAGE 172 ... The scene at which the prospectors brought the rocks from Owen Lake back into town is reported in the *Omineca Herald*. "The first excitement over a new discovery," *Omineca Herald*, June 14, 1912.

PAGE 173 ... "with their capital and mining experience": *Omineca Herald*, January 2, 1914.

PAGE 174 ... "part and parcel of everything that went to make up Hazelton": *Interior News* (Smithers), October 23, 1939, pp. 1 & 4.

PAGE 174 ... Horace loaned money to Loring, which Loring noted in his letter of January 4, 1904. Library and Archives Canada, Microfilm reel C-14857, Image 122.

PAGE 174 ... "Canada's land of opportunity": *Omineca Herald*, January 1, 1910.

PAGE 175 ... "New Strike at Silver Standard": *Omineca Herald*, March 28, 1913.

PAGE 175 ... "at the most enthusiastic": *Omineca Herald*, September 5, 1913.

PAGE 177 ... "yellow copper is coming in good": *Omineca Herald*, November 8, 1912.

PAGE 177 ... "The Federal Mining and Smelting Group": *Omineca Herald*, October 12, 1923; Annual Report to the Minister of Mines for the Year Ended 31st December 1923." Province of BC, 1924, p. A114.

PAGE 177 ... "The Silver Queen, owned by H.C. Wrinch": Annual Report of the Minister of Mines for the Year Ended 31st December 1927." Province of BC, 1928, p. C139.

PAGE 178 ... "referred to by mine management": Annual Report of the Minister of Mines for the Year Ended 31st December 1929." Province of BC, 1930, p. C173.

PAGE 178 ... "is right in every particular": Advertisement for Harris Mines in the *Omineca Herald*, October 27, 1911.

PAGE 179 ... "One thing is certain": *Omineca Herald*, June 6, 1913.

PAGE 179 ... "The directorate ... are men whose integrity": *Omineca Herald*, May 30, 1913.

PAGE 179 ... "Dr. Wrinch and Vic Procter": *Omineca Herald*, May 9, 1919.

PAGE 181 ... "Records broken at the Hospital": Headline in the *Omineca Herald*, February 27,1914.

PAGE 181 ... *Hazelton Hospital Herald* was reported on in the *Omineca Herald*, March 21, 1913.

PAGE 182 ... "As a result of the experiments Dr. Wrinch": *Omineca Herald*, July 10, 1914.

PAGE 183 ... "Everything to be had in the drug line": Advertisement in the *Omineca Miner*, November 2, 1912.

PAGE 184 ... "The danger of fire": Hospital Annual Report, 1906–1907, p. 1. In the author's collection. A selection of these annual reports is also held by each of the BC Archives, UCCA (Toronto and Vancouver).

PAGE 184 ... "Sir Richard McBride and his distinguished": *Omineca Miner*, July 20, 1912.

PAGE 185 ... Horace did obtain approval to sell part of the land the hospital owned that was surplus to its needs but at that time that did not make financial sense: H.C. Wrinch, Letter to Dr. Endicott, Mission Secretary, Toronto, April 9, 1914. UCCA (Toronto), Methodist Church Missionary Society. J. Endicott and J.H. Arnupp Papers, 1912–1913, 78.095C, Box 1.

PAGE 185 ... "believing you to be a friend": H.C. Wrinch, Letter dated January 30, 1913. BC Archives, GR-1549, Box 3, File 19.

PAGE 186 ... "Dr. Wrinch . . . is confident that the response": *Omineca Miner*, September 13, 1913.

PAGE 186 ... "Dr. Wrinch, who is making a personal canvas": *Omineca Miner*, October 25, 1913.

PAGE 187 ... "Encores were frequent": *Omineca Miner*, November 20, 1913.

PAGE 187 ... "which is less than one-third": H.C. Wrinch, Letter to Dr. Young dated September 30, 1913. BC Archives, Hospital Programs Administration Files–Hazelton, GR-1549, Box 3, File 19.

PAGE 188 ... "Next year, the report will be": *Omineca Herald*, January 30, 1914.

PAGE 190 ... "They came in the private entrance": Robert Bishop, Testimony. BC Archives, GR-2766, Box 13, Files 1–3. Mamukoff, Boris: bank robbery. There have been numerous descriptions of the two bank robberies. My primary sources have been the testimony taken at the time for the trial and the reports in the *Omineca Herald*.

PAGE 190 ... "I just had time to get the gun": R.W. Fenton, Testimony. Proceedings.

PAGE 191 ... "Dan tossed his .44 colt six-shooter": Eva MacLean, *The Far Land*. Prince George, BC: Caitlin Press, 1993, p. 158.

PAGE 191 ... "I saw a man, or just about half of him,": Dr. D.R. MacLean, Testimony.

PAGE 191 ... "We were shooting back and forth": B.A. Smith, Testimony.

PAGE 191 ... "They left the bank": B.T. Bishop, Testimony.

PAGE 192 ... "split and notched": *Omineca Herald*, April 17, 1914.

PAGE 192 ... A curious footnote: The only source for this story is the *Omineca Herald*, April 24, 1914.

PAGE 193 ... Servia: An old name for Serbia and used until about 1916 when it changed to Serbia.

PAGE 193 ... "Great Powers [are] On The Verge of War": *Omineca Miner*, August 1, 1914.

PAGE 194 ... "the most successful affair of the kind": *Omineca Miner*, August 1, 1914.

PAGE 194 ... "New Hazelton captured the banner": *Omineca Herald*, August 7, 1914.

PAGE 194 ... "Dr. Wrinch propelled the laggard": *Omineca Herald*, August 1, 1914.

Chapter 9: The War Years

PAGE 195 ... This story of Horace knitting socks in Old Hazelton is told by Jacqueline Burt in *Dr. Horace Cooper Wrinch: Pioneer British Columbia Physician*. 1966, p. 58. (Unpublished, 65 pages). In author's possession. Copies are available at the Hazelton Library and UCCA (Vancouver), Archives Reference Collection, Box 2093.

PAGE 196 ... "it is now almost universally looked for": *Omineca Herald*, August 14, 1914.

PAGE 196 ... "Kaiser is looking for peace": *Omineca Herald*, September 18, 1914.

PAGE 196 ... "patriotic speeches and songs": *Omineca Miner*, August 8, 1914.

PAGE 196 ... "In case of need, please enroll my name": *Omineca Herald*, August 14, 1914.

PAGE 198 ... "Canucks Made Brilliant Charge": *Omineca Herald*, April 30, 1915.

PAGE 198 ... "Great Slaughter in the West": *Omineca Miner*, September 9, 1916.

PAGE 198 ... "British Troops Again Smash German": *Omineca Miner*, September 16, 1916.

PAGE 201 ... "Hazelton is cheerfully bearing its part": *Omineca Miner*, January 22, 1916.

PAGE 201 ... "continue to a victorious end": *Omineca Miner*, August 11, 1917.

PAGE 202 ... "The service was excellent": *Omineca Miner*, April 6, 1918.

PAGE 202 ... "Dr. Wrinch . . . has joined the ranks": *Omineca Miner*, July 27, 1918.

PAGE 203 ... "had tried to climb the bank": *Omineca Herald*, January 6, 1922.

PAGE 203 ... "He favours speeding up slow drivers": *Omineca Herald*, December 19, 1924.

PAGE 203 ... "What was the most interesting crop": H.C. Wrinch, quoted in *Omineca Herald*, October 23, 1914.

PAGE 204 ... "I can remember my mother": Harold Wrinch, Recollections, based on family conversations and his written notes, and in part from an aural interview. BC Archives, Item AAAB2943, Component T 2693:001

PAGE 204 ... "surprised and gratified": *Omineca Miner*, February 12, 1916.

PAGE 204 ... "It will be impossible for this institution": *Omineca Miner*, January 12, 1918.

PAGE 204 ... "has been done by the use": Hospital Annual Report, 1916, p. 6. In the author's collection. A selection of these annual reports is also held by each of the BC Archives, UCCA (Toronto and Vancouver).

PAGE 205 ... "sincere acknowledgment of the overruling": H.C. Wrinch, Hospital Annual Report, 1914, p. 6. In the author's collection. A selection of these annual reports is also held by each of the BC Archives, UCCA (Toronto and Vancouver).

PAGE 206 ... "He was of course quite religious": Harold Wrinch, Aural Interview. BC Archives, Item AAAB2943, Component T 2693:0001.

PAGE 206 ... "finally, Dr. Wrinch made a proposition": J.H. White, *Western Methodist Recorder*, Vol. 17, No. 1, July 1917, p. 12; *Omineca Miner*, June 30, 1917.

PAGE 207 ... "Nothing finer is being done": J.H. White, p. 12.

PAGE 207 ... "he seemed very proud": Arthur H. Sager, *The Sager Saga: A Family History*. Self-published, 1998, pp. 37–47. (Available at Hazelton Library.) Horace had taken possession of his new car that week. The Sagers were in Hazelton while waiting for a posting as medical missionaries to China. However, in July 1917, after they had received their posting and while waiting in Vancouver for the ship to China, Hettie Sager put her foot down and refused to go. Will Sager therefore decided he could not accept the mission to China. In 1920, he took over as medical superintendent at Port Essington after Richard Large died.

PAGE 208 ... "Dr. Wrinch seemed to know": Arthur H. Sager, p. 40.

PAGE 209 ... "by a man not definitely": H.C. Wrinch, Letter to Dr. White, May 8, 1918. UCCA (Toronto). Board of Home Missions, Box 7, File 229.

PAGE 210 ... This fête was described in the *Omineca Miner*, July 7, 1917.

PAGE 211 ... Wipers, Valcartier, seam squirrels: "Wipers" was soldiers' slang for Ypres. Valcartier was the military training camp in Quebec. "Seam squirrels" were lice. Festubert was the battle on May 15–25, 1915, in which the 1st Canadian Division fought. Peggy was the nickname for Francis Pegahmagabow (1889–1952). A member of the Shawanaga First Nation, he was probably the most effective sniper of the First World War, being credited with killing 378 Germans and capturing 300 more. He was a member of the 1st Canadian Infantry Battalion. The Battle for Vimy Ridge (April 9, 1917 April 12, 1917) was only one part of the Battle of Arras. Hill 70 was a battle fought by the First Canadian Corps from August 15–25, 1917. Mud was a war all of its own, but particularly at the Battle of Passchendaele that was fought in it. A "dream of a blighty" was dreaming of a nice, clean wound that would send a soldier out of the front lines to somewhere green and safe. A "potato masher" was a German grenade. "The YMCA" was the name given to a particular dugout in the trenches. "Rum jars" were German mortar shells. Whale oil was used to deal with trench foot, a condition caused by standing in mud and water. Use of it was usually compulsory. Kinmel Park was a site in North Wales where, on March 4 and 5, 1919, some of the 15,000 Canadian troops waiting to come home mutinied. Five died and twenty were injured. The Pats are Princess Patricia's Canadian Light Infantry.

PAGE 212 ... "We are living on the lid": James Turnbull, Letter quoted in *Omineca Miner*, April 8, 1916.

PAGE 214 ... "The well are helping": *Omineca Herald*, October 26, 1918

PAGE 214 ... "The checking of the disease is credited": *Omineca Herald*, November 15, 1918.

PAGE 215 ... "being mindful of contagion": R.E. Loring, Letter to Indian Affairs Department, Ottawa, dated October 31, 1918. Library and Archives Canada, Film C-14857.

PAGE 215 ... "perfectly immune from the contagion": R.E. Loring, Letter to Indian Affairs Department, Ottawa, dated November 30, 1918. Library and Archives Canada, Film C 14857, Image 739.

PAGE 215 ... Loring's comments on flu and the First Nations: R.E. Loring, Report to Indian Affairs Department, Ottawa. December 26, 1918. Library and Archives Canada, Film C-14857, Image 741.

PAGE 215 ... "was often found asleep": Jessie Gould, 1977, statement in possession of the author. Also, *Omineca Herald*, October 8, 1936.

PAGE 215 ... "Uppermost in the thoughts of many": H.C. Wrinch, Letter, *Missionary Outlook*, April 1919.

PAGE 216 ... "Dr. Wrinch has always been worthy": *Omineca Herald*, November 22, 1918.

PAGE 217 ... "When the news came over the wire": *Omineca Herald*, November 15, 1918.

PAGE 217 ... The gala banquet for the returning soldiers was on Tuesday, July 22, reported in the *Omineca Herald*, July 25, 1919. Andrew Monour's death from his wounds was reported in the *Omineca Herald*, October 29, 1920.

PAGE 218 ... "beautifully decorated with greens and flowers": *Omineca Herald*, September 19, 1919.

PAGE 218 ... "Make the Returning Soldier Welcome": Government Advertisement (Repatriation Committee), *Omineca Herald*, February 21, 1919.

PAGE 219 ... "where Dr. and Mrs. Wrinch and the nurses": *Omineca Herald*, February 14, 1919.

PAGE 219 ... "The object today is to treat the largest number": *Omineca Herald*, February 21, 1919.

PAGE 220 ... "although he is still far": *Omineca Herald*, January 31, 1919.

Chapter 10: Brave New World

PAGE 222 ... "I never saw him ... without a collar": Harold Wrinch, Aural Interview. BC Archives, Item AAAB2943, Component T 2693:0001.

PAGE 222 ... "I am very glad I came to Rochester": *Omineca Herald*, March 21, 1919.

PAGE 222 ... "it being conceded, though": *Omineca Herald*, November 7, 1919.

PAGE 223 ... "very worthy move": *Omineca Herald*, November 7, 1919.

PAGE 224 ... "To Dr. Wrinch is due the credit": *Omineca Herald*, September 26, 1919.

PAGE 224 ... Gitxsan art, tools and cultural symbols: Over thirty-six years, Horace collected many objects of First Nations cultural significance. When he left Hazelton in 1936, he donated these to federal, provincial and municipal governments. He sent approximately 400 pieces to Ottawa, where three or four of them are displayed in the Canadian Museum of Human History, and about fifty to Victoria to the (Royal) British Columbia Museum. He also gave numerous pieces and some of his books to the Prince Rupert Museum. *Omineca Herald*, November 4, 1936. The

Victoria Daily Times, on October 26, 1923, p. 6, called his collection one of the finest private ones in the country.

PAGE 225 ... "Dr. Wrinch is remarkably well balanced": *Omineca Herald*, February 6, 1920.

PAGE 225 ... Telkwa Hospital: When Dr. Wallace moved from Hazelton to Telkwa to open a practice he intended to open a small hospital. It is not clear how far he got. A report in Vancouver newspapers mentions that he was in the process of establishing one, and an advertisement for the townsite suggests one was in existence. In any event, if it was established, it probably burned down in the disastrous fire of April 1914 that destroyed thirteen buildings, including those of Dr. Wallace. He joined the Army Medical Corps in 1915. The *Vancouver Daily Province* of December 16, 1910, reports on the hospital and Wallace being the Medical Superintendent. See also the advertisement for townsite lots in the *Vancouver Daily World*, December 9, 1911. There are also references in the *Omineca Herald*, April 22, 1911, and the *Victoria Daily Times* of September 8, 1910, p. 3.

PAGE 226 ... "This site could hardly be improved": H.C. Wrinch, Letter to the Provincial Secretary, April 9, 1920. BC Archives, GR-1549, Box 17, File 1. Telkwa Hospital. Floor Plans are at Item 15756A, Preliminary Plans, Telkwa Hospital.

PAGE 227 ... "lessening the efficiency of a hospital": *Interior News*, April 21, 1920.

PAGE 227 ... "lots of hospitals": L.B. Warner, Letter to C.G. Wood dated April 21, 1920. BC Archives, GR-1549, Box 17, File 1. Telkwa Hospital.

PAGE 228 ... "less likely to give effective": E.G. Arthur, Letter to Provincial Secretary dated July 2, 1920. BC Archives, GR-1549, Box 17, File 1. Telkwa Hospital

PAGE 228 ... The premier's opening of the Smithers hospital is set out in the *Interior News*, September 1, 1920.

PAGE 228 ... "a most complete and comfortable": *Omineca Herald*, January 30, 1925.

PAGE 230 ... "much relieved and concerned": R.E. Loring, Report to Indian Affairs Department, September 1919. Library and Archives Canada, Film C-14857, Image 789.

PAGE 230 ... "So Simon Gunanoot is dead": *Omineca Herald*, January 31, 1934.

PAGE 231 ... "Practically every person in town": *Omineca Herald*, July 18, 1919.

PAGE 231 ... "Almost nightly the justices of the peace": *Omineca Herald*, February 13, 1920.

PAGE 234 ... "the idea of a National Hospital Day": H.C. Wrinch, "Event Come To Stay," *Hospital Management*, Vol. 14, No. 1, July 1922, p. 40.

PAGE 234 ... "The Hazelton Hospital is regarded as part of the district": *Omineca Herald*, May 19, 1922.

PAGE 236 ... "The 'planes left Prince George": *Omineca Herald*, August 13, 1920.

PAGE 237 ... "Here in the great North a good soldier": *Western Methodist Recorder*, Vol. 18, No. 8, February 1919, p. 11.

PAGE 238 ... "This is the first church we have": J.H. White, *Western Methodist Recorder*, Vol. 22, No. 8, February 1922, p. 10.

PAGE 238 ... "an unobtrusive man, of few words": *Western Methodist Recorder*, Vol. 20, No. 11, May 1921, p. 9.

PAGE 238 ... "Any account of Dr. Wrinch's life-work": *Missionary Outlook*, May 1921, p. 98.

PAGE 240 ... British Columbia Hospital Association. There was another organization with the same name very different from the one set up in 1918. This one was set up in 1910 by a former barber, H.N. Snebber, as an association that offered extensive medical benefits to its members for $1 a month or $1.50 for a family of three. By 1912, it had 12,000 members in Vancouver. It thus had at least some similarities to Horace's ticket scheme at Hazelton Hospital. This organization, though, ran into numerous problems, including actions to close it down by the British Columbia Medical Association, which also stripped its four physicians of their licenses to practice. On appeal, the four physicians were reinstated. Snebber left the organization, which reportedly then changed its name to the Canadian Hospital Association.

PAGE 240 ... Malcolm T. MacEachern came from Argyle, Ontario, and qualified with a medical degree from McGill University. While at Vancouver General Hospital he was instrumental in persuading the authorities to set up a nursing school at the University of British Columbia. In 1923, after his time with VGH, he became director of the American College of Surgeons and had an important role in the administration of hospitals in North America. He left Canada in 1923 to become hospital director for the American Society of Physicians and went on to build for himself the reputation of being the "Founder of Hospital Administration in North America." He was appointed President of the American Hospital Association in 1924.

PAGE 240 ... Jessie MacKenzie (1867–1960), from Toronto, was one of the leading nursing administrators in British Columbia. She became lady superintendent of the Provincial Royal Jubilee Hospital in Victoria in about 1914. She led the drive to reform nursing standards and helped establish the legislative framework for the qualification of nurses.

PAGE 241 ... This evening at Capilano Canyon was recorded in the British Columbia Hospital Association's "Report of Proceedings of the First Annual Convention of the Hospitals of British Columbia," 1918, p. 100. (Accessible at Open Collections, University of British Columbia, Vancouver.)

PAGE 241 ... "spacious auditorium": The *Daily Colonist* used this description on June 27, 1918, p. 2. The auditorium was used by VGH for its annual meetings and was converted into an auxiliary hospital during the 1918 influenza pandemic.

PAGE 242 ... "becomes the function of our government": H.C. Wrinch, quoted in the *Omineca Herald*, August 1, 1919.

PAGE 242 ... "our most valuable national asset": H.C. Wrinch, Hospital Annual Report, 1921, p. 2. In the author's collection. A selection of these annual reports is also held by each of the BC Archives, UCCA (Toronto and Vancouver).

PAGE 243 ... "distressing financial conditions": Minutes of the Emergency Meeting of the B.C. Hospital Association held on February 11, 1921. Correspondence re BC Hospital Association, File 3104, BC Archives, MS-0313.9.1, Vol. 9, Folder 1.

PAGE 244 ... "Your statements with regard to the condition": Premier John Oliver, quoted in the *Vancouver Daily World*, February 12, 1921, p. 1.

PAGE 244 ... "Universal health insurance would": Ernest Hall, quoted in the *Victoria Daily Times*, December 28, 1916, p. 10.

PAGE 245 ... "the nationalization of the medical": Dr. J.W. McIntosh, quoted in the *Daily Colonist*, April 10, 1917, p. 7.

PAGE 245 ... "Many doctors are now ripe and ready": Dr. J.W. McIntosh, quoted in the *Daily Colonist*, April 10, 1917, p. 7. Dr. McIntosh was himself quoting a 1912 statement.

PAGE 246 ... "so far as may be practicable": Quoted in C. David Naylor, *Private Practice, Public Payment: Canadian Medicine and the Politics of Health Insurance, 1911–1966*. Kingston, Ontario: McGill-Queen's University Press, 1986, p. 42

PAGE 246 ... "A beneficent socialism that would": Dr. A.S. Munro, British Columbia Hospital Association. Report of Proceedings of the First Annual Convention of the Hospitals of British Columbia, 1918, p. 13. (Accessible at Open Collections, University of British Columbia, Vancouver.)

PAGE 246 ... "that all should have the inalienable": J.J. Bamfield, British Columbia Hospital Association, Report of Proceedings of the First Annual Convention of the Hospitals of British Columbia, 1918, p. 51. (Accessible at Open Collections, University of British Columbia, Vancouver.)

PAGE 247 ... "I am almost filled too full for utterance": H.C. Wrinch, British Columbia Hospital Association, Report of Proceedings of the Second Annual Convention of the Hospitals of British Columbia, 1919, p. 114. (Accessible at Open Collections, University of British Columbia, Vancouver.)

PAGE 247 ... "We have an assurance": J.W. McIntosh, British Columbia Hospital Association, Report of Proceedings of the Second Annual Convention of the Hospitals of British Columbia, 1919, p. 116.

PAGE 247 ... "Health insurance is an ideal condition": H.C. Wrinch, British Columbia Hospital Association, Report of Proceedings of the Second Annual Convention of the Hospitals of British Columbia, 1919, p. 119.

PAGE 247 ... "I wish to put myself on record": J.W. McIntosh, British Columbia Hospital Association, Report of Proceedings of the Second Annual Convention of the Hospitals of British Columbia. 1919, p. 120.

PAGE 248 ... On Thursday, March 6, 1919. Dr. J.D. MacLean moved the amendment: Journals of the Legislative Assembly of British Columbia. March 6, 1919. (Accessible at http://archives.leg.bc.ca.)

PAGE 248 ... As amended the resolution read: "Resolved That in the opinion of this House the early consideration by the Government of legislation with respect to State Health Insurance, Mothers' Pensions, and the broadening of the Workmen's Compensation is desirable."

PAGE 248 ... "Health begets happiness": Report of the Royal Commission on Health Insurance, March 18, 1921, p. 107. BC Legislative Library.

PAGE 249 ... On November 30, 1922, the Legislature did pass a resolution. Journals of the Legislature of British Columbia, November 1922. (Accessible at http://archives.leg.bc.ca.)

PAGE 249 ... "The tenor of the times had clearly changed": C. David Naylor, *Private Practice, Public Payment: Canadian Medicine and the Politics of Health Insurance, 1911–1966*. Kingston, Ontario: McGill-Queen's University Press, 1986, p. 46.

PAGE 249 ... "which would provide medical and hospital": *Omineca Herald*, December 18, 1925.

PAGE 250 ... "on account of the continued illness": *Omineca Herald*, June 16, 1922.

PAGE 251 ... "A long journey, a serious operation": *Christian Guardian*, Vol. 94, No. 18, May 2, 1923, p. 7.

PAGE 251 ... "The different tribes (six) sent representatives": *Western Methodist Recorder*, Vol. 22, No. 10, April 1923, p. 6.

PAGE 252 ... "The remains were conveyed from the residence": *Omineca Herald*, March 16, 1923.

PAGE 253 ... "Dr. Wrinch, and his family": *Omineca Herald*, March 23, 1923.

PAGE 253 ... "but perhaps a trifle cool for ice-cream": *Omineca Herald*, May 18, 1923.

Chapter 11: Stepping into Politics

PAGE 256 ... "punching a counter": Harold Wrinch, in conversation with Grant Edwards, 1996. In the author's possession.

PAGE 256 ... The Colfax School for the Tuberculous is sometimes referred to, incorrectly, as the Colfax School for Tuberculosis.

PAGE 256 ... "In addition to potatoes": Harold Wrinch, Recollections, based on conversations and his written notes, and in part from an aural interview in the BC Archives Item AAAB2943, Component T 2693:0001.

PAGE 257 ... Harvested seven tons: This amount is substantiated by a report in the *Omineca Herald*, September 25, 1925.

PAGE 257 ... "riot of bloom and colour": *Omineca Herald*, August 29, 1924.

PAGE 257 ... "at one point he was looking for a job": Harold Wrinch, Recollections, based on family conversations and his notes, and in part from an aural interview in the BC Archives, Item AAAB2943, Component T 2693:000.

PAGE 258 ... "R.S. Sargent presented the diploma": *Omineca Herald*, November 14, 1924.

PAGE 258 ... "a charming and hospitable manner": *Omineca Herald*, August 15, 1924.

PAGE 259 ... "I particularly want to meet": Governor General Lord Byng, as reported in the *Omineca Herald*, July 3, 1925.

PAGE 260 ... "Hazelton People to Bask in the Glow": *Omineca Herald*, September 18, 1925.

PAGE 261 ... Horace's nomination was described in the *Omineca Herald*, May 16, 1924.

PAGE 261 ... "The Fraser is fished out": The Assistant Commissioner of Fisheries, quoted in Margaret Ormsby's *British Columbia: A History*. Toronto, Ontario: MacMillan Company of Canada, 1958, p. 406.

PAGE 264 ... "The Liberals of Skeena have": *Omineca Herald*, May 23, 1924.

PAGE 264 ... "if he went to Victoria": *Omineca Herald*, May 30, 1924.

PAGE 264 ... "At every place Dr. Wrinch appears": *Omineca Herald*, June 6, 1924.

PAGE 265 ... "Oliver Government gave" and "Conservative Speakers": *Omineca Herald*, May 30 and June 13, 1924.

PAGE 265 ... "Late Hour Returns Show Liberals": *Omineca Herald*, June 20, 1924.

PAGE 265 ... "the candidates are as good friends today": *Omineca Herald*, June 27, 1924.

PAGE 266 ... The reception in the hospital grounds was described in the *Omineca Herald*, July 25, 1924.

PAGE 266 ... "This has been a wonderful day": William Lyon Mackenzie King, Diary entry for October 12, 1924. Library and Archives Canada. (Accessible at https://www.bac-lac.gc.ca/eng/discover/politics-government/prime-ministers/william-lyon-mackenzie-king/Pages/diaries-william-lyon-mackenzie-king.aspx.)

PAGE 267 ... "Dr. Wrinch told the Premier": *Omineca Herald*, October 17, 1924.

PAGE 267 ... "the Premier's sincerity": *Omineca Herald*, October 24, 1924.

PAGE 269 ... "had left much material for reflection": *Victoria Daily Times*, November 5, 1924.

PAGE 269 ... "The *Herald* liked the speech so much": *Omineca Herald*, November 14 and 21, 1924. The full text is set out in Appendix 1.

PAGE 269 ... "When opportunity came": *Western Recorder*, Vol. 2, No. 4, October 1926, p. 5.

PAGE 270 ... "The discursive debate was continued": *Vancouver Daily Province*, December 5, 1925, p. 6.

PAGE 270 ... "unless the minister of agriculture": *Omineca Herald*, November 20, 1925.

PAGE 272 ... "I have never seen in this House": Captain MacKenzie, *Daily Colonist*, February 25, 1927, p. 12.

PAGE 273 ... "soviet dictatorship under the control": Captain MacKenzie, *Daily Colonist*, February 25, 1927, p. 12. A general reference for this information is a history written by David Dendy, *The British Columbia Fruit Growers' Association 1889–1989*, to mark the occasion of its 100th anniversary. Published by the BC Fruit Growers' Association, 1990.

PAGE 273 ... "University training ... makes a man": H.C. Wrinch, quoted in the *Daily Colonist*, December 5, 1925, p. 20. See also *Omineca Herald*, December 11, 1925.

PAGE 273 ... "He should be invited": H.C. Wrinch, quoted in the *Daily Colonist*, December 5, 1925, p. 7.

PAGE 274 ... "in high spirits over the way": *Omineca Herald*, March 18, 1927.

PAGE 274 ... "For a number of years": Dr. E. H. Young, reported in the *Omineca Herald*, February 22, 1924.

PAGE 274 ... "Dr. Wrinch ... declared": H.C. Wrinch, quoted in the *Daily Colonist*, February 8, 1927, p. 3. See also the *Vancouver Daily Province*, February 28, 1927, p. 22.

PAGE 274 ... Colley and Wrinch's motion is referenced in the Legislative Journal of British Columbia, March 14, 1928. (Accessible at http://archives.leg.bc.ca); *Daily Colonist*, March 15, 1928.

PAGE 276 ... "emphatically that all recent experiments": H.C. Wrinch, quoted in the *Western Recorder*, Vol. 1, No. 3, August 1925, p. 10.

PAGE 276 ... "The only right thing to do": *Western Recorder*, Vol. 2, No. 8, February 1927, p. 8.

PAGE 277 ... "That young feller": Jimmy May, quoted in John Calam, editor. *Alex Lord's British Columbia: Recollections of a Rural School Inspector, 1915–1936*. Vancouver, BC: UBC Press, 1991, pp. 44–45.

PAGE 277 ... "about as low a condition as ever in its history": *Omineca Herald*, January 23, 1925.

PAGE 279 ... "The new residence is a handsome structure": *Omineca Herald*, March 26, 1926.

PAGE 280 ... "The Doctor was sailing serenely": *Omineca Herald*, June 19, 1925.

PAGE 281 ... Placer County Medical Society. California and Western Medicine. *Western Journal of Medicine*, Vol. 25 (2), August 1926, p. 241.

PAGE 282 ... "as per usual": *Omineca Herald*, May 13, 1927.

Chapter 12: Health Insurance Advocate

PAGE 284 ... "Dr. Wrinch would grace any cabinet": Duff Pattullo, in a speech quoted in the *Omineca Herald*, June 20, 1928.

PAGE 285 ... "The Doctor put up a good campaign": *Omineca Herald*, July 18, 1928.

PAGE 286 ... "That will or ought to keep the local member": *Omineca Herald*, February 19, 1930.

PAGE 287 ... "He argued ... that there was a disposition": H.C. Wrinch, quoted in the *Daily Colonist*, March 6, 1929, p. 1.

PAGE 287 ... "Dr. Wrinch is very highly esteemed": *Daily Colonist*, February 27, 1929, p. 5.

PAGE 287 ... Cato the Elder (234 BC–149 BC) was a farmer, soldier and statesman of Ancient Rome. According to Plutarch, the Latin words were *Delenda est Carthago*.

PAGE 288 ... "Wrinch to Insist on Health Action": *Vancouver Sun*, January 26, 1929, p. 2.

PAGE 288 ... "Dr. Wrinch ... said that he was glad": H.C. Wrinch, quoted in the *Vancouver Sun*, February 2, 1929, p. 1.

PAGE 288 ... "I am speaking now as a resident": Submission of H.C. Wrinch in Report of the Royal Commission on State Health Insurance and Maternity Benefits. Appendix H, Vol. 3, 1932. BC Archives, Series GR-0707 and GR-0707B, p. 772. See also *Omineca Herald*, August 20, 1930.

PAGE 289 ... "Dr. H.C. Wrinch was ... there with": *Omineca Herald*, October 12, 1932.

PAGE 289 ... "Dr. Wrinch, Skeena, sure started something": *Vancouver Daily Province*, October 5, 1932, p. 1.

PAGE 289 ... "Dr. Wrinch is one of the most useful": Bruce Hutchison, *Vancouver Daily Province*, March 8, 1932, p. 4.

PAGE 292 ... "one of the most influential members": *Vancouver Daily Province*, June 23, 1930, p. 1.

PAGE 292 ... "This was all very thrilling": Jane Eva Denison, *Caravaning to the Land of the Golden Twilight*, Diary, June 13th–July 1st, 1930. Quote from entry at Friday, June 20, 1930.

PAGE 295 ... "was not a joy ride": S.S. Hoskins, quoted in the *Omineca Herald*, December 31, 1930.

PAGE 295 ... The hospital was as much theirs: The address of H.C. Wrinch was reported in the *Omineca Herald*, December 31, 1930.

PAGE 296 ... As required by Duncan Campbell Scott: H.C. Wrinch, *History of Hazelton Hospital*, p. 11. Unpublished document in the author's possession. The original is in UCCA (Vancouver). The old hospital was taken down at that time. The Wrinch home though remained. Harold Wrinch recalled in 1996 that it was eventually sold to a man named Mero, who had been a carpenter in and around the hospital and who was a rancher or farmer. Mero moved the house and lived in it for many years.

PAGE 296 ... "specially prepared": H.C. Wrinch, *History of Hazelton Hospital*, pp. 10–11. Copy in the author's possession.

PAGE 296 ... "May You Enjoy Prosperity": *Omineca Herald*, December 25, 1929.

PAGE 296 ... "Stocks at N.Y. Just Escape": *Daily Colonist*, October 30, 1929, p. 1.

PAGE 298 ... "Human agencies, and not supernatural": H.C. Wrinch, quoted in the *Daily Colonist*, March 10, 1933, p. 6.

PAGE 298 ... "Resignations of Two Members": *Daily Colonist*, March 18, 1931, p. 1.

PAGE 300 ... "I will take the smile off his face": W.C. Shelley, quoted in the *Vancouver Sun*, March 18, 1931, p. 2.

PAGE 301 ... "The charge is frivolous": T.D. Pattullo, quoted in the *Vancouver Sun*, March 18, 1931, p. 2.

PAGE 301 ... "Then a member's character": H.C. Wrinch, quoted in the *Vancouver Sun*, March 18, 1931, p. 2.

PAGE 301 ... "Twaddle": A. Manson, quoted in the *Vancouver Sun*, March 18, 1931, p. 2.

PAGE 302 ... "not quite up to the mark for some time": H.C. Wrinch, Letter to Premier Pattullo, November 1, 1929. BC Archives, Thomas Dufferin Pattullo Fonds, Correspondence with H.C. Wrinch, MS 003.973, Reel AO 1802.

PAGE 302 ... "when he had to take a dose": *Omineca Herald*, November 2, 1932.

PAGE 302 ... "unbeautiful bruises": *Omineca Herald*, November 18, 1931.

PAGE 302 ... "Really the accident was not": H.C. Wrinch, Letter to Premier Pattullo dated December 8, 1931. BC Archives, Thomas Dufferin Pattullo Fonds, Correspondence with H.C. Wrinch, MS 003.849, Reel AO 1803.

PAGE 304 ... American Hospital Association Toronto Convention and award. *Omineca Herald*, October 14, 1931; See also *The Globe*, September 26, 1931, p. 13.

PAGE 307 ... "With regard to the future": Premier Pattullo, Letter to H.C. Wrinch dated November 6, 1930. BC Archives, Thomas Dufferin Pattullo Fonds, Correspondence with H.C. Wrinch, File MS 003.849, Reel AO 1803.

PAGE 308 ... "I hope ... this meets with your approval": H.C. Wrinch, Letter to Premier Pattullo dated July 13, 1932. BC Archives, Thomas Dufferin Pattullo Fonds, Correspondence with H.C. Wrinch, File MS 003.1092, Reel AO 1803.

PAGE 308 ... "If you desire to run again": Premier Pattullo, Letter to H.C. Wrinch dated July 19, 1932. BC Archives, Thomas Dufferin Pattullo Fonds, Correspondence with H.C. Wrinch, File MS 003.1092, Reel AO 1803.

PAGE 308 ... "Whether the boys will stay put": *Omineca Herald*, July 15, 1931.

PAGE 309 ... "could be re-elected ": *Victoria Daily Times*, March 10, 1933, p. 4.

PAGE 309 ... "You have given long": Premier Pattullo, Letter to H.C. Wrinch dated August 24, 1932. BC Archives, Thomas Dufferin Pattullo Fonds, Correspondence with H.C. Wrinch, File MS 003.1092, Reel AO 1803.

PAGE 309 ... "Dr. Wrinch has already done a great service": *Omineca Herald*, September 7, 1932.

Chapter 13: Last Years

PAGE 311 ... Mary E. Wrinch was elected the first female executive: *The Globe*, April 10, 1913. For references to Mary E. Wrinch see the following: Muriel Miller Miner, *Famous Canadian Artists*, Peterborough, Ontario: Woodland Publishing, 1984, Part IV, p. 100; Joan Murray, "Mary Wrinch: Canadian Artist," *Canadian Antiques Collector*, September 1969, pp. 16–19; "Celebrating Legacy: Mary E. Wrinch at the Ottawa

Art Gallery," National Gallery of Canada, July 20, 2015. Mary had started to exhibit before Horace left Toronto. She was in the 1896 annual exhibition of the Toronto Art Students' League (*The Globe*, November 30, 1896) and in 1898 she was in the tenth annual exhibition of the Women's Art Association of Canada (*The Globe*, April 19, 1898).

PAGE 311 ... "she had greater originality": A.J. Casson, quoted in Muriel Miller Miner, *Famous Canadian Artists*, p. 105.

PAGE 311 ... Frank Wrinch's murder was described in the *Fresno Bee*, August 30, 1934, p. 2 B.

PAGE 312 ... "It came, and quite suddenly": *Omineca Herald*, December 2, 1931.

PAGE 313 ... "In fact she could hardly tell": Annie Lawrence, *Omineca Herald*, August 15, 1934.

PAGE 313 ... "Hazelton Hospital needs more money": *Omineca Herald*, January 24, 1934.

PAGE 314 ... "The situation is somewhat as follows": H.C. Wrinch, Letter to R.B. Cochrane, dated December 29, 1933. UCCA (Toronto). United Church of Canada Home Missions Fonds, Series 2, Subseries 1, File 19-206, AC 83.050, Reel 15.

PAGE 315 ... "Our budget for expenditures": H.C. Wrinch, Letter to R.B. Cochrane, March 9, 1934. UCCA (Toronto). United Church of Canada Home Missions Fonds Series 2, Subseries 1, File 19-206, AC 83.050, Reel 15.

PAGE 315 ... "It is with much satisfaction": Hospital Annual Report for 1935, p. 1. In the author's collection. A selection of these annual reports is also held by each of the BC Archives, UCCA (Toronto and Vancouver).

PAGE 316 ... "'It is to be hoped,' he wrote to Harold": H.C. Wrinch, Letter to Harold Wrinch, dated January 12, 1936. In the author's possession.

PAGE 316 ... "It doesn't appear to be a very exciting": H.C. Wrinch, Letter to Ralphena Wrinch, dated March 18, 1934. In the author's possession.

PAGE 317 ... "Knowing the high respect": *Interior News*, May 2, 1934, p. 3.

PAGE 317 ... "Under its able chairman": Robin Fisher, *Duff Pattullo of British Columbia*. Toronto, Ontario: University of Toronto Press, 1991, p. 272.

PAGE 318 ... "We have two chief objects in view": H.C. Wrinch, quoted in the *Omineca Herald*, May 16, 1934.

PAGE 318 ... "no longer enough to have a strong back": H.C. Wrinch, quoted in the *Omineca Herald*, August 29, 1934.

PAGE 318 ... "What the government at Victoria ought": *Vancouver Daily Province*, September 4, 1936, p. 4. Carrothers was being accused of running a one-man show. *Financial Post*, May 23, 1936. Harry Morris Cassidy's early days with the CCF are described by Pierre Berton in *The Great Depression, 1929–1939*. Toronto: McClelland and Stewart, 1990, pp. 93, 133–134. Cassidy had a part in the drafting of the Regina Manifesto, p. 205.

PAGE 320 ... "Health Insurance Provided by the Hospital": *Omineca Herald*, February 6, 1935.

PAGE 320 ... "our modest and essentially conservative plans": H.M. Cassidy, quoted in Allan Irving, "The Doctors versus the Expert: Harry Morris Cassidy and the Health Insurance Dispute of the 1930s." *BC Studies*, No. 78, Summer 1988, p. 71.

PAGE 321 ... "Provincial Government has given": *Daily Colonist*, February 21, 1937, p. 1.

PAGE 321 ... "the Health Insurance Act on the statutes": *Daily Colonist*, December 4, 1937.

PAGE 322 ... "Merry Christmas! Today": H.C. Wrinch, Letter to Harold Wrinch, dated December 25, 1935. In the author's possession.

PAGE 323 ... "We are a little disappointed": H.C. Wrinch, Letter to Harold Wrinch, undated (1935?). In the author's possession.

PAGE 324 ... "I don't think I told you": H.C. Wrinch, Letter to Harold Wrinch, dated July 12, 1936. In the author's possession.

PAGE 324 ... "Dr. Wrinch has filled": Hazelton Hospital Board minutes. UCCA (Vancouver). Wrinch Memorial Hospital Fonds. Series Administrative Records, Box 2391, File 3.

PAGE 325 ... "Dr. Wrinch, accompanied by Mrs. Wrinch": *Omineca Herald*, October 8, 1936.

PAGE 325 ... "at 1.00 p.m. sharp": *Omineca Herald*, September 30 and October 8, 1936.

PAGE 325 ... "I had the fender straightened": H.C. Wrinch, Letter to Harold Wrinch dated September 4, 1936. In the author's possession.

PAGE 325 ... "No man has accomplished": *Omineca Herald*, October 8, 1936.

PAGE 325 ... "We have called upon": *Omineca Herald*, October 8 and 14, 1936.

PAGE 326 ... "at times men had to remove their jackets": *Omineca Herald*, October 14, 1936.

PAGE 326 ... "We are quite comfortable": H.C. Wrinch, Letter to Harold Wrinch dated December 27, 1936. In the author's possession.

PAGE 327 ... "In consideration of these facts": *Western Recorder*, Vol. 13, No. 10, April 1938, p. 14.

PAGE 327 ... "We had a good time in the East": H.C. Wrinch, quoted in *Interior News*, October 6, 1937, p. 1.

PAGE 328 ... "May and I are planning": H.C. Wrinch, Letter to Harold Wrinch dated June 22, 1939. In the author's possession.

PAGE 328 ... "My Dear Harold": H.C. Wrinch, Letter to Harold Wrinch dated July 14, 1939. In the author's possession.

PAGE 329 ... "no definite diagnosis": Robert Peers, Letter to Harold Wrinch dated November 9, 1939. In the author's possession.

PAGE 330 ... "I feel deeply grieved": Premier Pattullo, quoted in the *Daily Colonist*, October 22, 1939. Also *Vancouver Daily Province*, October 24, 1939, p. 12.

PAGE 330 ... "Dr. Wrinch, Horse [and] Buggy Doctor Dies": *Vancouver Sun*, October 20, 1939, p. 21. Also *Interior News*, October 25, 1939, p. 4.

PAGE 331 ... "He was ... a leader in many movements": *Omineca Herald*, October 25, 1939.

Afterword

PAGE 334 ... "medical service through ordinary channels": Commemorative Review of the Methodist, Presbyterian and Congregational Churches in British Columbia, 1925. UCCA (Vancouver), p. 81.

Appendix 1: Dr. Wrinch's Maiden Speech

PAGE 341 ... The *Omineca Herald* for these years and this speech is on the microfilmed copies of BC Historical newspapers in the BC Archives in Victoria.

Appendix 2: Recollections of Harold Wrinch, Dr. Wrinch's Youngest Son

PAGE 347 ... This account is in the author's possession.

Appendix 3: Receipts and Disbursements of Hazelton Hospital

PAGE 351 ... Information on the hospital finances comes from the *Omineca Herald* and *Omineca Miner* newspapers and from the Hospital Annual Reports, a selection of which is held by each of the BC Archives, UCCA (Toronto) and UCCA (Vancouver), and the author.

Appendix 4: Acquisition of Land for the Hospital in 1902

PAGE 353 ... The information in this appendix on acquisition of land for the hospital comes from numerous sources, including Horace's own reports and letters, the Crown Land grants (BC Archives, GR-3096, GR-3097, and GR-3139), and the letters of R.E. Loring who was the Indian Agent, as well as information on pre-emptions in the BC Archives (Inventory 15, Crown Lands).

PAGE 354 ... "lovely and ideal building site": R.E. Loring, Letter to Dr. Bolton dated July 21, 1900. Library and Archives Canada, Microfilm reel, Babine Agency, C-14856, Image 743.

PAGE 355 ... "it was found at the inception": H.C. Wrinch, Letter to Rev. Sutherland dated April 14, 1909. UCCA (Toronto).

PAGE 356 ... Map: On April 18, 1908, Horace wrote a letter to Rev. Sutherland of the Missions Board in Toronto about an application for a right-of-way over hospital land and he attached a map he had drawn of the hospital site. The shaded area (A, B, C, D) shows the thirty acres immediately to the east of DL 105 that the Gitxsan donated for hospital use. H.C. Wrinch, Letter to Rev. Sutherland dated August 18, 1908. UCCA (Toronto). Fonds 14, Series 2, Box 5, File 100, AC 1978.092C. Correspondence re the Hazelton Hospital, Skeena River. Also, Kitzegucla. Missionary: Horace C. Wrinch, M.D., Medical Superintendent. UCCA (Toronto). Larkworthy, who was in Ontario: Dr. Sutherland, Letter to H.C. Wrinch dated September 9, 1904. UCCA (Toronto). Fonds 14, Series 2, Subseries 2, 78.083C, Box 14.

PAGE 357 ... On October 11, 1902, Victor Spencer transferred both items of war scrip, each for 160 acres, to the Methodist Church for one dollar: Pre-emption Papers for DL 105, BC Archives, Inventory 15 Crown Lands.

PAGE 357 ... The Methodist Church had already applied for a Crown Grant for DL 105 on September 10, 1902: *BC Gazette*, October 30, 1902.

PAGE 357 ... A surveyor working for David Spencer then went and surveyed DL 105: Report of Surveyor Roberts on David Spencer's letterhead, October 3, 1902. The Missions Board formally approved the acquisition on November 3, 1902, and the Province executed the Crown grant two days later, on November 5, 1902: Dr. Sutherland, Letter dated December 15, 1902. UCCA (Toronto). Fonds 14, Series 2, Subseries 2, AC 78.083C. Correspondence re Hazelton Hospital, Skeena River. In 1906, the hospital transferred four and a half acres to Charleson, who then transferred half an acre to the hospital and paid an additional $132: Report of H.C. Wrinch to Dr. Sutherland, April 14, 1909. UCCA (Toronto). Fonds 14, Subseries 2, 78.083C.

PAGE 358 ... "A good building site, about one mile east": H.C. Wrinch, Report, *Missionary Outlook*, September 1903, p. 204.

PAGE 358 ... They had applied for this land on November 15: *BC Gazette*, October 30, 1902. Loring refers to the hospital to be built on the McCoskrie and Murray land south of the Larkworthy land: R.E. Loring, Letter, September 13, 1902. Library and Archives Canada, Babine Agency, Microfilm reel C-14856, Image 1192. See also UCCA (Vancouver). Methodist Missionary Society Reports, Microfilm 1902–1903, p. li.

PAGE 359 ... "to be built on Captain McCoskrie's": R.E. Loring, Letter to A.W. Vowell dated September 13, 1902. Library and Archives Canada, Babine Agency, Microfilm reel C-14856, Image 1192.

PAGE 359 ... "The Premier City in Northern British Columbia": *Vancouver Daily Globe*, January 13, 1906, p. 10

PAGE 361 ... "We, the undersigned chiefs and representatives of the Gitanmaax Indians": Resolution of September 1913. Library and Archives Canada, RG10, Vol/Box 4052, File 371968, Copied container C-10180.

PAGE 361 ... Vowell confirmed he was sending it on for approval by the Department of Indian Affairs on May 8, 1903, which replied on May 28, 1903, authorizing the Methodist Church to occupy the land for hospital purposes.

PAGE 361 ... "for mission purposes": The donation was confirmed by the Indian Department in November: Extract from a Letter of Superintendent of Reserves and Trusts, Indian Affairs, dated March 19, 1947. UCCA (Vancouver).

PAGE 362 ... Victor Spencer: BC Crown Land Grants. BC Archives, GR-3097. Victor Spencer had also pre-empted large areas of land at the Aldermere town site.

Appendix 5: Bridges across the Skeena and Bulkley Rivers

PAGE 365 ... The information on the bridges comes primarily from the *Omineca Herald*, government reports and the letters of R.E. Loring in the microfilm reel records of Library and Archives Canada. The extensive research done by Alan Pickard has also been most informative.

PAGE 366 ... Surveys had been done in 1908: *Omineca Herald*, January 2, 1909.

PAGE 366 ... Kispiox Settlers' Association: *Omineca Herald*, August 14, 1909.

PAGE 366 ... Kispiox bridge finished: *Omineca Herald*, July 23, 1910.

PAGE 366 ... Skeena bridge finished: *Omineca Herald*, December 24, 1910.

PAGE 367 ... Lach-al-sap bridge dispute: R.E. Loring, Letters of October 31 and December 30, 1893. Library and Archives Canada, Microfilm reel, Babine Agency, C-14855, Images 1740 and 1744. Lach-al-sap, also known historically as Moricetown, was renamed Witset in May 2018.

PAGE 367 ... Simon McGillivray's map: See Neil Sterritt, *Mapping My Way Home: A Gitxsan History*, Smithers, BC: Creekstone Press, 2016, pp. 107–108. Note also the map on p. 109; McGillivray, a Hudson's Bay Trader arrived at Hagwilget on June 20, 1833. "McGillivray's Map," *Northword Magazine*, March 29, 2013. Alan Pickard brought attention to this map in the Hudson's Bay Company's Archives. Also, Charles Horetzky, *Canada on the Pacific*, Chapter VIII, Montreal, Quebec: Dawson Brothers Publishers, 1874.

PAGE 368 ... "Not a single bridge was left standing": R.E. Loring, Report to A.W. Vowell dated June 30, 1897. Library and Archives Canada, Microfilm reel C-14856, Image 292; R.E. Loring, Report to A.W. Vowell dated July 31, 1897. Library and Archives Canada, Babine Agency, Microfilm reel C-14856, Image 332. Additional information is found in Loring's letter of April 30, 1896, when he wrote that the First Nations bridge was unsafe and he had to cross the river by canoe. R.E. Loring, Report, April 30, 1896. Library and Archives Canada, Babine Agency, Microfilm reel C-14856, Image 83; and again in his letter dated November 30, 1895, when he noted that the bridge was under repair, Image 856. There is a description of the First Nations bridges in the *Omineca Herald*, November 14, 1913.

PAGE 369 ... "proposed that they build": *Omineca Herald*, November 14, 1913.

PAGE 370 ... "Steps should be taken at once": *Omineca Herald*, October 3, 1913.

PAGE 370 ... "the government bridge across the Bulkley River": *Daily Colonist*, December 28, 1905. A description of its construction was set out in the Annual Report of the Department of Public Works for 1906/7. R.E. Loring also complained that the steep and long incline to reach the bridge was "exhausting to the horses and straining on the loaded wagons." R.E. Loring, May 31, 1913. Library and Archives Canada, Babine Agency, Microfilm reel C-14867, Image 489.

PAGE 370 ... "Three Bulkley River Bridges": *Omineca Herald*, October 17, 1913.

PAGE 371 ... Dismantled: *Omineca Herald*, May 9, 1924.

PAGE 371 ... "Unfortunately there is no road": *Omineca Herald*, October 17, 1913.

PAGE 372 ... The government reportedly bought the bridge for $12,000. Dirk Septer, "The Hagwilget and Walcott Suspension Bridges," *BC Historical News*, Summer 1994, p. 19.

PAGE 372 ... Orders would be given immediately: *Omineca Miner*, June 24, 1916.

PAGE 372 ... Destroyed and taken: Public Works Reports of 1939–1940, p. 24; and of 1942–1943, p. 28.

PAGE 373 ... "Why move bridge...": *Omineca Herald*, December 21, 1927.

PAGE 374 ... "You have not yet taken a stand": *Omineca Herald*, December 28, 1927.

PAGE 374 ... "I believe that now too many people": H.C. Wrinch, Letter in the *Omineca Herald*, January 11, 1928.

Appendix 6: Three Hazeltons and Two Railway Stations

PAGE 379 ... "As a member of the Board of Trade": H.C. Wrinch, Letter to Rev. T. Egerton. Shore, Methodist Missions Board, May 25, 1912. UCCA (Toronto). Shore Papers, 119. Indian Missions: British Columbia. Correspondence re Hazelton Indian Mission, 1911–1912.

PAGE 379 ... "New Hazelton is": *Vancouver Daily World*, January 2, 1912, p. 12. All the Vancouver newspapers at that time had advertisements promoting one of the townsites and inviting investors and speculators to buy land.

PAGE 381 ... "Only in the context of this town site": Frank Leonard, *A Thousand Blunders: The Grand Pacific Trunk Railway and Northern British Columbia*. Vancouver, BC: UBC Press, 1996, p. 233.

Selected Bibliography

Andrews, Margaret. "The Course of Medical Opinion on State Health Insurance in British Columbia, 1919–1939." *Histoire sociale — Social History* 16, No. 31 (May 1983): 129–41.

Barmer, Arthur. *Surgeon of the Skeena: A Brief Resumé of the Life and Work of Rev. Horace C. Wrinch, M.D., D.D., Hazelton, BC* (Hazelton, B.C.: Committee on Missionary Education, Woman's Missionary Society and the United Church of Canada, n.d.).

Bowen, Lynne. "Friendly Societies in Nanaimo: The British Tradition of Self-Help in a Canadian Coal-Mining Community." *BC Studies* 118 (Summer 1998): 67–92.

Burrows, Bob. *Healing in the Wilderness: A History of United Church Mission Hospitals* (Madeira Park, B.C.: Harbour Publishing, 2004).

Burt, Jacqueline. "Horace Wrinch–Pioneer British Columbia Physician." Unpublished manuscript, February 20, 1966. Available from some archives and libraries.

Hare, Jan, and Jean Barman. *Good Intentions Gone Awry: Emma Crosby and the Methodist Mission on the Northwest Coast* (Vancouver: UBC Press, 2006).

Huang, Alice Chi. *A Time to Heal: Medical Missions and Indigenous Medico-Spiritual Cosmologies on the Central Coast of British Columbia, 1897–1914.* MA thesis, Simon Fraser University, Vancouver, 2017.

Irving, Allan. "The Doctor versus the Expert: Harry Morris Cassidy and the British Columbia Insurance Dispute of the 1930s." *BC Studies* 78 (Summer 1988): 53–79.

Large, R. Geddes. *Drums and Scalpel: From Native Healers to Physicians on the North Pacific Coast* (Vancouver: Mitchell Press, 1968).

———. *The Skeena: River of Destiny* (Vancouver: Mitchell Press, 1957).

Lee, Eldon. *Scalpels and Buggywhips: Medical Pioneers of Central BC* (Surrey: Heritage House, 1997).

MacDermot, H.E. "A Short History of Health Insurance in Canada." *Canadian Medical Association Journal* 50, No. 5 (May 1944): 447–54.

MacLean, Eva. *The Far Land* (Prince George: Caitlin Press, 1993).

Monro, A.S. "The Medical History of British Columbia." *Canadian Medical Association Journal* 26, No. 6 (June 1932): 725–732.

Naylor, C. David. *Private Practice, Public Payment: Canadian Medicine and the Politics of Health Insurance, 1911–1966* (Kingston: McGill-Queen's University Press, 1986).

Ormsby, Margaret. *British Columbia: A History* (Toronto: Macmillan, 1958).

Shillington, C. Howard. *The Road to Medicare in Canada: The Story of the Development of Medical Care Insurance in Canada with Special Emphasis on the Role of the Physician Sponsored Non-Profit Prepayment Plans* (Toronto: Del Graphics Pub. Dept., 1972).

Sterritt, Neil J. *Mapping My Way Home: A Gitxsan History* (Smithers, B.C.: Creekstone Press, 2016).

Tomlinson, George, and Judith Young. *Challenge the Wilderness: A Family Saga of Robert and Alice Tomlinson, Pioneer Medical Missionaries* (Seattle: Northwest Wilderness Books, 1993).

Williams, David Ricardo. *Trapline Outlaw* (Victoria: Sono Nis Press, 1982).

Acknowledgements

The impetus for this biography came at a meeting in late September 2016 with my wife Alice and MaryJean Morrison, Past Chief Executive Officer of the United Church Health Services Society. MaryJean had come to see us about photographs and other Wrinch family papers in our possession. After reviewing our papers and photographs, MaryJean said, "someone should write the biography of Dr. Wrinch." I then saw four eyes looking at me expectantly. And so, a word of thanks is certainly due to MaryJean.

I particularly thank my wife Alice — Alice Mynett, née Wrinch — for her constant advice and encouragement and for her reading and re-reading the drafts as they emerged from notes into its present form, not to mention her patience with the writer's wandering sense of time. Many thanks to our sons Stephen and Peter for their encouragement and advice, and Stephen and his wife Annika Reinhardt for their invaluable help with my website — www.geoffmynett.com.

I owe a huge debt to Ron Hatch and Meagan Dyer of Ronsdale Press for accepting this biography for publication, for their advice on the manuscript and for their painstaking work on the publication process. I also thank Julie Cochrane for her inspiring work on the design of the cover and book.

I acknowledge with much gratitude the generous support of Dr. Peter Newbery, who read through a draft and gave me reassurance that I was on the right track. Thanks also to the residents of Hazelton for their hospitality and encouragement, especially Phil and Peggy Muir, Joe and Jan Francis, Eve Hope and Bruce Simms.

Neil Sterritt has been extremely helpful, not least for patiently answering my many questions. He read through the book in draft form and gave constant encouragement. Neil is the author of the prize-winning *Mapping My Way Home: A Gitxsan History*, Creekstone Press. He was President of the Gitxsan-Wet'suwet'en Tribal Council (1981–1987) and Director of Self-government and Land Claims for the Assembly of First Nations (1988–1991). He was one of the principal architects for the First Nations case in *Delgamuukw v. B.C.*, the precedent-setting Supreme Court of Canada case on Aboriginal title.

I cannot thank my first editor, Rowena Rae, of West Coast Editorial Services, enough for her careful reading of the early manuscript, catching many of my errors and suggesting many valuable changes. All writers should have such an editor. Morgan Hite of Hesperus Arts in Smithers, B.C., prepared the illuminating maps, and I am indebted to him for his accuracy, speed and efficiency.

To the writer Carol Shaben, I owe a special debt of gratitude for her sage advice and her exhortation to have fun writing this biography. I have taken her advice.

I am grateful to the many people who have been unstinting in their replies to my email inquiries. Archivists and other keepers of records have been unfailingly helpful and, in particular, those at the British Columbia Provincial Archives and United Church Archives, Blair Galston of the Bob Stewart United Church Archives in Vancouver and Elizabeth Mathew of the United Church Archives in Toronto. I also acknowledge the work of Alan Pickard, who has done thorough and extensive research on the bridges over the Bulkley River.

Without the advice and encouragement of such people, this project would never have reached fruition.

About the Author

Geoff Mynett was born in Shropshire, England. He qualified as a barrister in England. After immigrating in 1973, he re-qualified as a barrister and solicitor in British Columbia. He practised law in Vancouver until his retirement. A passionate believer in the importance of knowing our histories, he is also an artist. He is married to Horace Wrinch's granddaughter, Alice, and they have two sons. He and his wife live in Vancouver. Visit Geoff at www.geoffmynett.com.

Index